Science, Medicine and Culture

Science, Medicine and Culture

Festschrift for Fritz G. Wallner

Edited by Martin J. Jandl and Kurt Greiner

PETER LANG
Frankfurt am Main · Berlin · Bern · Bruxelles · New York · Oxford · Wien

Bibliographic Information published by Die Deutsche Bibliothek
Die Deutsche Bibliothek lists this publication in the Deutsche Nationalbibliografie; detailed bibliographic data is available in the internet at <http://dnb.ddb.de>.

Printed with support of the Bundesministerium
für Bildung, Wissenschaft und Kultur in Wien.

Cover illustration:
"Nike von Samothraki"
Courtesy of Kovac-Verlag.

ISBN 3-631-53652-6
US-ISBN 0-8204-7698-6

www.peterlang.de

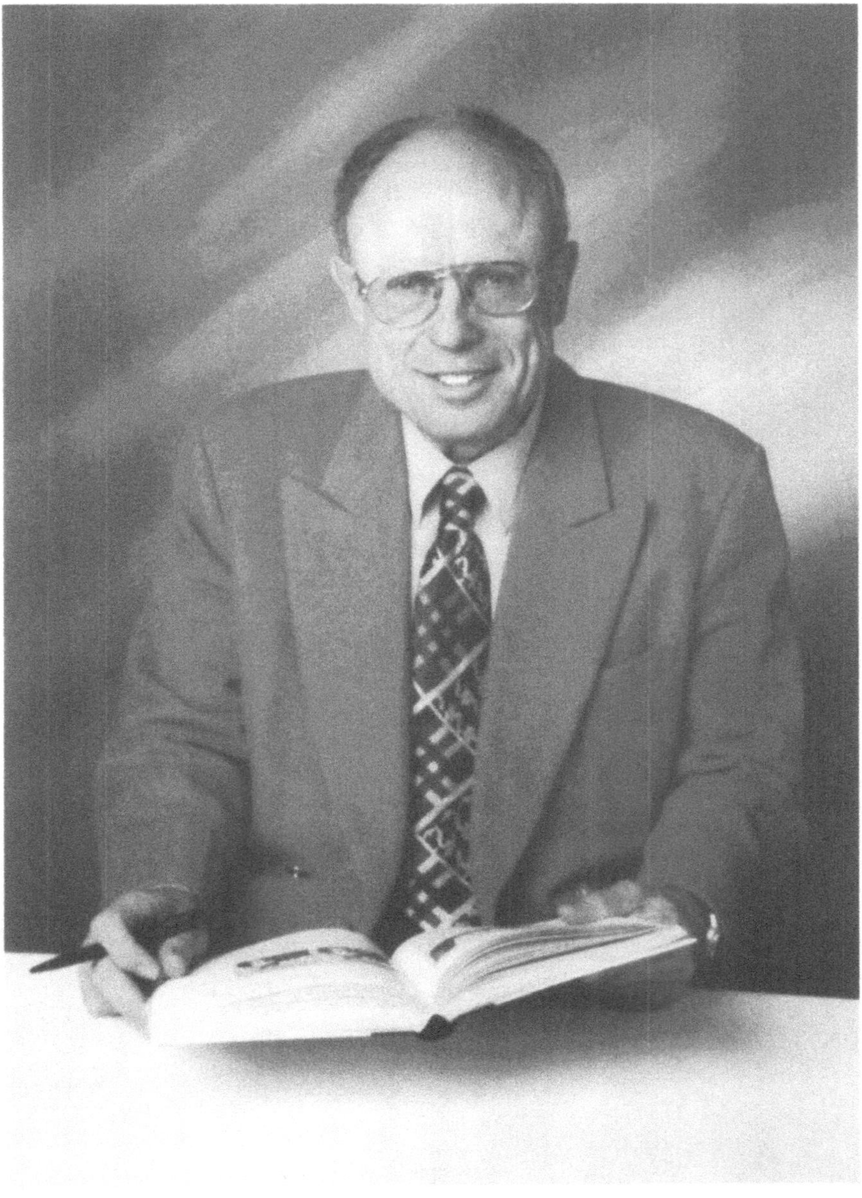

Friedrich G. Wallner

List of Contents

Editors' Preface

Two years ago we decided to publish a festschrift to honour Fritz G. Wallner's 60th birthday that will take place in July 2005. For this purpose, we invited many philosophers and scientists who know him personally because of mutual cooperation. Unfortunately, not everyone of the invited persons was able to write a contribution to this volume, but however, many friends, colleagues and scholars of Fritz G. Wallner took the chance to make him a very special gift. We both are happy and proud to be the editors of this interesting and worth reading volume. In this preface we will firstly give a sketch of Wallner's philosophical creation, famous as ›Constructive Realism‹, and secondly of the texts gathered in this volume.

In his lectures Fritz G. Wallner often tells a story of a crucial experience coining particularly his philosophical thinking: In his student's period in the 1960ies the assumption of natural laws valid for all possible worlds was self-evident (supported by the positivist and neo-positivist philosophy of science), but 30 years later this idea lost its powers of persuasion. This hints at the fact that in this time the claim of many scientists changed completely. This state of affairs must be accepted and offers epistemological chances at the same time. Wallner was aware of the fact that on the one hand many well-tried philosophical ideas must be cancelled, but on the other hand the gain is to formulate a philosophy of science opening a new approach to understand scientific research according to the current state of affairs. Thus Wallner shared the insight that the idea of the Western science is based on fictitious foundations. Traditional philosophy of science anticipates the features of science and knowledge before actual scientific research takes place; it must be thrown in the towel because these claims pertaining to natural laws and scientific research procedures are untenable. Hence a new draft of philosophy of science was required.

The necessity of a new philosophy of science became obvious vis-à-vis the development in natural sciences during the 1960ies referring early to a paradigm change of the notion ›natural science‹. Actually in many disciplines the theory development as well as the laboratory research was increasingly splintered off and differentiated. Correspondingly the possibility of the single scientist to understand his research activities in the overall horizon of his discipline decreased. This change has important consequences for the understanding of science: Theoretical systems adopt rather the role of action guidance and lose widely their claim to be the crystallisation points of insight into nature.

Hence, Wallner started to formulate a new philosophy of science in 1989. At this time he was a specialist on Wittgenstein (he still is) and employed at the

Viennese ›Department of Interdisciplinary Research and Further Education‹ and he was requested to give, so to speak, mentally homeless scientists new orientation. These scientists conceded frankly to be frustrated because they didn't know what they actually do when they create knowledge. The classical European ideology that natural sciences lead to true knowledge of an observer independent world was effectively destroyed in the view of these scientists and their need for a new self-image was immense. It was the starting point of dawning on scientists increasingly that obviously method and matter are determined mutually (the so called ›method-matter-circle‹ became increasingly obvious).

These were in short the reasons that made Wallner elaborating a reflection-theoretical system named Constructive Realism. By applying Constructive Realism scientists should understand their scientific activities and hence obtain knowledge. Constructive Realism is a procedure teaching scientists to understand their research, and hence Constructive Realism has a therapeutic (in the sense of Wittgenstein) service function.

In contrast to other constructivist approaches to science, Constructive Realism claims that scientists actually create knowledge. Constructive Realism counts on the ›working scientist‹, on his actions and the results produced by him, but Constructive Realism isn't orientated according to philosophical aprioris. Rather, in this philosophy of science two essential aspects are joined: (1) the claim of the occidental science to create knowledge and (2) the necessity to take into consideration the relativeness of knowledge. Wallner knew about the provocative effect of this double intention from the start, but joining these two aspects seems to be the squaring of the circle only at the beginning. He dissolved the seeming contrast by the sketch of a new ontology founding his philosophical idea of Constructive Realism. This ontology was simultaneously the frame in which scientists could grasp their actions when they create scientific knowledge.

The ontological kernel of Constructive Realism is, according to its founder, the differentiation of three ontological scopes. Wallner doesn't postulate them definitively, because like many Wittgensteinian philosophers he denies the senselessness of the development of new metaphysical ideas. These three scopes are grasped as regulative ideas (in the sense of Kant) necessary to obtain scientific knowledge by methodological means. These three scopes are (1) ›Wirklichkeit‹ (›environment itself‹ or ›given world‹), (2) ›Realität‹ (›reality‹), and (3) ›life world‹. However, the differentiation between ›Wirklichkeit‹ and ›Realität‹ respectively between two scopes of reality is very frequent in constructivist approaches. Wallner's feat is not the invention of this differentiation, but the combination of different constructivist approaches like the Bielefeld constructivism, i.e. ›radical constructivism‹ (represented by Foerster, Glasersfeld, Schmidt, et al.) and the Erlanger constructivism, i.e. ›Methodological Constructivism‹ (represented by Dingler, Lorenzen, Kamlah, Janich, Zitterbarth et al.) and the creation of a new philosophy of science based on Wittgensteinian ideas.

›Wirklichkeit‹ is the given world we live in and we live with. According to the sentence ›Real is whatever causes effects‹ (or in German making the play on words obvious: »*Wirklich* ist, was *wirkt.*« – this sentence traces back to Kurt Lewin), the given world is effective, but there is no sense in trying neither to prove nor to deny it philosophically. It's not possible to specify the given world more in detail, because it is the founding ground of the world, human existence and hence human knowledge, but its striking feature is its evading from being grasped by human mind. This scope is not to confuse with Kant's ›Ding an sich‹ (›object by itself‹), because it is not separated from the human mind, but the basis of the conscious actions.

Matter of knowledge is ›reality‹ entirely constructed and referring to the whole of scientific constructions. ›Wirklichkeit‹ is a *given* (or existing) world – the world humans are embedded in and part of; in sharp contrast, ›reality‹ is *produced* by humans. There would be no ›reality‹, if there were no humans. But there would be ›Wirklichkeit‹, if there were no humans (as it was before humans populated the earth). And hence reality is the ontological scope that is accessible for knowledge. Wallner adopts Vico's principle stating that humans are able to understand what they created – *verum et factum concertuntur*. Reality as the constructed world is conceived as the sum of all scientific theories. Wallner coined a new term for ›theories‹ aiming at avoiding the implications of the term ›theoria‹ tracing back to Greek philosophy hinting at the possibility of a spiritual (or mental) sight of the essence of matter, i.e. the ideas founding as invariabilities the possibility of human knowledge. In this new terminology of Constructive Realism scientists don't produce theories, but ›micro worlds‹. By a micro world a stringent structure is given to a mess of data, and this structure allows handling the data, especially to forecast events based on the assumptions of micro worlds. Hence, micro worlds are freely invented by scientists embedded in a specific technical terminology that cuts them off their life world; but micro worlds are connected with ›Wirklichkeit‹ as far as ›Wirklichkeit‹ is the source of data. We don't and can't know anything about ›Wirklichkeit‹, but since humans must survive in and with ›Wirklichkeit‹ they substitute it by outlining structures. As a consequence, forecasts of the not understandable ›Wirklichkeit‹ are possible. Micro worlds possibly don't work, so ›Wirklichkeit‹ remains an indirect instance. But if micro worlds work, then they will substitute ›Wirklichkeit‹ at least in some aspects. By doing so, humans build up a world that substitutes the not understandable ›Wirklichkeit‹ by their own artifacts that are principally understandable.

The sum of micro worlds constitutes ›reality‹, but not all humans are scientists. But all humans live embedded in a world built up by humans; no human being is confronted with ›Wirklichkeit‹ without being sheltered by society. Ontologically spoken, humans are embedded in life worlds as the third ontological scope of Constructive Realism. Wallner often stresses that his concept of life world is inspired by the works of Alfred Schütz, whereas ›Wirklichkeit‹ and ›reality‹ are inspired by the system theory especially of Humberto Maturana. According to Wallner, reality and life world penetrate mutually.

The question rises: How is it possible to understand micro worlds? Since micro worlds are conceived in a system theoretical perspective, it is not possible to know anything about a micro world as long as the scientist is a part of it. This question is also inspired by Wittgenstein who states that nobody can understand a language game as long as s/he ›plays‹ it. Thus, Wallner developed a methodological strategy leading scientists out of their technical language or their micro world, and this methodological procedure is called ›strangification‹ (in German: ›Verfremdung‹). It's easy to put the idea of strangification in words: to take a scientific micro world out of its original context (e.g. a physical micro world out of physics) and to set it into a different context (e.g. chemistry, biology, philosophy, etc.). The scientist performing strangification has to reformulate the doctrine of his micro world in this new context, and now the difficulties emerge; because implicit presuppositions of the micro world will no longer work. What was taken for granted before becomes now uncertain, and this new openness makes possible reflections of the micro world. In other words, the scientist has left his field and looks at the micro world from outside. By strangification the products of scientific actions can be understood and knowledge can be gained. Since it is matter of strangification to gain knowledge and since strangification is a procedure referring to a dialogue, in Wallner's Constructive Realism knowledge is not conceived as a monologue of the mind with the objective world, but as a dialogue of scientists embedded in an inter-subjective action field. This turn in the view of knowledge is important to grasp both the importance of strangification as a methodological procedure and the redemption of the occidental idea of knowledge (with different means). Wallner's Constructive Realism shows that relativism has no function and meaning in the context of micro worlds, but it enriches the inter-disciplinary context of interpretation of scientific language games, i.e. micro worlds.

The contributors to this volume were asked not to sing Wallner's praises, but to connect their research with the constructive-realistic doctrine. This theoretical effort is a much more interesting gift for a philosopher like Wallner who always aims at discussions with scientists and at the change of understanding of science.

In his contribution **Peter Janich** points out that Methodical Constructivism (or Cultural Constructivism) shifts the perspective of intellectual reflection from a metaphysical realism to action reality that is not understood as talking about action, but as action performance explaining the difference between performance and description perspective of acting. An operative foundation of science traces back to the production of scientific objects by actual action, by action performance – what is called ›prototheory‹. According to this view the founding chain of a theory is left where actions of questioning and answering, of defining and arguing are not in the focus, but life-world actions and their real performance. Janich applies the core idea of methodical philosophy that science is to be found by tracing back their objects to lifeworld action performances to communication theory and on this occasion he points out the action theory of Methodical Constructivism.

Daniël F. M. Strauss makes the effort to reflect both the constructive realistic ontology and the ›strangification‹-procedure in the light of the transcendental-empirical approach he stands for. Strauss emphasises the shift from Greek and medieval philosophy to nominalism in modern times that denies ›universalia ante rem‹ and ›universalia in re‹ transporting universals into the human mind, thus being the background of the modern idea of construction. As a consequence, the individual side of entities is lost because knowledge is grasped only as universal conceptual knowledge. Strauss, however, stresses that the universal and the individual side of entities are the two sides of one coin and that we must not lose the indiviual side of matters because the human experience of the world makes obvious that the universal and the individual side of entities are inseparably present at once. Strauss discusses Constructive Realism with regard to of these considerations and presents critical, but fruitful issues.

Tsugio Mimuro undertakes the attempt to compare Nishida's and Humboldt's philosophy. Nishida Kitarô is regarded as the founder of modern Japanese philosophy who points out his view of ›pure experience‹ in his famous book *A Study of Good.* The most intriguing feature of Mimuro's contribution is that Nishida – in sharp contrast to Humboldt – conceives (true) reality as a phenomenon of consciousness without referring directly to language. Mimuro reads Humboldt's definition of the touch of world and man as an electric shock that bursts language and his idea of language as ›energeia‹ in a fruitful way opening insights into connections and disconnections between these two philosophers and between Japanese and European philosophy.

Without a doubt, it is interesting for a historian to deal with Popper's thesis on historicism: **Helmut Reinalter** outlines Popper's idea of ›patchwork-technologies‹ founded on his belief that there is no law of development in the social field. Patchwork-technologies and patchwork-methodologies follow Popper's strong refusal of utopian social techniques and holisistic views. Reinalter emphasises that there is one important factor to understand Popper's viewpoint: his moralist-enlightened engagement in the sense of self-determination of humans leading to a system of values and norms of an ›open society‹ and forcing individualism and autonomy. According to Popper neither social scientists nor historians are prophets, but they have to search critically errors in the development of a society correcting them best in their initial stage.

Mathias Gutmann focuses on Cassirer's philosophy of symbolic forms that allows obtaining a definition of humans beyond the comparison with animals. Symbolic forms both generate the world and provide simultaneously the frame of human activity; they comprise and reveal structural aspects of human action as mediated form of world- and self-constitution. Gutmann points out that the concept of symbolic forms as the basis of a generic definition of human being as a developing entity leads from the narrow limits of substantialism towards the wide and seemingly unrestricted area of a functional characterisation of humans referring to the specific type of their activities and actions. The discussion of the architecture of symbolic forms yields the insight that the generation of objects is not a process of a secondary application of symbols and signs in order to schematise a pre-existing, with distinct objects equipped world, but that the difference of subjects and objects of their respective activities is generated within the symbolic system. According to this view, culture is not to be defined as trait of the species homo sapiens, but as a generic concept. Gutmann dwells on Cassirer's definition of technique as a form of human activity and draws the conclusion that experience is concrete and determined experience of something confronting humans with the resistance and resilience of the object of their action and activities. Finally, Gutmann reconsiders the consequences for the issue of nature-culture from the point of view that technique is a symbolic form claiming that nature is an aspect of the former cultural constitution defining nature as an aspect of technical self-production of the respective society.

Sandra B. Rosenthal shows that pragmatism rejects foundationalism or objectivism and avoids simultaneously the alternative of relativism or its equivalent dressed up new linguistic garb. Rather pragmatic philosophy rethinks the nature of foundations, and what emerges from this rethinking is a reconstructed realism housing a perspectival pluralism that avoids the perspectival closure of relativism, and that is a perspectival realism. According to pragmatism, humans are not mere passive spectators gathering ready made data, but rather creative inventors of theories entering into the character and organisation of the data grasped. The contextualism of pragmatic philosophy is rooted in a naturalism that both gives rise to interpretative activity and is the test of its adequacy. Hence, human interpretative activity emerges within and embodies organic activity and is grounded in a world not exclusively of human's own making. The fundamental, creative, interactive unity at the heart of lived experience is central to the spirit of pragmatic philosophy. Rosenthal points out that pragmatic naturalism demands realism, but demands as well to be reconstructed to rid itself of all vestiges of and trappings surrounding the spectator theory of knowledge and the concomitant corresondence theory of truth and fully structured reality of the traditional realism. Humans live through a reality with which they are interwined constituting experience. This primal interactive embeddedness in the world is something that can never be adequately objectified. Thus Rosenthal claims that truth is relative to a context of interpretation, not because truth is relative, but because without an interpretative context the concept of truth is meaningless – truth is not an absolute grasp, neither relative; truth is perspectival.

The starting point of **Julio Raúl Méndez'** contribution is the fact of human diversity, especially expressed in the great variety of languages. But asking the question how communication is possible, Mendez emphasises that the wrong approach is the belief that all humans reason in the same way, but express these similar thoughts using different signs and symbols. Hence he doubts the premise of formal logic that mental processes are absolute and claims that Aristotle introduces logic as a means of communication, not as a definition of the human mind. There is rather a multiplicity of ways of thinking obvious in the difference between European and Latin American thinking. Latin American thinking is estimative, that means that in contrast to European thinking there is no division between logos and eros. Mendez points out the distinct features of these both ways of thinking and draws the conclusion that the Latin American metaphysical thoughts do not treat the problems of the beginnings of reason, but the mysteries of the foundation of love.

Heinrich Beck analyses the development of the European idea of λογοσ from antiquity to modernity showing the good and bad sides of this concept. The European rational ability gave birth to the sciences and produced modern techniques. Hence an especial progressivity of European mind and culture developped. This consciousness confronting and dividing reality further included the evolution of individual rights of the human person as well as the construction of rational orders of society and economy. In these human values the possible contribution of the European culture to world's integration is grounded. But simultaneously this particular capacity of the λογοσ and of logical structuring of empirical reality seems to have been partially perverted into negative attitudes: in alienation, exploitation and destruction. Historical phenomena like rationalism, empirism, and positivism occur indicating the permanent danger and tendency of the European spirit to fall into a subject-centric nihilism. It is to be understood as a partial privation and perversion of the originally positive faculty and disposition signifying a deep crisis of the European culture. In its enlargement in the modern secular world civilisation it is a threat for mankind's survival and therefore a strong provocation. According to Beck, the task of overcoming this crisis demands a creative encounter with Asiatic and African cultural traditions which exactly embody those human values which could balance out the one-sidedness of the European access to reality.

In his first contribution to this festschrift **Martin J. Jandl** points out the idea of a non-intellectual understanding of language aiming at a linguistic embeddedness of humans. The core idea of the non-intellectual understanding of language is to refute the idea of language as transcendental means of world constitution. Jandl claims that the ›linguistic turn‹ took place in 1800 when Humboldt stated that language is the means by that humans form simultaneously themselves and the world. Although in the 19th century the mainstream of philosophical thinking developped in another direction (e.g. think of the German idealists Fichte, Schelling, Hegel), in the 1930ies the idea of non-intellectual understanding of language is reflected in Wittgenstein's Œuvre. Jandl points out the core idea of

Humboldt's and Wittgenstein's language conception and reads the one before the foil of the other. Especially the end of this text shows that the manifold of linguistic founded world views emerging from the refutation of a constitutive transcendental apparatus is a challenge for the issue of intercultural communication, and exactly this issue is one of the core issues in Constructive Realism.

The first author of the second section of this festschrift, **Zhu Ming,** compares two important medical systems, Traditional Chinese Medicine (TCM) and Western medicine. He starts this comparison by opposing the three famous medical schools of ancient Greek around 5th century BC (›Knidas‹, ›Sicily‹, ›Kos‹) to the three main medical schools in China (›Fu Xi‹, ›Su Nü‹, ›Shen Nong‹) almost in the same era. Zhu Ming finds remarkable similarities between the ›Five-Element theory‹ in TCM and the ›Four-Humor theory‹ in Western medicine and so he does between the idea of the unity of body and soul in TCM and the psychosomatic theory in Western medicine. Arguing in culture historical, science historical and methodological ways Ming finally shows that the medical holistic point of view is characteristic of TCM as well as of Western medicine.

The starting point of their analysis is the claim that Eastern culture is based on process theory: **Timon Cheng-Yi Liu, Jian-Ling Jiao, Xiao-Yang Xu, Jian Lu, Xiao-Yuan Deng & Song-Hao Liu** reflect a process from the viewpoint of quantum mechanics and put process-specific time forward to redefine *yin* and *yang* of traditional Chinese medicine (TCM) and extend *yin-yang* rules to systems of modern sciences such as cells, autonomic nervous system, and sports processes. Eastern culture draws its inspiration and insight directly from the perennial pattern of nature. TCM is a typical example of the Eastern culture taking *Qi* as its core conception to describe and summarize the life activities of the human body, and using *yin-yang* and the *Five Elements* as its basic models to establish a system of physiology, pathology, diagnosis, and therapy of diseases. The unobstructed flow of energy through the meridians (pathways of energy) is considered as a prerequisite for both a healthy body and mind. In this regard, ancient TCM views a disease in a holistic and dynamic way. Process theory in general seeks to elucidate the developmental nature of reality, emphasizing becoming rather than static existence or being. It seeks the-many-becoming-one in a sequence of integrations at every level and moment of existence, and that is why the authors claim that process theory has many affinities with the Chinese tradition. As TCM is an important part of Eastern culture and modern sciences are important parts of Western culture, this contribution shows that process theory should be an important candidate theory to bridge the gap between Eastern and Western culture.

In her contribution **Susanne Weigelin-Schwiedrzik** discusses the example of recent PRC scholarship on one of China's most prominent 20th century scholars Liang Qichao in the context of globalizing the historical discipline. In her opinion the historiography on Liang Qichao seems especially apt to perform this undertaking because last, but not least one can observe an upsurge of scholarly writings about Liang Qichao in the PRC. Nevertheless, neither Liang's notions on historiography as propelled in his early writings nor the arguments as proposed in his later writings, even though highly influential at the time of their first publication, seem to have had a long lasting effect on the concept of history writing in China. That is why Weigelin-Schwiedrzik finally analyses the reasons why even today Liang Qichao cannot serve as a model to define the rules of the game in the globalizing historiographical field.

In his contribution **Gustavo Bueno** discusses the discrepancies and historically emerged frontiers between medical sciences and biology. In a historical overview he especially refers to Feijoo, a Benedictine monk from the 17th century, to show the actuality of his visions for strangification. Unfortunately an English translation of his interesting text was not performed in the given timeframe; hence the reader will find Bueno's analysis in the original Spanish version.

In various agricultural regions of Siebenbürgen (Romania) **Hermann Schuster & Johann Muhr** made examinations of the local inhabitants, including the old Austrian population, in particular from a perspective of social and cultural studies. Schuster & Muhr define their project of ›regional science‹ as a kind of science related to a specific ethnic region that influences scientific insight and experience. In this connection the two authors relate their ethnological investigations to the constructive-realistic ideas applying Wallner's epistemological method for the qualitative empirical examination of the Lukas Hospital in Laslea. Especially in this way they show possible benefits of reflection by constructive-realistic strangification for the discipline of cultural anthropology.

In their paper **Martin Voracek, Oliver Bernecker & Gernot Sonneck** report on medical student's knowledge of suicides due to the fact that many suicide victims consult medical doctors prior to committing suicide.

Starting the third section of this festschrift, **Karl Klement** shows that a teacher needs a kind of thinking particularly suited to practical problems because the typical task of the teacher is a practical one. That's why action research in education, which can be defined as research designed to improve educational action, blossomed the last ten years. As an educational scientist Klement works with a kind of action research that is based on the so called ›interpretative research paradigma‹. He explains that interpretative researchers reject the positivist's view that the social world can be understood in terms of casual relationships expressed in universal generalisations. In their views human actions are based on social meanings, such as beliefs and intentions. Interpretative action researchers especially pay attention to the fact that people living together interpret the meanings of each other and they note as well that these meanings change due to social intercourse. Klement claims that Wallner's Constructive Realism is a very communicative method when using it for educational purposes in an interpretative way because it may offer possibilities, but no certainties, to understand what may be the outcome of future events.

In his contribution about learning processes **Kersten Reich** emphasises that we never just learn images in a situation which then are programmed comparable to a computer system. In contrast, we need to refer to a learning context which makes knowledge appearing relevant and meaningful as well as significant to us and our acting. Reich looks from a special methodological point of view called ›interactive constructivism‹ which opts, like Constructive Realism, for a context related and culturalist view. In this sense he describes three action levels of learning that can cause mutual strangification and shows that this circumstance can be well described by Wallner's theory of strangification.

Hans Rudi Fischer points out that since the time of Aristotle logicians have tried to separate valid forms of syllogistic inference from the invalid ones in order to pave the rational (royal) road leading human reasoning to true knowledge. Even today the psychiatric mainstream shares the view of philosophical logic that the ›laws of thought‹ embody fundamental principles of rationality and, consequently, speaks of ›disturbed‹, of ›paralogical‹ thinking. Fischer shows that human rationality not only cannot be reduced to the use of logical (apriori valid) patterns of inference but that it is, in most cases, not even tied to this particular form of ›logical laws‹. He is sure that if it can be shown that we all draw our inferences in precisely the same way as people who are alleged to be ›mad‹, then ›paralogical‹ inference will no longer be maintained as a rational criterion of irrationality. In this way Fischer contributes to the demystification of the myth of an exclusively logic-dependent rationality and shows that all our actual thinking is permeated by such paralogical figures of thought as have generally been ascribed to magical and mythological thinking and have also been considered to be characteristic of so-called schizophrenic thinking.

Focusing on the issue of quality control in psychotherapy **Vincent Shen** distinguishes between rationality and reasonableness. He makes this distinction for two reasons. Firstly, although it is true that all qualitative research and therapeutic treatment refer to ›reasonableness‹, yet the aspect of ›control‹ in the term ›quality control‹ implies certain element of rationality. Secondly, since therapy is an act of taking care to bring patients back to a life of sanity, this kind of caring should be an act of reasonableness rather than that of rationality. Obviously Shen tends to think that a life of sanity is a life of reasonableness. In this sense he considers that psychotherapy is a process of taking care which brings the mentally ill back to reasonableness. Moreover Shen claims that the process of psychotherapy itself must be reasonable rather than rational and so he emphasises that quality control in psychotherapy should rather be understood as self-control of psychotherapists within the range and to the demand of reasonableness.

It is no problem for **Cor van Dijkum** to have a look back to the common work with Wallner: They edited a booklet about ten years ago, and in his contribution to this festschrift van Dijkum firstly gives a view of the state of affairs in social science ten years ago pertaining to the application of computer simulation as a means of research. In this time Constructive Realims played a role because it was open for new ideas of cognitive science. Then van Dijkum ventures a look into the future: The application of computer simulation, Wiener's idea of feedback loops and self-organising systems in social science won't defeat the current widespread application of SPSS in social science, but perhaps the opportunity will emerge that the research founds will be shared between conventional SPSS research and innovative computer simulation research. In these research processes the constructive realistic method of strangification can play its role.

Kwang-Kuo Hwang who developed the Chinese indigenous psychology since the early 1980s realised that many of the ontological, epistemological and methodological disputes that have occurred in the progress of the indigenisation movement are essentially philosophical problems and that it is necessary to find a solid philosophical system to provide persuasive answers to the controversial issues related to the emergence of indigenous psychology. Although Hwang is convinced that Wallner's philosophical system can be used to serve such a function he claims that Constructive Realism may still be insufficient for solving the arduous problems encountered by non-Western scholars in developing indigenous psychologies. In his article he introduces his supplements to the main ideas of Constructive Realism for the sake of distinguishing two types of knowledge: that used in the life world and that of the scientific micro world. Finally Hwang explains how people in Chinese culture may use these two types of knowledge in different stages of life. In this way Hwang shows why it is necessary to develop indigenous psychology in non-Western countries.

Michael Weiss & Linda Roethlisberger stresses the service function of Constructive Realism given in the method of strangification. In metaphorical terms the authors circumscribe strangification as a travel into a strange country with a strange culture where the scientist becomes concious of the familiar within the unfamiliar: s/he starts to reflect on himself/herself and his/her personal and scientific settings. As a result of this process of strangification, the new context serves as a kind of mirror. The authors point out that strangification is a process of mediation, and ›medial reflection‹ is a method that enables everyone to reflect on himself/herself. The authors discuss the advantage of applying the so-called PsyQ® method to medial reflection claiming that the new produced (self-) knowledge gains authenticity and as a consequence the responsibility of the individual to the community and the responsibility of the scientist to science increase.

Martin J. Jandl starts his second contribution to this volume with some considerations pertaining to the definition of the psychological subject matter. Then he points out that Popper takes part of the subjectivistic (or mentalistic) definition of the psychological subject matter, but the discrimination of ›world 2‹ and ›world 3‹ prevents Popper from the individualistic fallacy because anchoring ›world 2‹ in ›world 3‹ is the opposite to the individualistic fallacy that anchors ›world 3‹ in ›world 2‹. Thus, Popper's definition of the psychological subject matter avoids a frequent mistake, but it will not show psychology the way out of a blind alley. In the following step Jandl discusses Popper's notion of the ›situational logic‹ and argues that this notion would be of great advantage to psychology, but however Jandl's argument is constructivistic referring to the ideas of Klaus Holzkamp. Finally, Jandl claims that an institutionalized division of basic and applied research in psychology may solve the tension between a subjectivistic definition of the psychological subject matter and an adequate definition of the psychological subject matter that avoids the subjectivistic reduction and the individualistic fallacy.

Opening the fourth section of this festschrift **Herbert Pietschmann** points out that only in the 20th century quantum mechanics replaced the Aristotelian frame of thinking (›either-or-logic‹) by the idea of complementarity. Pietschmann recognises the drawback in the fact that the Aristotelian approach leads all too often into a dilemma: Either we understand something scientifically or we just have (more or less) valueless opinions about it. In his essay the author shows that the Platonian way of thinking is much better suited for problems with complementary aspects. Compared with Aristotle Plato claimed that dialectic is less than science but more than (valueless) opinion and, above all, dialectic accounts the limitations of our knowledge. Because physicists are not trained in dialectic thinking, Pietschmann constructs a model serving as an introduction to the way complementary phenomena can be handled with and explains its application by quoting examples for the traditional way of physical thinking.

In his contribution **Kambiz Badie** points out that linking the contents of the frames of concepts can be viewed as an approach to strangifying one concept into another, and at the same time as an approach for generating new ideas. Badie shows that the process of strangification based on such an approach is principally capable of clarifying a variety of facts with respect to the possible roles that a concept may achieve toward the other concepts. He brings into prominence that strangification so far is important for a variety of real-world applications in the era of information & knowledge technology, such as cyber-learning, research and development, as well as cyber planning where the user needs some new ideas to be generated based on his desired application. This insight leads him to the conclusion that Wallner's method of strangification should not only be viewed as a strategy for understanding the inherent capabilities of the construct which is strangified, but as a systematic method for realising the inherent capabilities of the construct within which this process is performed.

In his contribution **Kurt Greiner** states that we all live in a high-tech life world but we are not able to recognise it because of the special existential indifference between us and our life world as long as we don't learn to dissociate ourselves from it. Therefore Greiner invites to a thought experiment concerning self-reflective intentions with regard to constructive knowledge of life world circumstances. For that purpose he suggests to view the own flat including the high-tech equipment as items exhibited in a fictitious museum of contemporary everyday life. From this consciously imagined perspective it should be looked at the usual things of our everyday environment. In this way the objects of everyday life leave the usual context of employment and dive into the contemplation context of the imagined museum. Greiner strangifies Wallner's special epistemological method of achieving knowledge (strangification) by transferring it in the context of life world existence. With his experiment Greiner shows a further applicability of strangification.

We, the editors, do hope that the reader will find interesting ideas in the manifold of issues discussed in this volume. Further we do hope that Fritz G. Wallner will highly enjoy reading this volume gathering texts written to honour his intellectual work.

Martin J. Jandl & Kurt Greiner
Vienna, in February 2005

A. Philosophy

Peter Janich

Performance and Description Perspective and the Problem of Scientific Transsubjectivity

Translated by Martin J. Jandl

Introduction

According to Wallner & Jandl (2002, p.260) instrumentalism undermines science because it destroys the commitment of scientific constructs. In a worth reading comparison of ›Methodical Culturalism‹ (see Hartmann & Janich 1996, 1998) and Wallner's ›Constructive Realism‹ the authors discuss the issue whether Methodical Constructivism (following H. Dingler and P. Lorenzen's ›Erlanger Constructivism‹) pleads for an instrumentalism that surrenders the commitment of scientific results. It seems likely that the authors emphasise Wallner's methodological procedure of ›strangification‹ and reject the idea of a normatively binding meta-language-game (see Wallner et al. 2002, p.277). This discussion should not be continued by showing that Wallner's attribution of commitment to the reconstruction of scientific terminology rightly expected by scientific results is a misunderstanding. Explicity and understanding of scientific terminologies obviously open for revisions is one of several means to guarantee transsubjective validity and, by the way, a recommendable remedy against talk without obligation. The issue at point aims at ›reality‹ that guarantees commitment of scientific results. However, pertaining to this issue Constructive Realism is noncommittal. But Methodical Constructivism shifts the perspective from a metaphysical realism in the sense of a ›super-observer‹ refused by all constructivisms to action reality (›Handlungsrealität‹). Action reality does not mean talking about acting (what is, by the way, by itself acting by performance) but action performance. Many contributions dealing with Methodical Constructivsm or Methodical Culturalism tend to oversee this important point – a mistake also to be found in Wallner's discussion of Dingler's approach.

Continuing the discussion with Constructive Realism pertaining to the commitment of scientific results that is – according to the commonly shared views of Constructive Realism and Methodical Culturalism – not to surrender I will explain the differences between the performance perspective (in German: ›Vollzugsperspektive‹) and the description perspective (in German: ›Beschreibungsperspektive‹) of acting concerning scientific transsubjectivity.

Nobody denies that sciences come to world by human action. The question is whether the consideration of sciences seen from this angle contributes to solve problems concerning the current understanding of science within cultural sciences, media sciences and communication sciences. To answer this question in the affirmative by reasons is the aim of this text. Firstly, in a first action-theoretical step I will introduce and discuss distinctions that assign to the neo-pragmatism in a methodical-cultural form. Secondly, I will apply these distinctions to the term ›communication‹ as a central term in communication sciences. Thirdly, I will answer the question of transsubjectivity as a postulate of scientificy.

1. Action perspectives

Due to phenomenological sociology the distinction between observer perspective and participant perspective has become a custom. A look at sciences in all shows that the discovery of the observer in physics precedes this sociological distinction. Classical physics of Galileo and Newton was methodologically naive because it restricted propositions to the field of matters like movement of bodies under the impact of power. With it conditions of observing, measuring, and experimenting with functioning instruments went unnoticed. The dependence of empirical data produced by measurement and experiment on artificially produced relevant features of instruments was overlooked. This naivety against the observer's role for experience in natural science attracted attention in physics as a defect when the incompatibility of classical mechanics on the one side and electrodynamics of Maxwell and Hertz on the other side was noticed and its dissolution by ether theory was rejected. The both basic concepts space and time emphasised as simultaneity of spatial remote events were (later on) interpreted as observer's discovery. (To discuss the scientific shortcut of the observer as a function of measuring instrument obeying the laws of nature is not possible here.)

In sociology and history it turned out that this type of observation in natural science (including distance between observer and observation matters) is not the only possibility to understand the relationship of the scientist with his research matters, but probably this type is a source of error: If the observer is at the same time a part of the investigated object (e.g. the sociologist as member of a society, or as a historian who investigates history that is the source of his science), then questions of self reference and objectivity of the investigation will emerge. In short, the observer perspective was confronted with a participant perspective that judges the membership of the scientist to the investigated matters not as surrender of the claim of scientificy.

Viewed from the action theory both observer perspective and participant perspective describe actions. The difference between these both perspectives consists of the existence or absence of self reference of description. This difference is considerable also from the view of action theory because actions of other agents must be interpreted by taking the observer view. But from the participant perspective the agent's authenticity and the privileged access to own intentions, aims, means selection, etc. open a broader and different knowledge about singular actions. In the difference of participant perspective and observer perspective classical philosophical problems of one's own inner (in German: ›Eigenpsyisches‹) and the other's inner (in German: ›Fremdpsychisches‹), the question of access to ›fremdpsychisches‹, the fundamental differences between introspection and behaviourism, the difference between mentalism and empirism, and even the difference between natural sciences and humanities emerge. That is the reason why the analysis of the difference between participant and observer perspective as two important description perspectives of human actions based on action theory is the cornerstone of neo-pragmatic considerations within Methodical Culturalism.

In spite of all points in issue it is indisputable that both perspectives focus on the description of actions. But the triviality that description itself is an action stays disregarded. And it is indisputable that the action of action description – whether from participant or description perspective – is itself not described, but performed. The difference (in contrast to differentiation) of participant and description perspective is put into world by action performances (›Handlungsvollzüge‹), namely of action descriptions. Thus nobody will claim that performance plays no part. However, performance usually is not reflected. I don't want to join in the intellectual play and shift from one linguistic level to the next one claiming that every description is an action that can be described on the next level. Rather I focus on the difference between theory and pratice. This difference – once again in the perspective of action theory – is both important and unnoticed. This difference splits the disputants in two sides when it is discussed – like in the controversy carried on by Methodical Constructivists and empirists who take a realistic view. In this controversy the empirists have strong support, and also non-empirical theorists who agree to the primacy of pratice but who nevertheless stay at the bright height of their conceptual constructions without granting control, falsification or even verification by pratice.

However, an operative foundation in a strong sense (i.e. foundation of geometry) traces back to the production of scientific objects by actual action, by action performance. The founding chain of a theory is left exactly where actions of questioning and answering, of defining and arguing are not in the focus, but lifeworld actions themselves – the production of objects science deals with. These maybe language free actions like craft production of spatial forms of solid bodies which is then formulated as a theory in geometry. The core idea of Methodical Constructivism is to develop foundational models tracing back to lifeworld action performances. The program of the so called ›prototheories‹ formulating this foundational claim makes a start with this idea. Out of action performances done by craftsmen's practices become established that are subsequently stylised to physics, chemistry, biology, and other sciences. Sure, taking the performance perspective in the sense of tracing scientific matters back to actual action performances concerns a perspective and by it a description. In a geometry founding text no bodies are grinded off and no planes, right angels, and parallel edges are produced, but discussed. Thus it is necessary to explain the difference between performance perspective and description perspective – the last one differentiated in observer and participant perspective. What are the features of performance perspective in action description?

In a first approach the definition reads: Action performance is the subject of action description from the performance perspective. This definition says at least that it is about a singular action performance of a special person at a special moment and not about an action type – in respect to the well know distinction by G.v. Wright differentiating between ›token‹ and ›type‹. In a second approach the performance perspective includes that questions at issue pertaining action description are only to be settled by recourse to actual action performance.

Let's have an exemplary look to requests lest validity problems block the view at action description. Nobody denies that the qualities of a cooking recipe or of instructions of use are best examined by doing, i.e. by action performances. With that a third feature of performance perspective in contrary to description perspective becomes obvious: Within the description perspective it is not possible to give an instruction, and that is neither possible in the participation perspective. Instructions are only described. But requests that are not simply discussed as examples of a text but performed as actions break through the borderline of staying within theory, language, and reflection – leading from theory out to the field of practice. The way out of theory to practice is gone – to name the fourth feature of performance perspective – not for the purpose of cooperation known from life-world contexts of requests being issued and followed but for the purpose of foundation. E.g., if a theory of geometry foundation is based on non-lingual production procedures of spatial forms of solids, then the prescribed action performances will not be given for the purpose to provide henceforth a (individual) drawing plane, a (individual) ruler etc. – like Robinson would do to produce drawing tools to construct a ship. Rather the actions are to perform in case of controversial questions to provide non-lingual actions as upholder of first exemplary special action predictors and with it first steps of securing definitions chains. (If a plane is defined by freely movable fittings of two casts that fit among each other freely movable, then will be non-lingual actions demonstrable to bring to touch solid tripels in pairs or to grind them off to fitting. By it the base vocabulary receives its interpersonally understandable semantics.)

To sum it up it can be said that the features of performance perspective in contrary to any description perspective is that speaking about action performances supports first steps of constructing a relevant terminology. Performance perspective resolves the initial problem of foundation (and thus it is a counter model to the ›Münchhausen-trilemma‹ of Critical Rationalism). In common carrying out of actions – just think of showing and imitating craft activities – the first steps of standardising the terminology relevant for this scope is provided. The reference to reality is anti-realistic in the sense of an independence of a hypostasified and human independent reality; rather it is pragmatic in the sense that reality results from human activity. Pointedly speaking, only the performance perspective serves the predicate ›pragmatic‹, whereas the description perspective of activity even in the participant perspective has nothing more in common with pragmatism as the speech of it.

2. Action – communication – science

In the following I will show the application of these action theoretical distinctions to ›communication‹. I see communication as base concept (and within the performance perspective as base subject matter). The grammar of ›communication‹ may be distrusted. Communication means both the process of communicating and its obtained result. It is both a description word of a practice as well as a reflection word in the theory of this practice. That is why I will use (generalising) the action predicator to communicate ›communicating‹ or respectively. This predicator represents a type of actions underrepresented in pragmatic and neo-pragmatic theories. To make this clear, I will make some further action theoretical distinctions. Actions can be assigned according to different aspects, and every assignment is as good as it serves as suitable means for certain assignment purposes. What I mean is that the following assignment scheme does not imply an ontology or exclusive claim. But I claim that talking about communicating without the following assignment is incomplete.

There are actions that can be performed only if several agents participate not casually, but intentionally in it. (The intention is: to participate in this activity.) E.g., it is not possible to make a race alone. Or, if an adult makes a race with a child and the adult let the child win for invigorating the childish self-confidence, so we won't speak about a race at all because the adult does not meet the condition to win the race. Actions of this type are called participation actions (›Teilnahmehandlungen‹). It is necessary to differentiate this action type from common actions (›gemeinschaftliche Handlungen‹). These actions will be successful only if several agents have a share in doing something (like lifting a heavy trunk). The distinction of participation actions and common actions is followed by a further important definition. The action performance can succeed or not succeed (gelingen‹ or ›misslingen‹). In contrary, achieving or missing an aim of an action is called success or failure (›Erfolg‹ or ›Misserfolg‹). The distinction of ›Gelingen/Misslingen‹ and ›Erfolg/Misserfolg‹ (that is, by the way, not easily translatable into English, because ›gelingen/misslingen‹ occurs only in German as a proper family of words, but not in other indogerman languages) corresponds to lifeworld experience – it is possible that an action succeeds (›gelingt‹) but fails its aim. If someone tends his garden carefully and thus is allowed to call his garden efforts as succeeded (›gelungen‹), but has to see the decay of his garden by reason of pest attacks or drought, will not state that his actions fulfil their aim (his actions are not ›erfolgreich‹). Whether an action performance succeeded (›gelungen‹) or did not succeed (›misslungen‹) is decided by the authentic actor in relation to his intentions or to rules (like in figure skating or in high diving the performance of the athletes is judged).

According to this distinction communicating is understandable as an action showing further aspects for communication sciences. First, communicating is a participation action. For communication at least two actors are necessary, and they must perform (or intend to perform) the communicating action simultaneously and addressed to each other. The non-succeeding (›Misslingen‹) of a communicating action results from disturbance of the succeeding (›gelingenden‹) standard. Unbearable noise, dramatic circumstances or the lack of a commonly shared language are such disturbances emerging and determinable if on easy terms communicating has been practised and marking the succeeding (›gelingenden‹) standard. In other words, succeeding (›Gelingen‹) of an action performance precedes in principle the definition of disturbances and non succeeding (›misslingenden‹) cases. ›Gelingen‹ is related to ›Misslingen‹ like true speech to lie: A person will be able to lie if he/she is able to say something differing from the believed truth intentionally. Sure, communicating as action predicator is rather undifferentiated regarding to lifeworld distinctions of speaking and listening, of the wish to be understood, and understanding. The speaker will judge the succeeding (›Gelingen‹) of his communicative action differently than the listener. It depends on the description purpose whether in judging the succeeding (›Gelingen‹) the speaker focus on grammatical correctness, on clear articulation, on apt expression according to his view or on another aspect of his speech. But the listener acts, too. His efforts of understanding may be exact listening, attentiveness, establishing of context relations etc.

A different kind of question is if we ask for the purposefulness success and failure (›Erfolg‹ and ›Misserfolg‹) of communicating in the perspective of a participation action. (And it's a further question whether communicating is judged as a common action in respect to ›Gelingen‹/›Misslingen‹ or in respect to ›Erfolg‹/›Misserfolg‹.) It depends on the purpose of the judgement whether ›Erfolg‹ and ›Misserfolg‹ of a speech action is granted by understanding and acknowledgement by the other. It is obvious that here dependencies exist within hierarchies of purposes because understanding must precede acknowledgement. Who agrees to a misunderstood assertion, or follows a misunderstood request, or answers a misunderstood question, or who reacts to a misunderstood performative speech act like begging, thanking, congratulating, condoling, etc., does not suggest the feeling of an aim reaching, successful (›erfolgreichen‹) speech act to the speaker.

The previous considerations were designed as if communicating has no purpose transcending the communication process. This is, so to speak, the type of talk-show communication or of talkativeness. Normally humans communicate to live together or, to speak more exactly, to organise cooperation. The methodologically most trivial case is a request issued by a speaker to a listener so that he fills with this request. It is a part of pragmatic understanding of requests to know which other responding actions are adequate, too. The understanding of the request by the listener granted, the listener is able to refuse to follow, or to question the legitimacy of the request, or to contest the feasibility to follow, etc. Analogously it is the case with questioning or asserting talking and with performative speech acts.

It depends on the description aim of the communication theorist what counts as success or failure, ›Erfolg‹ or ›Misserfolg‹ in a specific situation. In other words, the differentiation of communicative acts pertaining to the three pairs of action-theoretical distinction (participation action vs. common action; ›Gelingen‹/›Misslingen‹; ›Erfolg‹/›Misserfolg‹) by the communication theorist depends on his specific knowledge interests and must take into consideration the intentions and purposes of communicating persons if it is about an empirically applicable communication theory with adequateness conditions. A pragmatic point of the action-theoretical understanding of communication situations is to trace meaning and validity of lingual expressions back to the mentioned action-theoretical distinctions. If someone asks »Where is the railway station?« and gets as an answer »It is 5 o'clock« will proceed on the assumption that his communicative act didn't reach its aim (›erfolgreich‹), perhaps that it did not succeed (›misslungen‹). But if someone asks »What is the time?« and gets as an answer »It is 5 o'clock« at 10 o'clock, will proceed on the assumption that his communicative act succeeded (›gelungen‹), but didn't reach its aim (›erfolgreich‹). These hints, however, must be sufficient here. For a detailed elaboration of such a pragmatic foundation approach of meaning and validity of lingual acts see the literature (e.g. Janich 2001). Here I can only hint at possible ways of continuing these considerations.

On the one hand an information concept follows the pragmatic foundation of communication theory that is not subjected to dogmatic prerequisites known from the tradition emerging from Ch.W. Morris and, more general, from the Vienna Circle and that became famous as information concept of the ›mathematical theory of information‹ according to C. Shannon and W. Weaver. A merely syntactic information concept serving sufficiently for technical issues of messages transfer cannot be enriched additionally with semantics and pragmatics to transform signal patterns to succeeding (›gelingende‹) and aim reaching (›erfolgreiche‹) communication. Rather, according to the methodological order, first communication succeeds (›gelingt‹) and reaches its aim (›erfolgreich‹), and second it is possible to formulate and solve technical tasks to transport messages (›Kommunikate‹) through space and time applying technical means. At this point, structural aspects of coding and decoding, of canal capacity and disturbance suppression play a role. A further continuation of a pragmatic communication theory is to be found in linguistics that clears criteria of succeeding (›gelingenden‹), its aim reaching (›erfolgreichen‹) and ›good‹ knowledge transfer (see N. Janich 2002).

But instead of sticking to these ways of continuation I will dwell on the distinction of performative and description perspective. These considerations will found the following discussions concerning the problem of transsubjective or, so to speak, scientific validity of disciplines where communication always plays its role. It is so much obvious that it should not fall into oblivion: communication is an effect of action performance and not of description. Taking the performance perspective within a communication theory means that not the theorist's lingual acts, but the speaker's and the listener's object-linguistic utterances are the semantic starting points to construct an expert terminology methodologically. But let us focus on the action concept founding the considerations of performance and description. To speak exactly, we are dealing with the alternative of an authenticistic and an ascriptivistic action concept. An action concept will be authenticistic if the last authority to answer the question which action has been performed is the actor himself who answers authentically. This action concept will be applied if action is clearly distinguished from mere behaviour of a natural scientificly describable and explainable type by the condition that actions (in contrary to mere behaviour) can be omitted. (It is not possible to dwell on this action concept here.) The ascriptivistic action concept proceeds from the learning history of every actor in a culturally formed action and speech community (›Handlungs- und Redegemeinschaft‹) who then knows what is his/hers merit and blame – in contrary to mere behaviour that is not judged in this sense by fellow beings. Already little children know that scaring, stumbling, sneezing, becoming ill, falling asleep, waking up, etc. are assigned neither as merit nor as blame. Whether we act or not is assigned to us primarily in our learning history assigned by fellow beings – that's why I call this action concept ascriptivistic. Pertaining to the considerations about transsubjectivity of communication sciences it is important to emphasise that not a naturalised behavioural science in the sense of Quine's view of language acquisition is at issue, but an ascriptivistic action concept. We – the speakers of our language – learned that lingual actions are also assigned to us; that means we are responsible for being understood, truth, consequences, etc. of our speech acts and lingual actions (›Rede- und Sprachhandlungen‹).

This approach is pragmatic (or neo-pragmatic) because the performance of speaking and understanding are assigned to us in practice. In contrary, the description perspective of communicational action is not a specific pragmatic approach to communication because the specific feature lacks that distinguishes actions from mere behaviour. (To avoid misunderstandings I emphasise that the methodological approach to action differs from Habermas' theory. But, once more, I point to the literature.)

3. Transsubjectivity in communication science

Before intersubjectivity turned out to be the characteristic feature of science (especially under the influence of the Vienna Circle) objectivity of science was stressed. Objectivity was understood as dependence on the object in the sense of independence of a proposition in relation to space and time. Speaking more pointedly, the independence of the validity of a proposition in relation to the space and time point from which data were raised intended. This understanding of objectivity shows the common failure of the methodological naivety is to miss the distinction of matters and speaking about matters (and thus failing the criteria of meaning and validity). In this view the validity of propositions will be ›objective‹ if it is derivable from natural laws understood as invariant with respect to of space and time. Every ›observer‹ being within one inertial system will describe events (like pushing a billiard ball) in the same way because the spatial and temporal differences of relative motion between the (inertial) observers will be subtracted out.

The step from objectivity to intersubjectivity was to enlighten about this fact. The independence of the validity of a proposition from the individual subject and his position in space and time was in principle a precondition to formulate natural laws in lingual propositions. This was invested in the theory and not derived from it. This history of enlightenment concerning physics is also instructive for cultural sciences. It provides reasons for giving up the idea of objectivity in the sense of a deduction from the subject matter when we discuss the criteria of scientificy. At the same time it is not the end of an enlightenment history because the concept of intersubjectivity came across empirism. The mainstream nowadays understands intersubjective validity as a criterion of factual agreement and consensus between subjects with regard to a theory (or of a paradigma). Especially historising and socialising the philosophy of the Vienna Circle and Critical Rationalism by Thomas S. Kuhn made consensus within a scientific community a historical fact. Normative claims to be agreed or even a (relative) obligation to agree going beyond the historised and socialised intersubjectivity are not considered. That's why the concept of transsubjectivity is to prefer. The prefix ›trans‹ expresses the transcending of subjectivity as a validity claim in principle. To call a proposition transsubjective means to claim that in principle every person is able to agree and that it is possible to give understandable reasons for every person.

It is an ineradicable prejudice of empirism that (to speak logically) universal propositions are replaced by universal hypotheses possibly refutable empirically by an isolated case. According to empirism there are no other forms of universal or general propositions that are not defined within a mere formal system but claiming reference to reality. But lifeworld contradicts empirism. Especially requests are known and applied in everyday language with reference to reality establishing a kind of universality. Once more we can focus on such simple instructions like cooking recipe, instructions for use, and construction work that don't include a personal name of an addressed person and usually don't include a personal name of a situation or the object. In other words, a typical recipe (that means without proper name in a logical sense) formulates a universal ›following knowledge‹ (›Befolgungswissen‹) that is to be viewed from the perspective of action theory under the condition that someone follows the requests for realising aims connected with these requests. Thus transsubjectivity is a norm of scientificy in the sense of a universal, i.e. the individual subject transcending norm.

According to the differentiation of performance and description perspective of participation and common actions it is possible to specify that transsubjectivity makes sense as a norm only within the performance perspective. When transsubjectivity is described, it is just *described* and *not postulated* as a norm. That's why we must handle the words ›descriptive‹ and ›prescriptive‹, ›analytic‹ and ›normative‹ carefully because confirmed descriptivists and analysts *talk about* requests, action instructions, and norms captured from the descriptivist perspective as matters of their description that are true or false. But claiming a request or setting a norm and thus taking the performance perspective doesn't claim to be true or false. Rather there are validity claims in the sense of expectations to follow requests by performing and so creating reality by acting. Here you see once more the neo-pragmatic feature of my approach.

Let's reflect on the claim of transsubjectivity in the field of communication sciences. If physiology describes and explains the sensual perception of seeing or hearing (by structural and functional description of sense organs and central nervous system), then it will offer a scientific and empirical explanans (the explaining part of an explanation). But every explanans requires an explanandum in principle (i.e. something to be explained). In the case of physiology the explanandum is seeing or hearing. To speak methodically, first we must know what is seeing and hearing and it must also exist a consensus among the physiologists what it means to see or to hear in a particular case. In particular physiologists must be able to achieve to consensual propositions that are formulated semantically meaningfully only by laying claim to their own abilities of seeing and hearing. This short consideration makes plausible that scientific descriptions and explanations concern (at least in the most important cases) matters that are defined – what is called constitution since Kant. Defining the matters of a science means to constitute it. Definitions are not possible from description perspective neither in physiology nor in communication sciences. The communication scientist knows from the performance perspective which communication performances are meant. Or, in other words, the constitution of the communication sciences' matters emerges from the performance perspective. Thus I can answer the question of the introduction. To speak meaningfully of communication in the sense of communicating actions is possible only in performance perspective. First this constitution must be achieved and then it is possible to turn by scientific reasons to a description perspective (as an observer or as a participant).

So that this methodical beginning meets the claim to be transsubjective, the mere accidental fact that all communication scientists are members of the human culture community to which they owe their acting and speaking ability is not sufficient. Rather the claim of transsubjectivty must be kept explicitly, e.g. by putting elementary and if necessary stylised action performances to the methodical construction of a theory and, if there are controversies concerning the adequateness of descriptions in performance perspective *by performing itself*. This proposal is on the one hand methodical and on the other hand pragmatic. It claims a beginning and an ordered sequence of theory construction tracing back to practices (here the practice of communicating). These practices are not freely invented but in the view of actual lifeworld performance methodically reconstructed. The exact argumentation depends on the purposes of the intended communication science, but the critical potential of this approach against descriptivist, behaviourist, or naturalist misunderstandings of communication is obvious.

Reference

Hartmann, D., & Janich, P. (eds.).(1996). *Methodischer Kulturalismus. Zwischen Naturalismus und Postmoderne*. Frankfurt a.M.

Hartmann, D., & Janich, P. (eds.).(1998). *Die Kulturalistische Wende. Zur Orientierung des philosophischen Selbstverständnisses*. Frankfurt a.M.

Janich, N. (2002). *Richtig und falsch oder Anleitung zum Querdenken? Zur Frage des Anspruchs an Wissenstransfer*. Regensburg.

Janich, P. (1996). *Was ist Wahrheit? Eine philosophische Einführung*. München.

Janich, P. (1997). *Das Maß der Dinge. Protophysik von Raum, Zeit und Materie*. Frankfurt a.M.

Janich, P. (2000). *Was ist Erkenntnis?* München.

Janich, P. (2001). *Die logisch-pragmatische Propädeutik. Ein Grundkurs im philosophischen Reflektieren*. Weilerswist.

Wallner, F., & Jandl, M.J. (2002). Konstruktion und Verbindlichkeit. In M. Gutmann, D. Hartmann, M. Weingarten, & W. Zitterbarth (eds.), *Kultur, Handlung, Wissenschaft. Für Peter Janich* (pp.260-285). Weilerswist.

Daniël F. M. Strauss

A Transcendental-Empirical Interpretation of the »Verfremdung«-Procedure in Constructive Realism

1. Introduction

The title of this essay contains a number of terms familiar to anyone interested in the history of philosophy. Perhaps the only *strange* one is the German word for putting something in a *strange context*: *Verfremdung* (=»strangification«). Instead of using the English term »strangification« the italicized German word will rather be employed in our subsequent discussion.

Realism as philosophical stance already appeared in Greek antiquity and is primarily associated with Plato's theory of ideas and the subsequent Aristotelian-Thomistic metaphysics. At the cradle of Western philosophical speculation one certainly has to acknowledge Parmenides with his fundamental identification of *thought* and *being*.[1] Zeno's arguments against multiplicity and movement (*Achilles and the Tortoise*, the *flying arrow*, and so on), simply explore the basic position taken by Parmenides in his claim that *thought* and *being* are the same. Thought can only think what *is*, because it cannot contemplate what does not exist.[2] Veling remarks that it was Parmenides who inspired many later thinkers to pursue a *rational* search for »true reality« amidst what is *changeful* (Veling, 2000:29). Eventually this affirmation of the identity of thought and being emerged as the idea that reality itself has a *rational structure*. In the mean time the core issue in this legacy is centered in the notion of *universality* and the nature of *truth*. According to the ripened conception of medieval realistic metaphysics, as defended by Thomas Aquinas during the 13th century, *universalia* have a three-fold existence: (i) as *archè*-typical forms in the divine mind (*ante rem*), (ii) as the immanent (universal) essential forms inhering in entities (*in re*) and (iii) as the subjective universal concepts within the human mind (*post rem*). *Truth* was supposed to be based upon the correlation between *thought* and *being* (*adequatio intellectus et rei*). This realistic metaphysics assumed a *chain of being* according to the Platonic scheme of *essential form* and its *copy* (»Urbild« and »Abbild«), with God as the highest being (»*ipsum esse*«, die Form aller Formen«) at the top of the hierar-

1 Diels-Kranz I, 231; Parmenides, B. Fr. 3: »For thinking and being are the same«: (*τὸ γὰρ αὐτὸ νοεῖν ἐστίν τε καὶ εἶναι*).

2 Diels-Kranz I, 236; 28:18. Parmenides, B. Fr. 8: *οὐ γὰρ φατὸν οὐδὲ νοητόν ἔστιν ὅπως οὐκ ἔστι*. [»For it is neither expressible nor thinkable that (what-is) is not.«]

chy of being. Constructive realism (CR) questions this legacy. With reference to the thought of Plato's conception of reality (*Wirklichkeit*)[3] Wallner phrases the objection of CR as follows:

»Let us now look at the weak points in the Platonic concept of Wirklichkeit. In the first place it is taken as something fictional because it is imagined in one aspect only, namely that Wirklichkeit is something with an eternal and immutable persistence. This presupposed in this (originally Greek) conception of knowledge, even apart from the fact that it is impossible in principle to confirm this consideration in a sensory way, through experience (experience is only possible where change is also possible).« (Wallner, 1992: 71-72).

The first question to be addressed is the following one: what are the historically significant changes that took place in the transition from *metaphysical realism* to *constructive realism*? Answering this question will automatically enable us to investigate the way in which the term *transcendental* acquired a peculiar philosophical meaning in close connection with what is supposed to be given *empirically* and with what is currently known as *constructivism*.

2. The path from metaphysical realism to constructive realism

2.1 The disintegration of the medieval ecclesiastically unified culture

Early modern philosophy soon replaced the classical legacy of metaphysical realism with a *nominalistic* approach. The artificial synthesis between Greek antiquity and biblical Christianity – sustained by the societal power of the medieval Roman Catholic Church with its ecclesiastically unified culture – did not survive the disintegrating effects of the *nominalistic* movement emerging during the late 13th and early 14th century. John the Scott and William of Occam denied the primacy of the human intellect as opposed to the will and opened up an avenue for an *arbitrary creativity* by means of which the human intellect can acquire *control* over the surrounding world. Beck correctly points out that modernity caused a transformation in the understanding of human rationality. Human reason no longer *accepts* but rather *logically controls* nature as an object in service of the human spirit with its self-determination and self-understanding as pure *subject*, directed at the own ex-

3 Because the English language employs the same translational equivalent for the German words »Wirklichkeit« and »Realität«, namely »reality«, we shall specify in each case which German word is meant. The reason is that constructive realism attaches a distinctive theoretical significance to the two German terms – to be discussed later on in more detail.

perience of its power and freedom (Beck, 1999: 3).[4] In stead of looking at the world from the perspective of a pre-ordained hierarchical order of being with God as the highest being, the *nominalistic attitude* stripped reality (outside the human mind) of any and all forms of *order-determination* and of its *orderliness*. It thus leaves open a new domain of exploration manifested in the Renaissance urge towards the *rational control* and *mastery* of the world – which soon found a powerful ally in the rise of modern *natural science*.

2.2 From Plato to Descartes

In order to understand this development it should be noted that already Plato and Aristotle respectively unveiled two closely related features of our life-world (*Wirklichkeit*), namely the role of an *order for* or a *law for* entities (Plato) and an understanding of the *orderliness of* or *lawfulness of* entities (Aristotle). The former discovery was transposed into the speculative and transcendent realm as *static ideal forms of being* in Plato's thought, while the latter one was absorbed in Aristotle's problematic notion of *substance*. Aristotle also realized that *universality* plays a key role in human understanding, though in his *Categories* he starts with the strictly individual primary substance (*proten ousian*).[5] However, in its *individuality* it precludes conceptual knowledge – something Aristotle did not want to sacrifice. As a consequence he introduced the *secondary substance*, which is supposed to be the *universal substantial form* of an entity. This secondary substance is designated as the *to ti èn einai* (*De Anima*, 412b 16 and *Metaph*. 1035b 32). According to Aristotle a concept is always focused upon what is *general* or *universal*.[6] In this way he wants to safe-guard the universality of theoretical knowledge. But at the same time he restricted knowledge to *conceptual knowledge*. For Aristotle true knowledge is therefore always knowledge of the *universal form*. The counter pole of form, namely *matter* (which lacks any positive determination – cf. *Metaph*. 1029a 20-26) is therefore outside the reach of conceptualization. As such it is *unknowable*.[7]

---

4 »Ihr wurde nun nicht mehr die Aufgabe zugeordnet, einen Sinn-grund durch die Erscheinungen der Welt hindurch zu ver-nehmen, sondern vielmehr diese durch rationale Be-griffe gewissermaßen denk-technisch ›in den Griff zu nehmen‹, d.h. die Gegebenheiten der Erfahrung ›logisch zu beherrschen‹. Durch die Bestimmung und Ergreifung der Natur als reines Objekt zielte der menschliche Geist auf seine Selbstbestimmung und Selbst-ergreifung als reines Subjekt, auf Selbsterfahrung in seiner Macht und Freiheit«.

5 Compare Metaphysics 1031b 18ff.: *πρώτεν ούσιαν*, and *Cat.* 3b 10ff.

6 The Greek of this claim reads: *ὁ δὲ λόγος ἐστὶ τοῦ καθόλου* (Metaph. 1035b 34–1036a 1). Compare also Metaph. 1036a 8: *καθόλου λόγου*.

7 ὕλη ἄγνωστός καθ' αὑτήν (Metaphysics 1036a 2026).

Nominalism took a radical stance in opposition to this realistic metaphysical legacy by denying the existence (»reality«) of *universalia ante rem* and *universalia in re*. The place where nominalism allowed universality to prevail was *inside* the human intellect – either as *concepts* or as *words*. The world as such lacks any universal traits, it is populated by *individuals* only. Particularly Descartes, with his well-known methodical skepticism, exemplified the new spirit of the Renaissance and the post-Renaissance era by affirming the *autonomy* of the thinking subject as the ultimate starting-point for philosophical thought. He carried through the consequences of denying any universality outside the human intellect. The most important implicit consequence of this nominalistic orientation is that it does not acknowledge any *order* transcending the human being as such. A universal law-order for creatures and also the orderliness of such creatures (in their subjection to such laws), are transposed into the *human mind*. The seemingly innocent remark that »number and all universals are only modes of thought« (Descartes, *The Principles of Philosophy*, LVIII) demonstrates the radical reorientation caused by modern nominalism.

2.3 The new motive of »logical creation«

Without entering into a detailed analysis of the philosophical development from Descartes up to Kant one key-element ought to be highlighted, for it explains the background of the modern idea of *construction*. In the thought of Hobbes we already find a *new* motive, namely that of *logical creation* (*construction*). In his work on *Corporeal Things* (*De Corpore*) he introduces a thought-experiment by imagining that reality in its totality is broken down into a heap of chaos and that human understanding, with the aid of well-defined concepts, *creates* a new ordered cosmos. Being acquainted with Galileo's mechanics it is understandable that Hobbes employed the concept of a *moving body* as the basic tool in the logical *reconstruction* of reality. Cassirer explains that this stance no longer accounted for truth in terms of the relationship between *thought* and *being*:[8] »Truth does not inhere in the things, but is attached to the names and their comparison as they are employed in statements« (1971: 56).[9]

---

8 That the classical metaphysical correspondence theory of truth – adequatio intellectus et rei – is burdened by multiple problems is argued by Greiner (2003: 67-70).

9 »Die Wahrheit haftet nicht an den Sachen, sondern an den Namen und an der Vergleichung der Namen, die wir im Satze vollziehen: veritas in dicto, non in re consistit« (cf. De Corpore, Part I, Chapter 3, Par.7 & 8).

2.4 The Copernican turn in epistemology: Kant's »understanding« as a priori formal lawgiver of nature

Before Hobbes also Galileo formulated a thought-experiment and without taking account of any real sense-experience he arrived at his law of inertia.[10] Eventually Kant took the outcome of this thought-experiment further: Galileo derived a law and prescribed it to moving entities out of the pure understanding of the human being in its *spontaneous subjectivity*. This represents the crucial modern *epistemological turn*, known as the *Copernican turn*, in ascribing the primacy no longer to the object, but to the *subject*. Of course the problem was now to explain how the human subject inherently furnishes us with *universal* a priori form making possible our knowledge of the phenomena. Just compare the context where Kant wrote about the difficulty involved in this turn, namely to explain how »*subjective conditions of thought* can have *objective validity*, that is, can furnish conditions of the possibility of all knowledge of objects« (CPR, B 122). The solution given to this problem by Kant must be seen against the background of the ambiguous nature of modern nominalism. In spite of the radical differences between realism and nominalism, both orientations restrict knowledge to *universals*. This restriction of knowledge to *universals* is typical of what is known as *rationalism*. By contrast, one can define *irrationalism* as that epistemological approach that accentuates what is *individual* and *unique* (contingent) at the cost of any universal traits outside the human intellect. Against the background of these definitions of rationalism and irrationalism it is possible to see *nominalism* as being simultaneously *rationalistic* (concerning the universals – concepts or words – within one's mind) and *irrationalistic* (concerning the strict individuality of entities outside the human mind). Of course, this irrationalistic side of nominalism is self-contradictory, at least when one rejects the influential Aristotelian dichotomy between *quantity* (as a category of matter) and *quality* (as a category of form). A chair having *four* legs unmistakably possesses this definite numerical (quantitative!) *quality*! Therefore, the *being individual* of a plurality of (be it perceivable) things, manifests an inherent structural trait (i.e., something universal) of every particular entity.

But we still have to return to the above-mentioned problem formulated by Kant, namely how »*subjective conditions of thought* can have *objec*tive validity.« The way in which Kant tried to solve this problem illustrates that, in line with the thought-experiment of Galileo, he simply drew the radical modern *subjectivistic* conclusion: the laws of nature are *a priori* contained in the subjective understanding of the human being: »the categories are conditions of the possibility of experience, and are therefore valid *a priori* for all objects of experience« (CPR, B 161);

10 If a body is in motion and the path is extended into infinity the body will continue its motion indefinitely, unless some force affects it. Galileo realized that it is not motion, but only a change of motion that requires a cause.

»Categories are concepts which prescribe laws *a priori* to appearances, and therefore to nature, the sum of all appearances« (B 163); »Understanding creates its laws (*a priori*) not out of nature, but prescribes them to nature« (Kant, 1783, II §36, 320). In order to understand Kant's position better, it is important to realize that *nominalism* (also in its *conceptualist* variants, including Kant's own position), in fact *transposes* the universal side of entities (accounted for by Aristotle as the supposed universal substantial form of things) into the human mind (*understanding*). In our experience of the world we always encounter the universal and the individual sides of entities as being inseparably present at once. *This* atom is *an* atom – the individual side (»this«) and the universal side (»an«) are simply two sides of the same coin. The *being an atom* of this atom is nothing but the *universal way* in which this individual atom evinces its subjectedness to the *law-for-being-an-atom*. Consequently, by stripping an entity of its *orderliness* (its *universal side*), it is simultaneously stripped from its being subjected to the applicable *universal order* for its existence, i.e., stripped from its *orderliness*. What is left is *factual reality* in its (chaotic) *individuality* and *particularity*, *structureless* and without any *order-determination*. This very feature of nominalism enabled modern philosophy, from Descartes onwards, as driven by the new subjectivistic motive of *logical creation*, to *reconstruct* all of reality (in terms of natural scientific thought). Only the extreme consequences of this natural science-ideal, canceling in principle also *human freedom*, were questioned by Kant. But to him, within the restricted area of human understanding, limited by him to sensibility and appearances, the position of understanding had to acquire a firm foundation in the claim that it is the a *priori* lawgiver of nature.

Clearly, nominalism created an important *vacuum*, by leaving factual reality in its individuality *unstructured*. Kant indeed drew the ultimate subjectivistic conclusion to fill the gap of determination thus created. Human understanding took hold of this vacant position, since Kant promoted it to function as *the formal* (a priori) lawgiver of *nature* (given as chaotic sensory *material*). Consequently, Kant did not merely transpose the universal side of entities into human understanding, but in fact elevated human understanding to become the *conditioning order for things*. This made possible the above-mentioned belief of Kant that the thought categories of our understanding in a formal sense are not derived *from* nature but are *prescribed to nature* in an a priori way (1783: 320; §36).[11]

2.5 Constructive Realism

The constructive realism of Fritz Wallner relates to the history of philosophy on the basis of *continuity* and *discontinuity*. The restricted and misplaced view of the

---

11 »[D]er Verstand schöpft seine Gesetze (a priori) nicht aus der Natur, sondern schreibt sie dieser vor« (Kant, 1783: 320; §36).

Wiener Kreis, namely that the history of Western philosophy is simply the succession of bubbles of words, word shells and mistakes, is contrasted with a positive appreciation of the significance of the unbelievably genial ideas that are still made fruitful for a better understanding of contemporary problems.[12]

2.5.1 The Kantian distinction between transcendental and transcendent

Wallner is of the opinion that the Kantian use of the term *transcendental* does not have anything to do with what is *transcendent*: »Transcendental concerns the conditions for the possibility of an action; transcendent means supersensory« (Wallner, 1992: 34). This remark focuses only on the initial aim of Kant's *Critique of Pure Reason* (CPR) to uncover the a priori conditions for the possibility of an object. In the Introduction to the second edition of the CPR Kant writes: »I entitle *transcendental* all knowledge which is occupied not so much with objects as with the mode of our knowledge of objects in so far as this mode of knowledge is possible *a priori*« (CPR, B 25).[13]

Yet, when Kant discusses the *transcendental illusion* occurring when understanding reaches beyond the limits of experience, then the term *transcendental* acquires a meaning intrinsically related to that of the word *transcendent*. Kant now explains that although there is a difference between *transcendental* and *transcendent*, the basic propositions of pure understanding ought to be restricted to a merely empirical employment. That is tot say that they should not be used in a *transcendental* way, stretching beyond the limits of experience.[14] Here the word *transcendental* has the meaning of referring to that which is *transcendent* – and therefore it has *everything* to do with it. The importance of the connection between transcendental and transcendent in Kant's thought intimately coheres with

---

12 »Zu betonen ist also, daß die Verbindlichkeit hier im methodischen Sinn gemeint ist. In der Philosophiegeschichte könnte man diese beiden Arten in Verbindung mit Platon bringen. Eine methodische Anmerkung an dieser Stelle: wir sind nicht mehr so naiv wie der Wiener Kreis, dessen Vertreter wir zwar sehr schätzen, die jedoch glaubten, daß die Geschichte der abendländischen Philosophie eine Aufeinanderfolge von Wortblasen, Worthülsen und Irrtümern war. Die Geschichte der Philosophie war vielmehr eine unglaublich geniale Sache, eine Aneinanderreihung von genialen Ideen, und diese wenden wir an, um unsere gegenwärtigen Probleme besser verstehen zu können« (Wallner, 1992: 34).

13 Two secondary texts should be mentioned here: (a) Gideon, A. 1977 (1903) Der Begriff Transcendental in Kants Kritik der reinen Vernunft. Darmstadt (Marburg). (b) Duintjer, O.D. 1966. De vraag naar het transcendentale. Compare also Van Woudenberg 1991.

14 »Die Grundsätze des reinen Verstandes [...] sollen bloß von empirischen und nicht von transzendentalem, d.i. über die Erfahrungsgrenze hinausreichendem Gebrauche sein« (CPR, B 252-253).

the decisive distinction between »Ding and sich« (Thing in Itself) and »Erscheinung« (appearance). Surely, the distinction between »essence« and »appearance« is inherited from Greek philosophy, but in the CPR this distinction serves a dual purpose. On the one hand it is intended to *restrict* the (deterministic) meaning of *causality* to the domain of the natural science ideal, limited to the phenomena given as a chaotic sensory *material*. At the same time, on the other hand, this distinction serves the safe-guarding of human *freedom* which is not, like the sensory phenomena, subject to the categories of understanding (i.e., to human understanding as the *formal* law-giver of nature). Kant emphatically holds that the category of *cause and effect* (together with all the other categories) is only applicable to *appearances* and *not* to *things in themselves* (such as the free will of the human soul). In other words, Kant indeed realized that an *unrestricted* employment of the category of *causality* (of course understood in the deterministic sense of classical physics) inevitably entails the *abolition* of all freedom. That this motive of safe-guarding (practical ethical) human freedom ultimately directs Kant's entire CPR is already clear from his explicit statement in the ›Preface‹ to the second edition of the CPR:

»Now let us suppose that the distinction, which our Critique has shown to be necessary, between things as objects of experience and those same things as things in themselves, had not been made. In that case all things in general, as far as they are efficient causes, would be determined by the principle of causality, and consequently by the mechanism of nature. I could not, therefore, without palpable contradiction, say of one and the same being, for instance the human soul, that its will is free and yet is subjected to natural necessity, that is, is not free. For I have taken the soul in both propositions in one and the same sense, namely as a thing in general, that is, as a thing in itself; and save by means of a preceding critique, could not have done otherwise. But if our Critique is not in error in teaching that the object is to be taken in a twofold sense, namely as appearance and as thing in itself; if the deduction of the concepts of understanding is valid, and the principle of causality therefore applies only to things taken in the former sense, namely, in so far as they are objects of experience – these same objects, taken in the other sense, not being subject to the principle – then there is no contradiction in supposing that one and the same will is, in the appearance, that is, in its visible acts, necessarily subject to the laws of nature, and so far not free, while yet, as belonging to a thing in itself, it is not subject to that law, and is therefore free.« (Kant, 1787: B xxvii-xxviii)

Kant indeed *hides* his ultimate concern to safeguard the (autonomous) *freedom* of humanity behind this distinction between appearance and thing in itself. The primacy of the freedom motive in the thought of Kant indeed requires this distinction and determines its contents in his thought. This is also evident from the entire *Transcendental Dialectic*. In his discussion of the solution of the third cosmological idea he once more explains that we are not allowed to ascribe any absolute reality to appearances: »The common but fallacious presupposition of the *absolute reality* of appearances here manifests its injurious influence, to the confounding reason. *For if appearances are things in themselves, freedom cannot be upheld«* (my italics in the last sentence – DFMS).[15] The final remark of this subsection reveals the *basic motive* of Kant's whole CPR:

»My purpose has only been to point out that since the thoroughgoing connection of all appearances, in a context of nature, is an inexorable law, the inevitable consequence of obstinately insisting on the reality of appearances is to destroy all freedom. Those who thus follow the common view have never been able to reconcile nature and freedom.« (I am italicizing, A 537, B 565)[16]

2.5.2 The »world« subdivided in Wirklichkeit and Realität

In the constructive realism (CR) of Wallner a distinction is drawn between *Wirklichkeit* and *Realität* (see Wallner, 1992: 13, 18-19, 43, 48, 72, 74, 78).[17] The existence of *Wirklichkeit* cannot be doubted, but what we construct as *Realität* is something different from it, as that within which life is possible. What we construct as knowledge-world could best be designated as »Realität« while that with which we live is »Wirklichkeit« (Wallner, 1992: 18).[18] This position entails that

15 Kant, 1787, B 564 »Denn, sind Erscheinungen Dinge an sich selbst, so ist Freiheit nicht zu retten«.

16 Dooyeweerd in a penetrating and encompassing analysis argues that the inherent tension between nature and freedom (natural science ideal and personality ideal) is indeed operative in modern philosophy since Descartes as the deepest direction-giving ground-motive of modern philosophy (see Dooyeweerd, 1997-I: 188-495; and pp.325-402 for the dialcetic of the science ideal and the personality ideal in the three Critiques of Kant).

17 There may be a similarity with the late 19th century German mathematician and logician, Gottlob Frege in this regard. When something can act as a causal agent Frege calls it ›wirklich‹. Dummett argues convincingly that it should not be taken to mean real as opposed to ideal, but rather be understood as his »manner of distinguishing between what present-day philosophers usually call ›concrete‹ and ›abstract‹ objects« (Dummett, 1995: 80); and numbers belong to the class of »objects« which are objective but not wirklich (Dummett, 1995: 81). Since, as we shall see, Wallner conceives of Wirklichkeit as something unknowable he may concur that numbers are not Wirklich, but he may differ from Frege's view that they are objective because they are apparently constructed by the human subject. We shall return to this issue below when we argue for the acceptance of ontic modes or aspects of Wirklichkeit.

18 »Wir gehen im Gegenteil davon aus, daß es Wirklichkeit als etwas, dem man nicht entgeht, zweifellos gibt, daß aber dasjenige, was wir als Realität konstruieren, etwas anderes ist als die Wirklichkeit. Das ist jene, in der Leben möglich ist. Das was wir als Erkenntniswelt kontruieren, nennen wir am besten ›Realität‹, dasjenige, mit dem wir leben, ›Wirklichkeit‹«.

one should give up the idea that science *describes* the world (*Wirklichkeit*) (Wallner, 1992: 19; see also 37, 41, 45, 47, 61, 65). The world (*Wirklichkeit*) functions like a Kantian »Ding an sich«), because CR *accepts* as *given* an object that is not *known*.[19] Of course the critical question is: if we do not *know* the Gegenstand, how do we know (!) that it is a Gegenstand? Kant had his own solution to this problem, given in his account of ideas of reason (*Grenzbegriffen*). He argues that in order to *think* the unknowable »Ding an sich« a thought-form is required in which one can think it as unknowable – and this thought-form is the (regulative) transcendental idea (as *Grenzbegriff*).[20] But in the case of Kant, as we have seen, this distinction between *concepts of the understanding* and *ideas of reason* runs parallel with the demarcated domains of the science ideal and the personality ideal – where the former is (constitutively) restricted to sensory impressions and the latter (regulatively) directed towards the supersensory domain of ought to be [where the human being functions as an aim in itself (*Selbstzweck*)].

At this point, something ambiguous surfaces within the position taken by constructive realism. It rejects with good reasons traditional metaphysical views almost to the point of denying a given *Wirklichkeit*. But although the given world (*Wirklichkeit*) is not »known« and although science does not describe it according to the view of CR, this world (*Wirklichkeit*) it is not *denied* either. In opposition to the traditional ontological convictions CR intends to replace them with an alternative *ontology*. It argues that on the one hand it does make sense to say that scientific labour is a construction of reality (*Wirklichkeit*), while on the other it does not lead to a relativization of science (Wallner, 1992: 36). But something more is »known« about the *unknown* »Wirklichkeit« in CR, for the *way* in which *Wirklichkeit* is made into an object (*Gegenstand*) is designated as *reality* (*Realität*) (Wallner, 1992: 48). Wallner eventually explains that the higher (Genus) concept »Welt« (world) is subdivided by CR into *Wirklichkeit* and *Realität* (Wallner, 1992: 72). The latter is what is *constructed* by human beings for there is no *Realität* without human beings. But there is *Wirklichkeit* without humans (Wallner, 1992: 74). In other words, we do »know« that the »unknowable« *Wirklichkeit* is *constructible* and *objectifiable*! However, if *Wirklichkeit* concerns what »there« *is* without the presence of human beings, this view approximates what traditionally is understood under *nature*. What is certain in respect of *Wirklichkeit*, nonetheless, is that it does display an inherent *durability*. This *trait* of *Wirklichkeit* is affirmed while holding on to the dialectical formulation that we cannot *argue* about it.

19 »Hingegen nimmt man im Konstruktiven Realismus einen Gegenstand als gegeben an, den man nicht kennt, ...« (Wallner, 1992: 42).

20 Cf. Hartmann, 1957: 311: »Denn bei Kant ist es nicht so, dass etwa das Ding an sich bloss Idee wäre; umgekehrt, da wir das Ding an sich nicht erkennen [...], wohl aber denken können, so muss es eine Denkform, eine Art des Begriffs geben in der es – eben als unerkennbares – gedacht wird. Das ist die ›Idee‹.«

Wallner says that it is not that absurd to compare the constructive realistic understanding of *Wirklichkeit* with the view of Plato, for the »moment of durability« (»das Moment des Dauerns«) is also contained in the concept of *Wirklichkeit.*[21]

Moreover, if our concept of *Wirklichkeit* includes (alongside *constructability* and *objectifiability*) also the moment of *persistence* (durability), the claim that no knowledge of *Wirklichkeit* is possible becomes eroded more and more. After all it does seem to be possible to obtain *conceptual knowledge* of *Wirklichkeit*! When Wallner states that when we disregard all constructions *Wirklichkeit* constitutes a *borderline experience* (*Grenzerfahrung* – 1992: 73), he implicitly alludes to *Wirklichkeit* as the *limit* (border; boundary) of *experience*, similar to the way in which the *horizon* delimits our visual field in normal daylight. *Wirklichkeit* in its persistence and endurance forms the *horizon* of the constructive and objectifying possibilities of humankind. But it seems as if we may venture to expand the constructive realism of Wallner in two respects: (a) regarding its notion of *experience* and (b) regarding the implicit reduction of *Wirklichkeit* to nature.

2.5.3 Expanding the Wirklichkeit of constructive realism

Remark (a): *The supposed* sensory *nature of* experience

Wallner holds the view that *experience* is *sensory* (*sinnlich* – 1922: 71), but at the same time states that *experience* is only possible if *change* is possible. The first problem is that no further analysis is provided of what the idea of *change* entails. Already early Greek philosophy challenged the assumption that static being (Parmenides) is all there is by arguing that whatever is, is taken up in constant *flux* (see Heraclitus, B Fr.90). It was Cratylus, a younger contemporary of Socrates and associate teacher of Plato, who caused the latter to come to a radical and one-sided view of the ideas of Heraclitus. He took Heraclitus to claim that the world of the senses is caught up in a process of *change* and that it therefore is *unknowable.* In his dialogue *Cratylus* Plato portrays the latter as holding that since we cannot say »what is not« we are also unable to say what is *false.* Cratylus indeed understood *change* in such a *radical sense* that he even questioned references to »sameness.« The alleged statement of Heraclitus, namely that *one cannot step into the same river twice*, is therefore taken yet one step further: one cannot step into the same river even *once* (see Freeman, 1949: 285).

Plato, who found himself confronted with this thought-climate, assumed that *change* belongs to the world of the *senses* – almost literally reiterated by the

21 »Vergleichen wir nun die ›Wirklichkeit‹ unserer Überlegungen mit der bei Platon, so ist das nicht so absurd, wie es im ersten Moment erscheint, denn das Moment des Dauerns ist auch in unserem Konzept der Wirklichkeit enthalten, nur kann man darüber nicht reden« (Wallner, 1992: 73).

above-mentioned statement of Wallner that *change* enables *experience.*[22] This emphasis on *change* caused Plato to struggle with distinctions helping him to account for the *possibility* of *knowledge*. He did realize that *knowledge* always depends upon something *more basic* than *change*. Having learned from Heraclitus that all things accessible to *sensory perception* exist in an ever-fluctuating state, the conclusion apparently must be that it is therefore impossible to *know* these things. Yet, Plato's intention to uphold the nature of knowledge caused him to question the assumption that the existence of everything is exhausted by a state of *change*. If this was true, knowledge would have been cancelled. Whenever a knowledge-claim is made, it is at once uprooted, because what is assumed to be known the next moment will change. It will become something *not yet known* – in fact it will turn into something *unknowable*! In order to secure the *possibility of knowledge* Plato then postulated the *enduring essential being* of things (their static *eidos*) – which is supposed not to be subject to *change* (Cratylus, 439c- 440a). Without an awareness of *endurance* (*persistence*) the very notion of *change* becomes problematic, for the difficult question then is: »what« changes? For example, an ageing person can only claim to be ageing because there is a constant reference to the *same* person! One can detect *changes* only on the basis of *constancy*. This is indeed the valuable insight of Plato's theory of ideas positively appreciated by Wallner when he conceded that his *concept* of *Wirklichkeit* entails the moment of *durability* (1992: 73). While we may distance ourselves alongside constructive realism from the speculative (metaphysical) construction of *transcendent ideal forms* (static essences), we all still have to take serious the brilliant Platonic insight that *change* rests on *constancy.*[23]

At this point we have to assess the limitations of *sensory experience*. First of all, if *Erfahrung* (experience) pre-supposes change and the latter pre-supposes constancy, then experience is pre-supposing constancy as well. Perhaps a positive interpretation of the position taken by constructive realism is to take it as affirming that experience pre-supposes both constancy and dynamics (change). But since the human sensory apparatus is geared to »sense« entities (and events encompassing entities), the *property-terms* employed in *describing* what has been

---

22 »Erfahrung ist nur möglich, wo auch Veränderung möglich ist« (1992: 72). In passing we may ask the question whether the emphasis on change is not responsible for Wallner's questioning of the principle of contradiction (see 1992: 72 ff., 78, 79, 81, 82) as well as for his rejection of the idea of truth. Of course one may ask whether his statement »that the idea of truth« has to be »relinguished« (»[die] Idee der Wahrheit wird aufgegeben« – 1992: 84) itself is true!? Agnese alludes to Davidson's remark that truth is the clearest and most basic concept we have and also to the fact that truth is relative to a language (1999: 46-47).

23 This insight recurred in Galileo's formulaiton of the law of inertia and in Einstein's special theory of relativity where the velocity of light in a vacuum is postualted as a constant, implying that whatever moves is moving relative to this constant!

sensed, refer to a *Wirklichkeit* transcending sense experience. If I have observed a (one) big *cheetah* (apparently the fastest animal on land), then the numerical, spatial and kinematical terms used in this statement (number, size and speed) are not themselves phenomena open to sense perception. One cannot describe the *colour* of the quantitative aspect of *Wirklichkeit*, one cannot *weigh* the spatial aspect, someone cannot *taste* the kinematical aspect, and so on. The same applies to the human experience of *time*. With which sense is time experienced? Can anyone *smell* time? Is it possible to *touch* time? Or can one *hear* it? Though I am sure that a constructive realist will concede that we do have an experience of time, these questions demonstrate that our experience of time transcends the senses! Experience therefore must be more encompassing than *sensory* experience.

Remark (b): *The reduction of* Wirklichkeit *to nature*

In our preceding argumentation *constancy* and *change* appeared as belonging to two aspects of ontic reality (*Wirklichkeit*), namely the kinematic aspect of pure (uniform) movement and the physical aspect of energy-operation. Aspects such as these do not concern the concrete *what* of entities, but merely their functional *how*. When certain events occur it is always possible to discern various aspects or modes of functioning of such events. Of course the *articulation* of any specific mode of being (mode of functioning) involves the human subject and the *constructive* input of the latter. But the pre-constructive *datum*, making *possible* any and all articulations of human constructions, ought to be acknowledged in its *ontic* givenness.

For that matter, the meaning of *motion* is constituted by a *spatial* and *quantitative* (functional) foundation, for *speed* depends on a ratio between *distance* and *time*, expressible in *numerical* terms.[24] Epistemology traditionally is well at home with *sensory perception* (»sense data«) and with the ontic status of (at least: *physical*) entities (usually simply referred to as »objects«). But when *Wirklichkeit* is assigned to (physical) entities only, it should not surprise us that the *quantitative nature* of number is transposed into the domain of thinking – as constructions of the human mind.[25] The outcome of this conviction is that only concrete entities are real (in the sense of *wirklich*) and that their properties are *human constructions*. The fundamental question to be addressed to this belief is the following one: are there not, prior to any human *intervention* or *construction*, a *given multiplicity* of aspects or functions of *Wirklichkeit*? Hao Wang remarks that the famous mathematician, Kurt Gödel, is very »fond of an observation that he attributes to

24 If a material entity (and not the mental human construct of it) covers 30 km in two hours, then the average speed with which it travells is 15 km per hour.

25 We have noted that Descartes (1596-1650) already claimed that »number and all universals are mere modes of thought« (*Principles of Philosophy*, Part I, LVII).

Bernays«, namely »[T]hat the flower has five petals is as much part of objective reality as that its color is red« (quoted by Wang, 1982: 202; see Strauss, 2002).

Gödel introduces the idea of »semiperceptions« when it concerns »mathematical objects.« Next to a physical causal context within which something can be »given,« Gödel refers to data of a second kind which are open to »semiperceptions.« The data of this second kind »cannot be associated with actions of certain things upon our sense organs« (quoted by Wang, 1988: 304). Gödel says:

»It by no means follows, however, [that they] are something purely subjective as Kant says. Rather they, too, may represent »an aspect of objective reality« (my emphasis – DFMS), but, as opposed to the sensations, their presence in us may be due to another kind of relationship between ourselves and reality.« (quoted by Wang, 1988: 304)

Wang is »inclined to agree with Gödel«, but he does »not know how to elaborate his assertions« (Wang, 1988:304). He says that he »used to be troubled by the association of objective existence with having a fixed ›residence‹ in spacetime«, but he now feels »that ›an aspect of objective reality‹ can exist (and be ›perceived by semiperceptions‹) without its occupying a location in spacetime in the way physical objects do« (Wang, 1988: 304). Clearly, Gödel and Wang contemplate the »reality« of »ontic« (designated by them as: »objective«) »aspects of reality« which are not like »concrete entities« occupying »a location in spacetime«. It therefore seems that some of the most prominent mathematicians of the 20th century indeed wanted to acknowledge the *ontic status* of the quantitative and spatial modes (aspects) of reality (understood as *Wirklichkeit*).

Wallner also leaves open the possibility to speak about *aspects of reality* (in the sense of *Wirklichkeit*) – even though he will add that the *human involvement* with such »ontic aspects« will always entail an element of *construction* (and therefore the creation of *Realität*).[26] From the fact that Wallner attributes the »moment of durability« to *Wirklichkeit* one can also argue that implicitly he does show an awareness of the *ontic* meaning of *uniform motion* in the sense of the

26 »Rekursive Tätigkeit des Beobachters heißt, daß bei der Erkenntnis die Beobachtung und die Wirklichkeit im Gegensatz zum traditionellen Modell nicht ident sind, und wir zwischen verschiedenen Beobachtern unterscheiden, die ganz bestimmte Konstruktionen entwerfen, die ganz bestimmte Aspekte aus dem, was geschieht, herausarbeiten (Realität), die insofern mit Wirklichkeit in Beziehung stehen, als sie als Lebewesen zur Wirklichkeit gehören und zusätzlich die Deformationen, die sie von der Wirklichkeit zugefügt bekommen - wie Maturana sagt -, unter verschiedenen Verfahrensweisen verarbeiten. Erkenntnis wird als Deformationsverarbeitung verstanden, als die Verarbeitung von Deformation. Was sich dabei ergibt, ist die Realität« (Wallner, 1992: 47).

kinematical aspect (phoronomic aspect). (Just compare the way in which Janich draws a clear distinction between *phoronomic* and *dynamic* statements.[27])

But if one is willing to argue for the ontic status of certain (pre-constructed) aspects of nature, such as the numerical, spatial, kinematical and physical, why then not expanding the scope by considering the biotical and sensitive modes of nature alongside those aspects that typically condition the possibilities of human beings in a truly *normative* sense as well? I want to argue that Wallner will enrich the potential and scope of his constructive realism if it contemplates the acknowledgement, not only of ontic modes belonging to natural reality (*Naturwirklichkeit*), but also of *ontic normativity*.

2.5.4 The normativity of human life

Humans are *normative* beings in a fundamental sense. They have to respond to the normativity of human life – either by conforming to or by rejecting (violating) the norms guiding human endeavours. When Wallner writes about what it means to be civilized and well-educated, he categorically states that an educated person (»gebildeter Mensch«) cannot be a *relativist* (Wallner, 2003a: 50). The example given on this page concerns a young engaged woman (mis-)interpreting the *egoism* of her friend as a sign of *male strength*. He then correctly remarks that when they do get married, the marriage may not last. Implicit in this example is an awareness of the normative meaning of human life – also pertaining to the moral relationship obtaining between husband and wife in a marriage.

In his questioning of the meaning of *contradiction* Wallner expresses the view that it is incorrect to assume that reality (as *Wirklichkeit*) is without any contradictions (»widerspruchsfrei«) (Wallner, 1992: 79). It is not clear why he claims that subscribing to the view that an antinomy (*Widerspruch*) ought to be avoided entails that one adheres to the theory that language *copies* reality (»daß Sprache Wirklichkeit abbildet«). Without the implicit (ontic) reality (*Wirklichkeit*) of logical normativity, it would be altogether impossible to speak about »contradiction« at all. For that reason humans indeed are able to discern *truth* from *falseness* and

---

27 »Die Tragweite einer strengen Unterscheidung phoronomischer (im Folgenden kinematisch genannt) und dynamischer Argumente möchte ich an einem Beispiel erläutern, das [...] aus der Protophysik stammt. Die Aussage ›ein Körper kann seine Geschwindigkeit nur stetig ändern‹ kann von der modernen Physik nur dynamisch verstanden werden. Geschwindigkeitsänderungen sind Beschleunigung, d.h. als Zweite Ableitung des Weges nach der Zeit definiert. Zeit wird von der Physik als ein Parameter behandelt, an dessen Erzeugung durch eine Parametermaschine (»Uhr«) de facto bestimmte Homogenitätserwartungen geknüpft sind ... Bezogen auf den Gang einer angeblich so ausgewählten Parametermaschine kann ein Körper seine Geschwindigkeit deshalb nich unstetig, d.h. mit unendlich großer Beschleunigung änderen, weil dazu eine unendlich große Kraft erforderlich wäre« (Janich, 1975: 68-69).

that they do have an awareness of what is *logically sound* and what is *illogical*. Similarly they know the difference between what is *beautiful* and what is *ugly*.[28] This normative fibre of our shared humanity naturally spans across multiple dimensions of normativity, exemplified in considerations such as:

- Humans are extremely sensitive to the difference between *justice* and *injustice*.
- They are aware of the benefits of *frugality* as opposed to the sorrows of *wastefulness*.
- Their experience of lingual ambiguities is filled with examples of correct and wrong *interpretations*.
- They know what the worth of *courtesy* is and what the effects of *impoliteness* may be.

Similarly, humankind has heroic and heartbreaking stories to tell about what is *norm-conformative* in a historical sense and what is *historically antinormative* or *un-historical* (for example: what is *reactionary* or what is *revolutionary* as opposed to what is *reformational*).

Every inter-human encounter brings to expression this *normative dimension* and takes place under its »supervision«; is played out within this cosmic theater of human beings as *norm-observing agents*. Although individuals oftentimes have diverging understandings of what *truth*, *logicality*, justice, *love*, *frugality*, *interpretation*, *courtesy* and *norm-conformative historical actions* are, they cannot side-step this »norm-determinedness« of human life. For that reason even in every antinormative action the human being is constantly haunted by the underlying and presupposed normed awareness of what »ought to be« – aptly captured by an age-old legacy which designates it as the uniquely human *conscience*.

Remark: *The opposition between description and construction*

Wallner opposes description and construction when he states that the natural sciences do not describe something since it is always constructive.[29] Although he is certainly justified in his rejection of a naïve realistic correspondence claim that views »natural laws« as fixed representations of a unique homogeneous *Wirklichkeit*, he does not distinguish between human theoretical artifacts (»theories« and

---

28 Normativity as such, commonly manifested in contraries like logical – illogical, historical – unhistorical, clear – ambiguous, polite – impolite, thrifty – wasteful, beautiful – ugly, legal – illegal, moral – immoral and certain and doubtful – in fact can only exist on the basis of the logical principle of non-contradiction.

29 »Naturwissenschaftliche Arbeit stellt Konstruktion von Welten dar. Naturwissenschacftliche Arbeit stellt nich eine Beschreibung von etwas dar, sondern ist immer konstruktiv« (quoted by Greiner, 2003a: 88).

»theoretical law-statements«) on the one hand, and the ontic *orderliness of* (and *order for*) *Wirklichkeit*.

For example, when Newton *formulated* his law of gravity[30] the formulation of this law is a human *construction* – but one pointing *beyond itself* to a *physical reality* (*Wirklichkeit*) given in an *ontic sense*. The incredible scope of this discovery is best demonstrated by the story about the discovery of Neptune. With the aid of his newly designed powerful telescope W. Herschel succeeded in discovering the planet Uranus in the year 1781. However, there was a problem because the *path* of this planet did not conform to the predictions made for it. Alexander Bouvard thought that this deviation was caused by another planet not yet discovered. Various attempts were launched to find this unknown planet. Only in 1845 a young student from Cambridge, J.C. Adams, on the basis of Newton's law of gravity, succeeded in calculating an accurate estimate of the mass, position and path of this unknown planet. He sent his calculations to Sir George Airy at the »Royal Astronomical Observatory« in Greenwich. The latter did not value the importance of these calculations and that gave a French student, J.J. Leverrier, the chance independently to come up with practically the *same* calculations. He communicated his findings to the German astronomer, Johann Galle, who received them on September 23, 1846 – the latter discovered Neptune that very evening – with a deviation of only 55 minutes off the path as predicted by Leverrier. Kline is certainly justified in asking the question how one can doubt the *predictive power* of a mathematical-astronomical theory that manages to make predictions accurate up to one ten thousandth of a percentage point (cf. Kline, 1980: 62-63).

Because physical entities also *function* within the numerical aspect of *Wirklichkeit* a theoretical *disclosure* (not »copy«) of the meaning of this aspect makes possible the mathematical formulation of gravity. Therefore physical theories are both involved in a disclosure (more than a mere description) of the meaning of an ontically given *Wirklichkeit* while at the same time they are examples of *constructive* human responses to what is ontically given.

3. A transcendental-empirical interpretation of »Verfremdung«

Against this background I now want to give a brief sketch of what I will call a transcendental-empirical interpretation of *Verfremdung*.[31] The constructive realistic orientation introduced the method of *Verfremdung* in order to understand what

30 The law of Gravity states that F = G times *mM* divided by r^2, where F is the force of gravity, G a constant, *m* the mass of the one physical body, *M* the mass of the other one, and *r* the distance between the two bodies.

31 Perhaps the word *alienation* is a more appropriate translational equivalent for *Verfremdung* than »strangification«.

scholars do. The aim of this method is to put the statements and theories of a scholar within a context totally foreign to it (Wallner, 1992: 27). One possibility is to describe the operation of a physicist with the aid of the conceptual apparatus of a psychologist – and when it is done physics is *alienated* (*verfremdet*) (Wallner, 1992:36). Another perspective is given in what Greiner highlights as leaving aside the *mode of thinking* of a specific scientific discipline – in which case *Verfremdung* also takes place.[32] In terms of the perspective of ontic *modes* inherent to the world (as *Wirklichkeit*), one can show that every distinct scholarly discipline explores its own delimiting *mode of explanation*. The basic laws of thermodynamics obtain for every possible physical entity – these laws hold universally for all material entities. They differ from the specific laws applicable to certain *kinds* or *types* of laws (type-laws) that are only delimiting a limited class of entities.[33] The fact that modal functional laws – such as those of quantum physics – hold for all possible »objects« is clearly seen by Von Weizsäcker: »Quantum theory, formulated sufficiently abstract, is a unversal theory for all Gegenstandklassen (classes of objects)« (von Weizsäcker, 1993: 128). When he explains, on the next page, that one cannot deduce the *kinds of entities* of experience from the *universal scope* of quantum theory, he clearly has in mind what we are calling *type-laws*.

Kant's basic concern in his CPR was to prevent an unlimited application of the category of *causality*. Suppose now we take the original physical concept of causality and place it within a strange context, within a different universe of discourse, such as that of *jurisprudence*. The only (quite important) step to be given is to refer back to the (pre-constructive) ontic givenness of functional modes of existence, in this case the physical aspect of reality (*Wirklichkeit*) on the one hand and the jural aspect of reality (*Wirklichkeit*) on the other. The question to be answered then simply is: does it make sense to restrict the employment of causality to the physical aspect only? The remarkable practice is indeed that disciplines dif-

32 »Aus diesem neuen und heterogen-strukturierten Kontext wird schließlich das ursprüngliche Satzsystem betrachtet, beurteilt etc. STRANGIFICATION bedeutet somit das Verlassen der Denkweise einer wissenschaftlichen Disziplin« (Greiner, 2003a: 90).

33 Whereas the law of energy conservation and the law of non-decreasing entropy encompass all physical entities, the law for being-an-atom merely applies to atoms. The type-law for an atom is specified – it holds only for atoms – and at the same time it is universal since it applies to all atoms. But because not everything in Wirklichkeit is an atom, its type-law is restricted only to those entities known as atoms. In passing we may note that this distinction runs parallel to Kant's distinction between (universal) a priori laws and so-called »empirical laws« (1783: 320; §36): »Wir müßen aber empirische Gesetze der Natur, die jederzeit besondere Wahrnehmungen voraussetzen, von der reinen oder allgemeinen Naturgesetzen, welche, ohne daß besondere Wahrnehmungen zum Grunde liegen, bloß die Bedingungen ihrer notwendigen Vereinigung in der Erfahrung enthalten [...].«

ferent from physics in fact do speak about causality, albeit every time within a different (»strange«) context. Just consider the connection between the premise and conclusion of an argument – an instance of *logical* causality. Or think about the book written by the sociologist McIver on »Social Causality« (1942). The same applies to the science of law, where there are prominent theories defending different views of jural causality – such as the *conditio sine qua non* theory (von Buri), the theory of adequate causation (von Kries) or that of the »typical causal course« (Traeger).[34]

A systematic and comprehensive theory of the uniqueness and interconnectedness of the various ontic modes of reality (*Wirklichkeit*) is needed if a meaningful account is required of the *basic concepts* of the various disciplines. First of all the dimension of modal aspects ought to be acknowledged as an integral part of the experiential horizon of the human embeddedness within *Wirklichkeit*. These modal aspects are not human constructions – they belong to the ontic structure of the world (*Wirklichkeit*) in which we live. They should not be confused with our provisional and fallible human account (»constructions«) because they *make possible* such projects to begin with. Whatever we can experience as human beings is co-conditioned by this dimension of ontic modes.[35] The neo-Kantian Marburg school in legal philosophy, for example, claimed that the human experience of jural relationships is made possible by our *concept of law* (Stammler, Radbruch, Kelsen). But this view is subjectivistic and constantly struggles with the basic problem of all subjectivism already clearly apprehended by Kant, namely how subjective conditions of thought (in the case of neo-Kantianism: subjective concepts) can obtain objective (universal) validity. We have mentioned that Kant wrote about the difficulty involved in explaining how »*subjective conditions of thought* can have *objective validity*, that is, can furnish conditions of the possibility of all knowledge of objects« (1787, B 122).

If we understand the term *transcendental* in an *ontic sense*, namely with reference to the delimiting and enabling horizon of human *experience* making possible whatever we are and can do within the *Wirklichkeit* in which we live, we have already embarked on applying the *transcendental-empirical* method. This application gives a new meaning to *Verfremdung* insofar as the latter relates to different (»strange«) disciplinary universes of discourse, because at once it highlights the inevitable *connectedness* between those ontic domains, evidenced in the innumerable *modal analogies* present between them. If every modal aspect of reality is indeed *distinct* then our language must contain words (terms) reflecting this unique (and irreducible) meaning of each particular aspect. For example, when it

34 See the penetrating analysis of Dooyeweerd where he discusses the issue of jural causlity in depth – 1997: 39-70.

35 The time dimension and the dimension of entities are also conditioning human experience.

comes to functional »property-terms«, such as causality, life, power, multiplicity, and wholeness, one has to specify the *original modal seat* of these terms. Where the core meaning of the physical aspect is given in energy-operation the original modal seat of the term *causality* is clearly found within the *physical* aspect. *Life* finds its modal seat within the biotic aspect of reality (*Wirklichkeit*). Similarly, *power* relates to the free formative fantasy of humankind located within the cultural historical aspect of reality. *Multiplicity* and *wholeness* reside respectively within the quantitative and the spatial aspects of reality.

Suppose we start (almost like the Pythagoreans who overstated their case in claiming that everything *is* number) with the meaning of multiplicity, i.e., with the *one* and the *many*. Then our most basic intuition is an awareness of one, another one, yet another one, and so on indefinitely, infinitely. The core meaning of *discrete quantity* entails the most basic understanding of infinity in the sense of the *successive infinite*. Suppose that we now want to alienate (*verfremdet*) this arithmetical vocabulary by placing it within a context *different* from the numerical, namely the *spatial*. Spatial figures are extended and they present themselves *at once*. If all the parts of a spatial figure are not given simultaneously, it is lacking. The three sides of a triangle cannot be given in succession; they ought to be present at once for otherwise we simply would not have a triangle at hand. Although we are now operating within a universe of discourse different from the numerical, the remarkable outcome of a scrutiny of what happens here is that the meaning of spatial extension intrinsically coheres with the meaning of number, for otherwise we cannot explain the descent of our (analogical) awareness of *multiplicity* evinced within the structure of *spatial* relations. First of all space is extended in different (more than one) dimensions and in order to designate these dimensions we need to employ the natural numbers 1, 2, 3 and so on. Furthermore, the factual extension of any specific spatial figure – be it in one, two or more dimensions – once again shows the interconnection between space and number, because one dimensional extension is normally designated as length, two dimensional extension as surface, and so on (every time specified by using a particular number, for example when reference is made to 2 inches, 3 square feet or 5 liter). The *differences* between any two aspects are always seen in their *similarities*. The *successive infinite* within the numerical aspect – endlessness in the literal sense of the word – is similar to what is found in a spatially extended figure, for the latter always allows for a *successive infinite number* of divisions. Yet in this similarity a fundamental *difference* is seen, for the succession beyond all limits is now turned »inwards« – captured in the *infinite divisibility* of any spatial continuum. Compared with the nature of *physical space*, this original modal meaning of space once again evinces both a moment of *similarity* and of *difference*. Both physical space and mathematical space are *extended*, but whereas mathematical space is both continuous and infinitely divisible, physical space is neither continuous nor infinitely divisible.[36] The meaning of an aspect may also be *deepened* or *disclosed* in the case where it refers or points beyond itself to an aspect which is less basic than the aspect under consideration. For example, when the numerical meaning of the successive infinite is deepened under the guidance of our spatial intuition of *at once* then the deepened and disclosed meaning of infinity is met in the form of the at *once infinite.*[37] Logical analysis (identification and distinguishing) may be deepened by the frugal meaning of the economic aspect – evinced in the logical principle of the economy of thought (historically also known as »Occam's razor«). In this case the meaning of the logical aspect is deepened by its interconnection with the economic aspect of reality.[38]

The transcendental-empirical method of analyzing the interconnections between different modal aspects thus reveals that although every aspect is unique its *meaning* can only come to expression in its *coherence* with all the other aspects of reality. Within the various disciplines this interconnectedness manifests itself in the inevitable employment of basic concepts and ideas referring to all those aspects *differing* from the one delimiting the field of investigation of the discipline under consideration.[39] Whereas *Verfremdung* may highlight the *difference* between the contexts of different aspects, the inherent connectedness evinces an intimate bond or relation between different aspects and in this sense *Befreundung* constitutes the other side of the *Verfremdung* coin.

4. Concluding remark

Insofar as this contribution searched for points of connection to an expanded understanding of the ontological foundations of constructive realism it attempted to appreciate many facets of the thought of Fritz Wallner positively. But insofar as this expanded understanding articulated a few critical reservations and even instances of immanent criticism, it is meant to stimulate the thought of this creative and respected philosophical colleague. Because I can identify pretty well with his struggle against enemies such as metaphysics, the over-estimated role of technol-

36 Hilbert, the foremost mathematician of the 20th century, explained this remarkable situation in his commemorative article on the infinite. See Hilbert, 1925: 164.

37 Traditionally, with a less intuitive appeal, these two kinds of infinity were designated as potential infinity and actual infinity (or: incompleted and completed infinity).

38 Naturally it by far transcends the scope of this article to explain the general theory of modal aspects in more detail, but its first formulation is still accessible in the Collected Works of the Dutch philosopher Herman Dooyeweerd (see Dooyeweerd, 1997a, Volume 2, pp.3-426).

39 An example of the application of the transcendental-empirical method within the natural sciences is found in the comprehensive work of Stafleu (1980), and within the humanities in the equally penetrating works of Hommes (1972, 1976 and 1986).

ogy, the limitations of cognitive science, and so on, I do hope that my portrayal of the intellectual background of modern constructivism may inspire him to some second thoughts in this regard. I did not explore his idea that intellectual endeavours are *activities* and I also did not interact with his idea of the constructive role of contradiction and antinomy (apparently derived from Vaihinger's philosophy of »as if«).

But it is clear that the challenge posed to contemporary philosophy of science by the approach of constructive realism will generate fruitful discussions in the future.

Reference

Agnese, B. (1999). *Konstruktion und Metapher. Der Metapher-Begriff zwischen Sprachphilosophie, Literatur und Wissenschaft.* In Wallner (1999).

Beck, H. (1999). *Metaphysische Implikationen im Konstruktiven Realismus.* In Wallner (1999).

Cassirer, E. (1971). *Das Erkenntnisproblem in der Philosophie und Wissenschaft der neueren Zeit* (Volume 2, 3rd edition). Darmstadt: Wissenschaftliche Buchgesellschaft.

Greiner, K. (2003). *Pädagogische Intention und Importanz des konstruktiven Realismus.* In Wallner (2003).

Greiner, K. (2003a). *Vacation, Strangification and Self-Knowledge – Versuch einer epistemologischen Verhältnisbestimmung von Alltag und Urlaub.* In Wallner (2003).

Dooyeweerd, H. (1997). *The modal structure of jural causlity*, in *Essays in Legal, Social and Political Philosophy. The Collected Works of Herman Dooyeweerd, Series B, Volume 2* (General Editor D.F.M. Strauss). Lewiston: The Edwin Mellen Press.

Dooyeweerd, H. (1997a). *A New Critique of Theoretical Thought. The Collected Works of Herman Dooyeweerd, Series A, Volume 1-4* (General Editor D.F.M. Strauss). Lewiston: The Edwin Mellen Press.

Dummett, M.A.E. (1995). *FREGE, Philosophy of Mathematics* (second printing). Cambridge: Harvard University Press.

Freeman, K. (1949). *Companion to the Pre-Socratic Philosophers.* Oxford: Basil Blackwell.

Hartmann, N. (1957). *Kleinere Schriften. Volume II.* Berlin.

Hilbert, D. .(1925). Ueber das Unendliche. In *Mathematische Annalen*, Vol. 95, 1925 (pp.161-190).

Hommes, Van Eikema. (1972). *De Elementaire Grondbegrippen der Rechtswetenschap.* Deventer: Kluwer.

Hommes, Van Eikema. (1976). *De Samengestelde Grondbegrippen der Rechtswetenschap.* Zwolle: W.E.J. Tjeenk.

Hommes, Van Eikema. (1986). *De Wijsgerige Grondslagen van de Rechtssociologie.* Zwolle: W.E.J. Tjeenk.

Janich, P. (1975). *Trägheitsgesetz und Inertialsystem.* In Thiel (1975) (pp.66-76).

Kant, I. (1781/1787). *Kritik der reinen Vernunft* (first edition 1781, second edition 1787). Hamburg: Felix Meiner (1956).

Kant, I. (1783). *Prolegomena einer jeden künftigen Metaphysik die als Wissenschaft wird auftreten können* (ed. by Karl Vorländer). Hamburg: Felix Meiner.

Kline, M. (1980). *Mathematics. The Loss of Certainty*. New York.

Stafleu, M.D. (1980). *Time and Again. A Systematic Analysis of the Foundations of Physics*. Toronto: Wedge.

Stafleu, M.D. (1987). *Theories at Work: On the Structure and Functioning of Theories in Science, in Particular during the Copernican Revolution*. Lanham: University Press of America.

Strauss, DFM (2003). Frege's Attack on »Abstraction« and his Defense of the »Applicability« of Arithmetic (as Part of Logic). In *South African Journal of Philosophy, 22(1)* (pp.63-80).

Thiel, C. (1975). *Frege und die moderne Grundlagenforschung*. Meisenheim am Glan: Verlag Anton Hain.

Van Woudenberg, R. (1991). *Transcendentale reflecties, Een onderzoek naar transcendentale argumenten in de contemporaine filosofie, met bijzondere aandacht voor de transcendentale pragmatiek van Karl-Otto Apel*. Amsterdam: VU Boekhandel Uitgeverij.

Veling, K. (2000). *Ruimte voor de rede, Filosofie als systematische reflectie*. Kampen: Agora.

Von Weizsäcker, C.F. (1993). *Der Mensch in seiner Geschichte*. München: dtv.

Wallner, F.G. (1992). *Acht Vorlesungen über den Konstruktivismus*. Vienna: Universitäts-Verlagsbuchhandlung.

Wallner, F.G. (1999). *Konstruktion und Verfremdung* (edited by Wallner, F.G. & Agnese, B.). Vienna: Universitäts-Verlagsbuchhandlung.

Wallner, F.G. (2003). *Konstruktion und Erziehung, Zum Verhältnis von konstruktivistischem Denken und pädagogischen Intentionen* (edited by Wallner, F.G. & Greiner, K.). Hamburg: Kovač.

Wallner, F.G. (2003a). *Bildung, Ethik und Konstruktion*. In Wallner 2003 (pp.37-58).

Wang, Hao (1988): *Reflections on Gödel*. Cambridge MA: MIT Press.

Tsugio Mimuro

Nishida's Concept of ›Pure Experience‹ and Language with Special Reference to Humboldt's View of Language

Translated by Martin J. Jandl

Nishida Kitarô (1870-1945) is regarded as the founder of modern Japanese philosophy, and his book *A Study of Good* (*Zen no Kenkyû*) first published in 1911 is considered without doubt as the most famous and the most important work in the history of Japanese philosophy. Nishida tackled intensively the Western history of thought in philosophy, the humanities, and mathematics, but this dealing was critically orientated according to the Japanese tradition of reasoning.

His work is founded on the concept of ›pure experience‹. Nishida intended to explain everything with pure experience as the only reality. »What is reality?« is a question he asked for a long time. Although Nishida's trains of thoughts modify partially or sometimes radically during his philosophical reasoning and deepened, the concept of pure experience is the core notion in his philosophy. Nishida himself considered the concept of pure experience as the ›foundation‹ of his philosophy. Very intensively he aimed at clearing up the structure of the true reality and of the true self until death. Because of that Nishida's philosophy is after all a ›philosophy of nothingness‹ broadening in contrast to Western ›philosophy of being‹ new horizons and attracting global attention. Nishida's philosophy is known as ›Nishida-philosophy‹, and his scholars at the Kyoto University established the Kyoto School where his philosophical views were adopted and developed.

Nishida's *A Study of Good* deals with reality understood as phenomenon of consciousness without referring directly to the issue of language. In the following I will reflect Nishida's concept of pure experience from the perspective of Wilhelm von Humboldt's ideas of language to examine the relation of pure experience and language, why Nishida didn't conceive language as subject matter of his philosophy, and whether his conception of reality as pure experience can be considered as an issue of language.

1.

A Study of Good commences with the following words: »To experience means to know events precisely as they are. It means to cast away completely one's own inner workings, and to know in accordance with the events. Since people usually include some thought when speaking of experience, the word ›pure‹ is here used to signify a condition of true experience itself without the addition of the least thought or reflection.« (Nishida 1988, p.1) According to Nishida the view of matter and spirit as separated entities conceiving matter as object and mind as subject – as often found in Western philosophy – is »only hypothesised by the demands of our thought« (Nishida 1988, p.38). E.g. here is a table. Nishida asks: ›What is the desk that is now before my eyes?‹ The table has a special shape, a special colour, and if I touch the table, I will feel a special resistance. From it Nishida draws the conclusion that shape and colour are perceptions of my eyes and the feeling of resistance is a perception of my hand. That means: »Even such things as the form and condition, size, position, and movement of matter – all that which we directly perceive – are not the objective states of matter itself.« (Nishida 1988, p.39) The matter itself will not be perceived if it is separated from our consciousness.

Nishida claims that understanding the true reality requires to drop all artificial hypothesis and to take »direct knowledge which allows no doubt« (Nishida 1988, p.39) as starting point. Direct knowledge »consists only of events of our intuitive experience, or, in other words, it resides only in knowledge concerning phenomena of consciousness« (Nishida 1988, p.39). »Intuition is not seeing the latter as a judgement of the former; it is merely knowing events just as they are.« (Nishida 1988, p.40) This state of consciousness is the unity of knowledge, feeling, and volition in which subject and object are not separated, in which knowledge and its matter are absolutely one. That's what Nishida calls ›pure experience‹ that is as base experience to equate with direct experience. Nishida assumes that the starting point of all knowledge is direct knowledge of events in consciousness respective in events of direct experience. Direct experience concerns not only perception. For Nishida our reasoning is a phenomenon of consciousness. We cannot recognise the nature of matters by reason. »When we wholly cast away our ego and become one with the object of our thought, namely our problem, or if we speak even more appositely, when we have submerged our ego in the midst of it, we first see the operation of thought.« (Nishida 1988, p.12) The judgement has its source in demands of our reasoning and is achieved after the distinction between subject and object: It arises the dissecting of the direct experienced. Even our bodies are »nothing more than a part of our conscious phenomena« (Nishida 1988, p.43). There are only conscious phenomena. »Our world is composed from the facts of conscious phenomena.« (Nishida 1988, p.45) »In the ordinary meaning, even though there is no thing, seen from the point of intuition which destroys the distinction between subject and object, still a consciousness of ›nothing‹ truly exists.« (Nishida 1988, p.47)

Nishida emphasises the original uniformity of consciousness. It is a system in all and unfolds itself spontaneously and systematically because our conscious functions are structuring and active and accordingly the true reality is totally dynamic. »The basic form of reality lies in the fact that while it is one it is many, while it is many it is one, in the midst of equality it maintains distinctions, and in the midst of distinctions it maintains equality.« (Nishida 1988, p.60) True reality consists of unity and opposition or contradiction. »Red things are established in opposition to colours which are not red, and things which operate are established in opposition to that which receives such operation.« (Nishida 1988, p.59) Thus »true reality is the free development arising from one thing's internal necessity« (Nishida 1988, p.61). True reality is the unfolding of conscious contents till completion. It is the active force of volition working in the inner of the conscious system that searches for a greater unity. The conscious system unfolds itself – like all organisms – according to an order in accordance with this force until its unity is completed. Nishida stresses this constantly working unifying force that he also calls ›a certain unifying thing‹, ›a certain unifying and unchangeable element‹, or ›the generality‹. This unifying force transcends the individual. If we assumed the self as subject hidden behind this unifying force, we would be caught in solipsism: »It is not that since there is the individual there is experience, but rather that since there is experience there is the individual.« (Nishida 1988, p.19)

Namely Nishida supposes that in the background of all reality there is ›the generality‹ working with its dialectic relatedness. An event of pure experience is the so-called generality realising itself (see Nishida 1988, p.17). The structure of reality consists of the generality as unseparated reality and the reality as the diversity evolved of the self realisation of the generality. The same principle is guilty for reality and consciousness: Reality as unifying side and consciousness as unified side emerges from the same principle of unifying force underlying all things and of the conscious inner. Nishida assumes that the force of our consciousness and the unifying force of all cosmic phenomena are identical. Our spirit as unifying function fills the whole reality in which unity prevails. E.g., if we are looking at a thing, we will grasp a homogeneous certain something in his unity, the whole reality in its unity.

In this way Nishida explains the emergence of all things and all reality by the unifying force of the self resulting from the unifying force of the spirit. According to him nature is constituted by this eternal, unchangeable, and endless unifying force of the self. Pure experience is the direct perception both of the self and the universe, and the advance of the will is the completion of this intuitive unity (see Nishida 1988, p.36) – the completion of the will is the realisation of the true self. In this self-realisation of the self ›the good‹ is to be searched. Thus the good is the manifestation of man's innate nature (see Nishida 1988, p.134) and reconciles with the true reality of the self (see Nishida 1988, p.135). It is about to know the true self (see Nishida 1988, p.156). Nishida (1988, p.69) emphasises that actually it is not that there is a self apart from matter, but rather that our self is directly the unifier itself of the reality of the universe. The knowledge about the true self units us with the general good of mankind, with the substance of the universe, and with God's will. »The law of knowing the true self and of uniting with God lies only in becoming aware of the force of the union of subject and object.«

(Nishida 1988, p.156) Thus God is both the foundation of the universe (see Nishida 1988, p.167) and the unity of the universe (see Nishida 1988, p.177). According to Nishida we can thus view God in this sense as »one great intellectual intuition at the foundation of the universe« (see Nishida 1988, p.175) and we can see Him as the unifier of pure experience which embraces the universe.

By determining reality as a phenomenon of our consciousness and as an event of pure experience based monisticly on direct perception Nishida fights against the artificial dualistic hypothesis and tries to overcome solipsism. Ultimately Nishida's philosophy of pure experience starting with concrete facts and events achieves the issue of moral and God.

2.

As an example for pure experience Nishida (1988, p.50) names the moment »when our hearts are captured by sublime music, one's self and things are both forgotten, and the whole universe becomes only one melodious sound, at this moment so-called true reality is present«. The thought is a vibration in the air; or: Saying ›It's me listening to the music‹ would pull us out of true reality. A thought emerges a reflection that does not share the true occurrence of reality. The thought refers to that moment »of seeing a colour or hearing a sound which occurs not only before one has added the judgement that this seeing or hearing relates to something external or that one is feeling this sensation, but even before one has judged what colour or what sound it is« (see Nishida 1988, p.1).

The true pure experience is according to Nishida without importance; no matter how complex pure experience is, however, at the moment of its happening it is always one simple event (see Nishida 1988, p.2). He states: »True, pure experience can exist only in present consciousness of events as they are without attaching any meaning to them at all.« (Nishida 1988, pp.1) The meaning arises if conscious leaves the present unity and relates to a different conscious content. With it experience is not any longer present and pure. »That which appears within meaning or judgement is a part which has been abstracted from the original experience.« (Nishida 1988, p.7) Nishida claims that in the severe unity of the present and concrete consciousness lies the truth and that criteria of truth are comprised within the state of pure experience. And he stresses that »perfect truth is not that which must be expressed in words« (Nishida 1988, p.28). True reality as an event of pure experience like true meaning of arts can't be communicated from one person to another one. »The true state of this kind of reality is something which we must only apprehend and not something we must reflect upon, analyze, or must be able to express in words.« (Nishida 1988, p.53)

Nishida's concept or pure experience offers us an approach to the issue of language. Normally we suppose that we describe our experiences linguistically.

What is captured by language is usually called experience. Nishida (1988, p.1) replies to this view that people usually include some thought when speaking experience. Thus language includes some thought. And so we can state that Nishida's concept of pure experience aims at a conscious state that is before or above language and that can't be conceived as subject of linguistic consideration. In the second appendix of the collected lectures at the Kyoto University titled *Pure Experience* Nishida writes: »The event of true unmediated experience does not mean that we recognise it. It is no question whether *we* recognise, but simply a question of *cognition*. But that's not exactly the point. That's how it is: Red is red. If you say that something is red then you will judge – what is no longer the event of true unmediated experience. The event of true unmediated experience is just the event of red that can't be conceived linguistically.« (Nishida 1966^2, p.180) It concerns not the designation ›red‹ that is a categorised colour name, neither a state possibly designed with ›red‹ because recognised it is the result of a judgement. The point is the event ›red‹, the moment in which we recognise the event as so-being. In this moment the recogniser and the recognised is one, the recogniser and the recognised meets without being one the subject and the other the object. In this moment world and human comes in touch.

Wilhelm von Humboldt who is regarded as the founder of modern linguistics because of his investigations of diverse languages and because of his reflections on language states: »Die Berührung der Welt mit dem Menschen ist der elektrische Schlag, aus welchem die Sprache hervorspringt. [The touch of world and man is the electric shock which bursts language.]« (Humboldt 1968^2, p.204) We have to scrutinise whether Humboldt's electric shock leads directly and immediately to the bursting of language, how he conceived the development of language and whether he thought of something that transcends language.

In general language is viewed as historically developed social institution that is given to us with birth, and we express our thinking and feelings by means of language. To speak, to talk about something means to use the acquired language to express our thoughts and feelings. By means of acquired words we express ourselves and communicate with others. But Humboldt does not aim at the use of language or the employment of words. Contrarily he states: »Language cannot indeed be regarded as a material that sits there, surveyable in its totality, or communicable little by little, but must be seen as something that eternally produces itself, where the laws of production are determined, but the scope and even to some extent the nature of the product remain totally unspecified.« (Humboldt 1988, p.58) Humboldt claims that intellectual activity of the mind is connected inseparably with language and thus he calls language as »the formative organ of thought« (Humboldt, 1988, p.54). Language, indeed, arises from a depth of human nature which everywhere forbids us to regard it as a true product and creation of peoples. It possesses an autonomy that visibly declares itself to us, though inexplicable in its nature, and, seen from this aspect, is no production of activity, but an involuntary emanation of the spirit, no work of nations, but a gift fallen to them by their inner destiny (see Humboldt 1988, p.24).

His often quoted definition of language reads: »In itself it is no product (*ergon*), but an activity (*energeia*). Its true definition can therefore only be a genetic one. For it is the ever-repeated *mental labour* of making the *articulated* sound capable of expressing *thought*.« (Humboldt 1988, p.49) And he continues: »In a direct and strict sense, this is the definition of *speech* on any occasion; in its true and essential meaning, however, we can also regard, as it were, only the totality of this speaking as the language.« (Humboldt 1988, p.49) According to Humboldt (1988, p.59) the word is »a copy, not of the object in itself, but of the image thereof produced in consciousness.« Words are signs of concepts, and without concept there is no object for consciousness. Thus there is no concept without language. Words compromising meaningfully articulated sounds and concepts are the true elements of speech. But for Humboldt speech is not compounded by words emerging the speech, but conversely words emerge the totality of speech. »It is impossible to conceive the origin of language as beginning with the designation of objects by words, and then proceeding to put them together. In reality, speech is not compounded out of words that have preceded it; the words, on the contrary, emerge from the totality of speech.« (Humboldt 1988, p.70) Language arises in the moment when ›reflection‹ supervenes: »Speech flows on, indeed, with unbroken continuity, and until reflection on language supervenes, the speaker is contemplating therein the totality only of the thought to be designated.« (Humboldt 1988, p.70) Before reflection there is the totality only of the thought to be designated. »Within the soul, what we distinguish in reflection is undividedly one.« (Humboldt 1988, p.85) In his first work on language young Humboldt (1961[1], p.581) wrote: »Die Sprache beginnt [...] unmittelbar und sogleich mit dem ersten Akt der Reflektion. [Language rises immediately with the first act of reflection. – Translation by M.J.]« He conceived reflection as distinction of the thinking person and the thought. To achieve distinction the soul in its ongoing activity must come to a standstill, grasping this notion (›Vorstellung‹) achieved in the standstill in a unity, and so confronting itself as an object. The nature of reasoning is to make sections in its own course.

It is obvious that Humboldt thought of a moment concerning the emergence of language at which the ongoing mind comes to a standstill and until this standstill the notion (›Vorstellung‹) is not a unity of subject and object. Up to the moment of standstill thinking and thought are not separated – there is no distinction of subject and object without language. Humboldt's view of a pre-reflective state reminds one of Nishida's pure experience although there is a difference between Humboldt's and Nishida's view. According to Humboldt the first act of reflection as the first impulse arouses man out of dullness of lust in that the subject engulfs the object and thus leads man to consciousness. Humboldt does not make the pre-reflective state to a matter of his considerations because language starts immediately and instantly with the first reflective act: By it the totality of the thought to be designated or the inseparable unity in the inner of the soul is distinguished (separated), articulated in separate words, and made to speech. In the totality of this mental process as concrete speaking – as speech – Humboldt conceives the nature of language. According to Humboldt speaking means the ›production‹ and the ›formation‹ of language. The »language proper lies in the act of its real production« (Humboldt 1988, p.49). That is a constantly language producing intellectual activity giving rise to the genesis of language. That is the reason why Humboldt views language as ›*energeia*‹ and why he claims that its definition must be a ›genetic‹ one.

3.

In a note possibly written at the time of *A Study of Good* that has been published after his death and titled by the editor as *Fragments of Pure Experience* Nishida writes: »Pure unmediated experience is a state without judgement. When wind rustles this *rustling* is the event of unmediated perception. It is no question whether it is *the wind*. This event has neither subject nor object. « (Nishida 1966[1], p.283) Usually both the wind's rustling and the listening is assumed to be experience. Ueda Shizuteru who holds as descendant of Nishida's philosophy the view of the Kyoto School assumes that the ›I‹ doesn't hear the rustling, but that the rustling represents an infinity as totality of perception without split of subject and object. The event of rustling is the basic event that is simply given. Besides the rustling there is no ›I‹. That is the reason why the ›I‹ is the rustling itself without an ›I‹ (see Ueda 1988, p.42).

Sure, Nishida is influenced by Buddhism, especially by Zen Buddhism. Indeed Nishida was instructed in Zen meditation by suggestion of his primary school friend Suzuki Titarô Daisetsu (who is a globally known Zen philosopher and a spiritual master) through a period of nearly 10 years starting in his mid-twenties. According to the Buddhist doctrine consciousness is the true source of the mind, and all modes of being and phenomena owe their existence to the activity of consciousness. »There is [in Buddhist doctrine], indeed, one complete undivided whole world and nothing else.« (Suzuki 1948, p.6) This one whole world is a mental world that exists without the conception of an ›I‹, a world containing everything indiscriminate, indeterminate, undistinguished, and undifferentiated. It is the absolute world of non distinction. In Buddhism contrary concepts merge on a spiritual level: »It is to become Prajña itself where there is no distinction between the subject and the object of intuition, and yet there is a clear perception of the distinction – that is the distinction of non-distinction and the discrimination of non-discrimination.« (Suzuki 1948, p.15) Suzuki continues: »Prajña is thus *achintya*, ›beyond thinking‹, or ›no-thinking‹. All thinking involves the distinction of this and that, for to think means to divide, to analyse. *Achintya*, no-thinking, means not to divide, that is, to pass beyond all intellection, and the whole Buddhist teaching revolves about this central idea of no-thought, or no-thinking-ness, or no-minded-ness, or *achintya-prajña*, showing that no spiritual truth could be grasped by ratiocination.« (Suzuki 1948, pp.14)

Nishida's concept of pure experience relates to the basic level of consciousness where the linguistic determination of experience is broken. As long as the linguistic determined world is the horizon of our experience it may happen – according to Ueda – that a certain event breaks the linguistic determination and thus deprives us of language. The appearance of this event creates again language that designates this event and opens us a new and wider world. Ueda describes this double process as follows: »Out of language, into language.« According to him pure experience is nothing else but this dynamic process – a process melted into both the process ›Out of the self, into the self‹ and the process ›Out of the world, into the world‹. This process is a basic event recreating the originality of experience and simultaneously creating language (see Ueda 1991, p.42).

By breaking the frame of subjectivity and objectivity by a certain event the totality appears immediately in consciousness comprising the moments of true reality, of true self, and of the universe. Thus it is an opening of the world to the infinite in which human leaves himself behind and loses language. In other words, human is in a state of de-articulation (›Entsprachlichung‹) that opens as a start point the possibility of a new articulation (›Versprachlichung‹): At this point the world is opened as a meaningfully structured linguistic horizon and language arises. Indeed, we experience this process in every day life. E.g., Mori Arimasa (1911-1973) who was a philosopher studying Descartes and Pascal and who lived for a long time in Paris where he taught as a university professor writes in an essay after seeing his native country after a surgery: »I felt pleasure so that nature itself got into my perception nakedly without any disturbance by the names or sentences made up by man. No, to speak more exactly, it was the state before what is called pleasure. Only subsequently I call this state by ›pleasure‹.« (Mori Arimasa 1976^2, p.100)

Like Nishida Mori assumes that the so-called reality is our experience itself and that experience founds the ›I‹. The individual is made of experiences based on the immediate relation of perception to matters (see Mori 1976^1, p.56). This immediate relation of perception to matters is a frequent subject of short poems in Japan – like a Haiku made of 17 syllables or a Tanka (short poem) made of 31 syllables. Matsuo Bashô, a well known Haiku poem who lived in the 17th century and is famous until our days explained the art of Haiku to a scholar in the following way: »Our teacher said: ›Everything that concerns the pine learn from the pine itself; what concerns the bamboo learn from the bamboo itself.‹ That means: ›Free yourself from your own will!‹ […] ›To learn‹ means in this context: If you are confronted with things and if you look at them, then you will reveal their subtle life. If you conceive it with your heart, then it will appear in a poem immediately.« (Hattori 1961, p.398)

If you let something appearance directly at the surface of a poem then, according to Bashô, the thing and the self are separated. »Take hold of the flash in that a thing appears with words before it vanishes in the heart.« (Hattori 1961, p.401) The situation in that appears a flash of something should be captured by a poem. Nishida, too, views in the Haiku the character of the Japanese way of life and its particularity to grasp the infinite within reality (see Nishida 1966[3]). He wrote many short poems in his life assuming that they are appropriate for the designation of the inner. In the form of the short poem the writer conceives life from the centre of the present, from the point of moment (see Nishida 1966[4], p.131). One of Nishida's short poems reads:

The gloomy, long rain	Urasaburu
Has stopped.	Nagaame harete
Down at the fence	Kaki no Ne ni
Flowers shine.	Moezuru Hana no
And how fresh their colour!	Iro no Sayakesa

Nishida saw after a long period of rain suddenly the beauty of flower shining under the fence, and he grasped it by words. As Bashô said Nishida took »the light making things shining by words until it vanishes in the heart«. Enthusiastic about the beauty his self dissolves in it and he was freed from his own will. In other words, in this short poem pure experience as de- articulation (›Entsprachlichung‹) is articulated (›versprachlicht‹) by the poet. This is the Zen method, and, as Suzuki writes, the Zen approach is to enter right into the object itself and see it, as it were, from the inside: »To know the flower is to become the flower, to be the flower, to bloom as the flower, and to enjoy the sunlight as well as the rainfall. When this is done, the flower speaks to me and I know all its secrets, all its joys, all its sufferings; that is, all its life vibrating within itself. [...] By losing myself in the flower I know my Self as well as the flower.« (Suzuki 1960, pp.11)

4.

Nishida views the structure of true reality in the self development of the conscious content. He describes the emergence scheme of the independent, self determining true reality with as follows: »First the whole appears ›implicity‹, and from his content differentiatingly develops; and when this differentiating development is concluded, the whole of reality has been realised and is completed.« (Nishida 1988, p.54) These words hint at the three moments of pure experience. Firstly the basic phase before the subject-object-split in that the totality appears implicitly. Secondly the differentiation of the totality content by that self consciousness becomes structured in itself, develops, and becomes aware of itself as one reality. And thirdly, the final unity in the differentiation of the conscious content as realisation and completion of reality. Nishida conceived this process abstractly; at least he was searching the reason for the self development of the conscious content in the infinite power of universe unifying reality. Thus Nishida comes by metaphysics.

The three phases of pure experience are interpretable pertaining to Humboldt's view of language like this: In the first phase – the pre-reflective phase – the totality to be designated by words appears as unite whole in the inner of the mind. In the second phase begins the first act of reflection distinguishing the thinking person from his object, separating the totality, and the impression of the image produced in the soul by this object becomes a word and is meaningfully articulated. In the third phase following the second one immediately the word or language emerges as emancipation of mind. For Humboldt (1988, p.70) results from this view: If we picture language as a second world, that man has objectified out of himself from the impressions he receives from the true one, then words are the sole objects therein for which the character of individuality must be retained, even in form. But Humboldt (1988, p.157) also adds: If the feeling truly awakens in the soul, that language is not just a medium of exchange for mutual comprehension, but a true *world* which the *mind* must insert, by its own inner labour, between itself and *objects*, then it is on the right road towards continually finding more and depositing more in its language. But this presupposes two things: a feeling that there is something which the language does not directly contain, but which the mind, spurred on by language, must supply; and the impulse, in turn, to couple everything felt by the soul with a sound (see Humboldt, 1988, p.157). He continues: »Both arise from the living conviction that the nature of man has intimations of a region that *transcends* language, and is actually constricted by language; but the language in turn is the only means of exploring and fertilizing this region, and that precisely by technical and sensuous improvement it is capable of assimilating an ever larger proportion thereof to itself.« (Humboldt 1988, p.157)

Nishida's considerations are obviously accompanied by this ›feeling‹ or by these ›intimations‹. He makes the field transcending language to the starting point of his understanding of true reality to understand the true face of universe and life. To use Ueda's words, Nishida's point is leaving language, whereas Humboldt defines human as a linguistic determined being: »Man is only man because of language.« (Humboldt 1997, p.12). Humboldt is interested in the development of language, in the coming-into-language. Because of Nishida's view that human is being-above-language instead of being-in-language he tries to break the frame of language as a second world in the Humboldtian sense and to grasp the most basic foundation transcending language because Nishida is convinced that human touches world in its true originality by his consciousness becoming one with it. From the perspective of language Nishida's concept of pure experience is an articulation (›Versprachlichung‹) of super-articulation (›Über-Sprachlichung‹) and de-articulation (›Ent-Sprachlichung‹).

Reference

Hattori, Dohô (1961). *Akasôshi. In Rengaronshû, Haikuronshû*. Tokyo: Iwanami-Shoten.

Humboldt, Wilhelm von (1988). *On Language. The Diversity of Human Language-Structure and its Influence on the Mental Development of Mankind* (translated by P. Heath). Cambridge, New York, New Rochelle, Melbourne, Sydney: Cambridge University Press.

Humboldt, Wilhelm von (1997). *On the Comparative Study of Language and its Relation to the Different Periods of Language Development*. In W. v. Humboldt, Essays on Language (edited by T. Harden and D. Farrelly). Frankfurt am Main, Berlin, Bern, New York, Paris, Wien: Peter Lang.

Humboldt, Wilhelm von (1968[1]). *Über Denken und Sprechen*. In Wilhelm von Humboldts Gesammelte Schriften. Bd. VII. Berlin: Walter de Gruyter.

Humboldt, Wilhelm von (1968[2]). *Ueber die Verschiedenheiten des menschlichen Sprachbaues*. In Wilhelm von Humboldts Gesammelte Schriften. Bd. VI. Berlin: Walter de Gruyter.

Mori, Arimasa (1976[1]). *Henbô. In Shisaku to Keiken o megutte*. Tokyo: Kôdansha.

Mori, Arimasa (1976[2]). *Kigi wa Hikari o Abite. In Shisaku to Keiken o megutte*. Tokyo: Kôdansha.

Nishida, Kitarô (1988). *A Study of Good* (translated by V. H. Viglielmo). Tokyo: Yushodo.

Nishida, Kitarô (1966[1]). Junsui Keiken ni kansuru Danshô. In *Nishida Kitarô Zenshû. Vol. 16*. Tokyo: Iwanami-Shoten.

Nishida, Kitarô (1966[2]). Kôgi. Tetsugaku Gairon. In *Nishida Kitarô Zenshû. Vol. 15*. Tokyo: Iwanami-Shoten.

Nishida, Kitarô (1966[3]). Kokugo no Jizaisei. In Nishida *Kitarô Zenshû. Vol. 12*. Tokyo: Iwanami-Shoten.

Nishida, Kitarô (1966[4]). Tanka ni tsuite. In *Nishida Kitarô Zenshû. Vol. 13*. Tokyo: Iwanami-Shoten.

Suzuki, Daisetsu Teitarô (1960). Lectures on Zen Buddhism. In D. T. Suzuki, *Zen Buddhism and Psychoanalysis*. New York, Hagerstown, San Francisco, London: Harper & Row, Publishers.

Suzuki, Daisetsu Teitarô (1948). *The Essence of Buddhism*. Kyoto: Hozokan.

Ueda, Shizuteru (1991). *Nishida Kitarô o yomu*. Tokyo: Iwanami-Shoten.

Ueda, Shizuteru (1998). *Nishida Tetsugaku eno Michibiki*. Tokyo: Iwanami-Shoten.

Helmut Reinalter

Karl R. Popper's View of History

Translated by Martin J. Jandl

Popper's first work dealing with history titled *The Poverty of Historicism* was published in 1957 (in German: 1964). This title is, as Popper emphasises in the preface of the English edition, an allusion to Marx' work *The Poverty of Philosophy*[1]. As thesis Popper states that the doctrine of historical necessity is pure superstition regardless whether it is covered up as scientific, because it is not possible to predict historical events rationally[2]. Popper criticises the pseudo-scientific, pseudo-historical and mythological character of historical philosophy, and Popper names this mainly philosophical-methodological criticism a ›criticism of the historicistic philosophy of history‹ (ibid, p.VIII). Nevertheless, Popper breaks this frame by discussing the widely branched out connection between historicistic and utopian views. This critical approach leads to a criticism of utopian planning and planned economy that starts with the logic viewpoint of its realisation and considers the human consequences to make possible the impossible (ibid.). The idea of a utopian social planning misleads and thus Popper postulates to give up dreams of making the world happy. These dreams plunge human beings into misery. Popper confronts this erroneous belief with the method to search constantly for mistakes and to correct these mistakes early so that little mistakes won't rise (ibid, p.IX). This early correction of mistakes is according to Popper an ethical duty to permanent self-criticism and to permanent learning. He states: Because we are able to learn from our mistakes, thus it is our duty to learn from our mistakes (ibid). This approach became famous as Critical Rationalism. Popper's criticism of historicism includes an exact determination of the view in social science claiming that historical predictions are its main objective and that achieving this goal is possible by discovering patterns, laws, or trends founding historical development (ibid, p.2).

---

1 see Popper, *Das Elend des Historizismus*, Tübingen 1964 (preface of the English edition: 1959), p.XIII. This paper is based on the 7.edition, Tübingen 1979. – To Popper's work in general see e.g. Eberhard Döring, *Karl Popper*, Hamburg 1987; B. Magee, *Karl Popper*, Tübingen 1986; Eberhaft Döring/Waltern Döring, *Philosophie der Demokratie bei Kant und Popper*, Berlin 1955.

2 ibid., preface, p.VII

1.

Popper summarises his most important objections in two examples – the anti-naturalistic doctrines and the pro-naturalistic doctrines. Historicism claims that some physical methods are not applicable to social sciences because of differences in physics and sociology. With that historicism fights against methodological naturalism in sociology (ibid, pp.5ff). Historicism emphasises the validity of physical laws (or laws of nature) – in nature dominates a system of physical regularity that is apparently spatially and temporarily invariable. In contrast to this sociological laws characteristically differ pertaining to places and time. Regularities in social life differ fundamentally from regularities in nature because historical developments and cultural differences form social life that thus depends on these presuppositions. Historical relativism prevents the application of physical methodologies on sociology because of the historicistic view of generalisation, experiments, and complexity of social phenomena, exact forecast, and the meaning of methodological essentialism that is discussed by Popper (ibid, pp.6ff).

As mentioned, historicism is anti-naturalistic in principle although it does not refuse the view that there is a common element in natural sciences and social sciences. As Popper points out historicists support the view that sociology and physics are disciplines that proceed theoretically and practically at the same time (ibid, p.9). By means of theories or general laws sociology explains and even forecasts events, and simultaneous sociology is founded by experiences and represents events in form of observable facts. Finally observation supplies the criterion whether a theory is accepted or not. »Sprechen wir vom Erfolg der Physik, dann denken wir an den Erfolg ihrer Prognosen: und dann kann man sagen, daß der Erfolg ihrer Prognosen gleichzusetzen ist mit der empirischen Bewährung der physikalischen Gesetze. [If we talk about the success in physics, then we will think about the success of its forecasts: and we can state that this success is equate with empirical trial of physical laws.]« (ibid)

According to Popper, success in sociology also results in principle from trial of forecasts. That's why it is possible to conclude that special methods like forecasts based on laws and scrutiny of laws by observation is a common ground in physics and sociology (ibid). Popper refuses special trends of this views, especially all the prerequisites of anti-naturalistic doctrines like comparison with long-term forecasts, observation base, social dynamic, historical laws, prophecies of history, social techniques, and the theory of historic development respective interpretations in stead of planning of social change (ibid, pp.30ff). Popper does not rule out that historicism as methodology or the historicistic method that he criticises arised as a part of a comprehensive world view[3]. His guess is confirmed by

3 ibid, p.43f; see also: *The Open Society an its Enemies*.

the idea that methodologies are – not logical, but historically viewed – by-products of philosophical opinions (ibid, p.44).

2.

The third chapter of *The Poverty of Historicism* Popper discusses critically anti-naturalistic doctrines. In this context he judges the historicistic method – the ›methodological poverty of historicism‹ (ibid, p.47) – very negatively and labels it as a poor method that is not able to yield the expected results (ibid). In Popper's terminology successful methods are called ›patchwork-technologies‹ (ibid, pp.47ff) by which means (connected with critical analysis) practical results are yielded best in social sciences and natural sciences: »Die Sozialwissenschaften verdanken ihre Entwicklung in sehr großem Maße der Kritik sozialer Verbesserungsvorschläge, genauer gesagt, versuchen, festzustellen, ob damit zu rechnen ist, dass eine bestimmte wirtschaftliche oder politische Handlungsweise ein erwartetes oder erwünschtes Ergebnis herbeiführen wird. [Social sciences owe its development to a high degree to the criticism of social suggestions of improvement, pointedly spoken to the attempt to find out whether it is to reckon that a specific economical or political way of acting brings about an expected or desired result.]« (ibid, p.47)

This is exactly Popper's method when he speaks about technologically orientated patchwork-social-technology. It's obvious that Popper emphasises the practical-technological perspective, but simultaneously he indicates that theoretical problems resulting from the analysis of practical considerations must not be settled. The technological orientation proves desirable because it shows problems and disciplines speculative inclinations; the more it subjects theories under the clarity and practical examination (ibid, p.48).

Patchwork-technologies must be distinguished from ›utopian social techniques‹ and ›holism‹ (ibid, pp.57ff. and pp.61ff). Popper pleads for patchwork-technologies, but technological historicism interprets itself as holistic (ibid, p.58). Moreover historicism is connected with ideas that are characteristic for holistic-utopian social techniques like a new order of society or central planning (to be found in the works of Plato or Marx) both strongly suspected as ideologies. Historicism is not very interested in aspects of historical development, but rather deals with the development of society as a whole. Popper criticises that wholeness is no subject of scientific research. Historicism and utopianism share the problematic idea that final objectives of historical developments are not subject of choice or moralist decision, but subject to scientific discovery. »Sowohl der Historizist als auch der Utopist glauben, die wahren Endziele der Gesellschaft etwa dadurch finden zu können, daß sie deren historische Tendenzen feststellen oder die Forderungen der Zeit diagnostizieren.« (ibid, pp.59f)

In this context differences between Popper's patchwork method and historicism or utopianism becomes obvious. Popper starts his criticism with historicistic doctrines, and one of them is holism (ibid, pp.61ff). Apart from the ambiguity of ›wholeness‹ Popper emphasises that wholeness in the sense of totality never is subject to scientific research – a fact ignored by holistic philosophers. Moreover the concrete structure of social reality is not comprehensible (ibid, pp.62f).

But Popper aims at an even more important aspect of holism that broadens the study of society as a whole based on a problematic method and that leads to endeavours to control society as a whole and to rebuild it (ibid, p.63). At the bottom of that is a totalitarian world view. As an example for the holistic foundations of utopianism and of historicism Popper quotes Karl Mannheim: »Wir waren nie gezwungen, das gesamte System der Natur so vollständig zu bilden und zu lenken, wie wir es heute mit unserer Gesellschaft tun müssen, und deshalb mußten wir nie in die Geschichte und Struktur der individuellen Naturwelten eindringen. Die Menschheit schickt sich an, [...] ihr ganzes soziales Leben zu regeln, obwohl sie nie versucht hat, eine zweite Natur zu schaffen [...].«[4] For Popper this view and the method at its bottom is an erroneous belief. Holistic philosophy is especially disastrous because of its influence on the historicistic theory of social experiment stating that a social experiment is useful only if it is realised in holistic scale. Popper argues that with this doctrine the patchwork experiments are ignored and that holistic experiments can't contribute to experimental knowledge[5].

Popper reflects on the problem of social experiments also pertaining to sociological laws, especially to generalisation. In this context he refuses the historicist's thesis that in social science the validity of generalisations is limited to special historic epochs in which the observations are made (ibid, p.78). It is a fact that during a fast social change seemingly definite laws lose their validity. But the historicist overestimates the difference between historic epochs and underestimates the scientific inventiveness. Popper supplies evidence for his view by referring to Kepler and Newton (ibid, pp.79ff). According to Popper sociological theories are valid for all historic epochs. Thus he refuses emphatically the historicist's thesis that it is not possible to discover a real universal law in social sciences because of its invalidity in different epochs. That thesis does not understand proceedings of science because scientific methods always aim to search laws with an unlimited range of validity (ibid, p.81).

---

4 Karl Mannheim, *Men and Society in an Age of Reconstruction*, pp.175f. (quoted in: Popper, ibid., p.65)

5 Popper, *The Poverty of Historicism*, ibid, p.68

3.

In the last part of *The Poverty of Historicism* Popper points his criticism of pronaturalistic doctrines out (ibid, pp.83ff). These chapters deal with the question concerning a possible law of development, a question denied by Popper. The description of the development of life on earth and of the human society is no law but just a singular historic proposition (ibid, p.85). The research of the law of a irrevocable development order is not the task of the scientific method. Popper justifies this view with the words: »Wir können nicht hoffen, eine universale Hypothese prüfen und ein für die Wissenschaft annehmbares Naturgestz finden zu können, wenn wir dauernd auf die Beobachtung eines einzigartigen Prozesses beschränkt sind. Auch kann uns die Beobachtung eines einzigartigen Prozesses nicht bei der Voraussicht seiner zukünftigen Entwicklung helfen [...].« (ibid, p.86)

Trends or tendencies are assessed similarly by Popper, bearing in mind that Popper views trends not as laws, but only as statistical aids. Thus there is a great difference between trends and laws. There are no laws defining the dynamic succession of events, but there are trends with a dynamic characteristic, like population growth (ibid, pp.90ff). According to Popper historical successions laws are no laws, at best trends supplying no base for scientific forecasts (ibid, p.94). Only if a trend is traced back to a system of laws it will be used as a base for forecast like laws are used. This reduction or inverse deduction maybe will overcome the gap between trends and laws. The problem in historicism is its confusion of trends and laws what is scientifically not tenable (ibid, p.95). Historicism ignores that trends depend on margin conditions and uses trends like laws. Historicism postulates that there are universal (absolute) trends and that development laws turn out to be absolute trends. »Wie die Gesetze sind sie nicht von Randbedingungen abhängig und reißen uns unwiderstehlich in eine bestimmte Richtung in die Zukunft. Sie bilden die Grundlage von unbedingten Prophezeihungen« contradicting the cautious forecasts of natural sciences (ibid, p.101).

But according to Popper there is an even more serious mistake of historicism: It confuses interpretation with theory. Historicists avoid a selective point of view because they strive for objectivity that they won't achieve. They adopt a point of view without cognition and thus they ignore that it is impossible to reflect on one's own point of view without beeing aware of having taken a point of view (ibid, p.119).

4.

In the sense of Popper historicist reasoning can be designated as exaggerated opinion of reason pertaining to the human capacity to discover the laws determining history what would allow precise forecasts about social developments. This reproach is directed against all ideological trends in history, but especially against Marxist theory of history[6].

At the base of Popper's criticism of historicism is his philosophical interest in the methodology of social science – and this interest is influenced by his ideas on methodology worked out in *The Logic of Scientific Discovery* (1934)[7]. According to Popper historicism is a view of history based on the assumption that social development is determined by universal laws. This view is strongly influenced by the conception of laws in natural sciences. But the historicist is not fixated on natural sciences because of the differentiation in a pro-naturalistic and anti-naturalistic version[8]. Popper's concept of historicism means a miss-conception or a miss-version of social sciences; it is not a methodological criticism of special form of social sciences, but a critical approach starting with normative prerequisites. Popper's criticism seems to be characterised more by a vague humanism than by method rationalism. The thesis of the impossibility to make historical forecasts is connected with two premises: The way of history is strongly determined by growth of human knowledge and the future growth of scientific knowledge is not predictable by any method. Both assumptions result from Popper's philosophy (ibid, pp.93ff). In this context Popper's viewpoint can be characterised as a methodological individualism. Institutions have some importance, sure, but ultimately social events must be explained by individual actions.

Beside the mentioned philosophical interests in methodologies of social sciences there is one more factor important to understand Popper's viewpoint: his moralist-enlightened engagement in the sense of self-determination of humans. It leads to a system of values and norms of an ›open society‹ and forces individualism and autonomy (ibid, pp.104ff). Both *The Poverty of Historicism* and *The Open Society and Its Enemies* are connected. In *The Open Society...* Popper deals with the main exponents of historicism[9]. In the first volume Plato is the centre of Popper's criticism, in the second volume Hegel and Marx are discussed. Popper's criticism of these ideologies is very sharp, because these approaches are according to Popper totalitarian philosophies justifying state tyranny[10].

---

6 see Kurt Salamun: *Das Ethos der Aufklärung im kritischen Rationalismus*. In: *Moral und Politik aus der Sicht des Kritischen Rationalismus*, edited by Salamun, Amsterdam/Atlanta 1991, pp.95ff; Karl-Ernst Bühler/Hans-R. Fischer: *Vom Elend des Historizismus zur biographischen Methode*. In: *Karl Popper – Philosophie und Wissenschaft*, edited by Fritz Wallner, Vienna 1995, pp.125ff; Johann Dvorak: *Dialektik, Logik, Materialismus. Zum Verhältnis von Marxismus und kritischem Rationalismus*, ibid., pp.141ff.

7 see Karl Popper: *Logik der Forschung*, Wien 1934.

8 See the interpretation of Lothar Schäfer: *Karl R. Popper*, München 1992, pp.91ff

9 Popper: *Die offene Gesellschaft und ihre Feinde*, ibid; see also Herbert Keuth: *Die Philosophie Karl Poppers*, Tübingen 2000, pp.244ff

10 ibid, see also Schäfer: Karl R. Popper, ibid, pp.104ff

5.

According to the historicistic view of history a possible objective of historiography is to report on the historical development as it actually occurred. Popper refuses this view because of the necessary selection and interpretation of data. A key formulation in *The Poverty...* pertaining to Popper's understanding of history reads: »Wie die Naturwissenschaft muß auch die Geschichtsforschung selektiv sein, wenn sie nicht unter einem Wust von wertlosem und zusammenhängendem Material ersticken will [...]. Der einzige Ausweg aus dieser Schwierigkeit ist [...] die bewußte Einführung eines vorgefaßten selektiven Standpunkts in die historische Forschung, d.h. wir schreiben die Geschichte, die uns interessiert. Wenn ein solcher selektiver Standpunkt oder Brennpunkt des historischen Interesses nicht als prüfbare Hypothese formuliert werden kann, werden wir ihn als historische Interpretation bezeichnen.«[11] But historicism confuses these interpretations with theories. Thus Popper concludes that historiography is a subjective historic interpretation. Universal history as lining up events would be problematic[12].

Popper's view of history is determined by the attitude of a social engineer and by the thesis of interventionism confronted with the historicistic determination. »Weder die Natur noch die Geschichte kann uns sagen, was wir tun sollen [...]. Wir sind es, die Zweck und Sinn in die Natur und Geschichte einführen [...], und obwohl die Geschichte keinen Sinn hat, können doch wir ihr einen Sinn verleihen [...].«[13] Historic developments turn to the better not because of a necessary historic process but only if the historian takes side of the better. »Statt als Propheten zu posieren, müssen wir zu den Schöpfern unseres Geschicks werden. Wir müssen lernen, unsere Aufgaben zu erfüllen, so gut wie wir können, und wir müssen auch lernen, unsere Fehler aufzuspüren und einzusehen.« (ibid, p.347)

According to Popper historicism is a special attitude to social sciences postulating that historical forecasts are the main objective to be attainable by discovery of laws or trends basing historical development. »Der Historizist stellt sich [...] die Soziologie als theoretisch-empirische Disziplin vor, deren empirische Basis allein von Chronik der geschichtlichen Fakten gebildet wird und deren Ziel es ist, Voraussagen, möglichst Großprognosen, zu formulieren.«[14] The historicist's mistake is the restriction of data and the postulate of general forecasts. The limitation in social sciences to the validity of all generalisations is also the centre of criticism pertaining to historicism[15], expressed in the historicist assumption that

11 Das Elend des Historizismus, ibid., pp.117ff

12 Schäfer, ibid., p. 120; see also Rudolf Lüthe: *Zur Rolle von Interpretation und Imagination bei der Bildung historischen Wissens. Überlegungen im Anschluss an Karl R. Poppers Historik*, in: *Karl Popper – Philosophie und Wissenschaft*, ibid, pp.119ff

13 *Die offene Gesellschaft und ihre Feinde*, ibid, p.344

14 *Das Elend des Historizismus*, p.32

15 To this criticism see also Keuth: *Die Philosophie Karl Poppers*, pp.233ff.

there are absolute trends like a general historic tendency of progress that is not limited to special epochs. In this argumentation the fact is ignored that trends depend on margin conditions. Historicists trust blindly in progress because the ignore changes in conditions of developments (ibid, p.234). Thus, the main thesis of Popper's criticism on historicism reads: »Die Lehre von der geschichtlichen Notwendigkeit [ist und bleibt] der reinste Aberglaube, wie sehr sie sich auch als ›wissenschaftlich‹ gebärden mag, und daß man den Lauf der Geschichte nicht rational voraussagen kann.«[16]

16 *Das Elend des Historizismus*, ibid, p.VII

Mathias Gutmann

Humans as Self-Developing Entities. Some Remarks on Cassirer's Concept of Symbolic Forms

1. Introduction

The definition of humans usually refers to a comparison with animals. Compared, e.g., with primates, humans are defined as *ζoov λoγov εχηov*, *animal sociale* or *tool-making animals*. From a methodological point of view this definition of humans shows a predicative scheme, the naturalisation of which seems to be inevitable. An alternative can be gained by characterising the »form of human action« as a starting point of reflection. Following Cassirer's approach of *symbolic forms* the form of human action is to be understood as intrinsically double-barrelled: referring to the respective symbolic forms it literally *generates* »world« and »world-access«. At the same time symbolic forms provide the conceptual framework for the reconstruction and reflection of the products as well as the form of human activities itself. Symbolic forms comprise and reveal the »structural« aspects of human action as a *mediated* form of world- and self-constitution. They are the *media* for the constitution of human action and the self-expression and self-interpretation of this action. This concept of humanity finally leads to a developmental theory of culture as reflection and reconstruction of the comprehensive self-unfolding and self-differentiation of humanity within which even natural sciences and their descriptions of human beings can be relocated. The *manifest image* of humans becomes to be the (historical as well as conceptual) self-expression and self-development of humanity. From this point of view, the defining characters of a predicative conceptualisation, such as language, tool-making etc. are themselves the *media* of human self-development and one of the main sources of human self-conceptualisation. As a result of this dialectical reinterpretation a new methodological starting point for the understanding of the *development* of human abilities and skills is gained, by avoiding the naturalistic shortcomings of the comparison of animals and humans.

2. Criteriological approaches

Following a criteriological approach, humans are described in a substantialist framework ascribing specific character to the entity »homo«. Thus, the animal-human-comparison gains a central position insofar as this comparison allows us to determine the characters we are looking for. Typical descriptions of homo as the result of this ascriptive procedure can be found throughout the entire history of philosophy and the natural sciences, summarised in Scheler's paradigmatic list:

»l'homme machine, homo faber, homo pecans et redivivus, homo sapiens, homo mechanicus, homo sensitivus, homo negans et patiens, homo patheticus et divinans, homo curans, homo vitalis (homo oeconomicus, homo politicus, homo libidinosus) super-homo, homo geometricus« (Scheler 1988: 22f)

An excellent example of criteriological approaches provides Gehlen's concept of humans' second nature. Following Plato's Prometheus/Epimetheus-myth in the dialogue *Protagoras*, humans are defined by their deficiency compared with animals. Animals are equipped either with special weapons or with skills and abilities that allow the defence against other animals or at least successful escape, whereas humans show a significant lack of natural equipment. Additionally, humans show neotenal ontogenesis with an extremely prolonged phase of »hatching«. They are born and raised as extremely immature beings what could be called a »physiological premature birth«. Following Herders description of humans as »deficient entities« (mängelwesen), Gehlen gives this description a biological interpretation. Humans as mängelwesen are to be considered as a biological problem insofar as they are *biologically* deficient: But in contrast to Herder, who understands this difference between the natural equipment of humans as the starting point for a specific development of freedom, Gehlen uses this description as basis for the explication of the specific biology of humans. In accordance with Uexküll's theoretical biology, a regular organism is surrounded by its self-constituted umwelt, into which it is embedded. Organisms are intergrated strictly into their environment (they are wedged into their environment to use Darwin's metaphor here). From this point of view, humans cannot even be considered to be »complete animals« and this result of the human-animal comparison is the basis for Gehlen's further considerations. In very contrast to animals, humans are incomplete. Gehlen explains this idea referring to their instinctual equipment. Whereas animals are guided in all relevant aspects by their instincts, this is not the case for humans: The lack of instincts becomes obvious and is expressed by the specific form of human activity namely by human »action« (handlung). Humans are *urged* to act, they cannot (and must not) behave (instinct-driven) but they have to act intentionally. And in contrast to animal behaviour, actions are not self-regulated, but must be guided and regulated externally. This guidance and regulation cannot be found within human's *biological* nature itself.

3. The cultural nature of humans

Uexküll's theory of the organism provides a basis for the comparison of humans and animals, and it leads to the conclusion that humans do not have an environment (umwelt), but only a world (welt). They are »world-open« (weltoffen). This character, understood as a *deficiency*, implies that Uexküll's concept cannot be adequate for the description of humans in respect to their world-constitution: The essential character of humans must be seen in its »second nature« that is culture: Humans *have* culture *by* nature. But despite the fact that Gehlen excludes a direct application of Uexküll's theory, this structure of humans »second nature« allows at least an indirect application. This is possible by defining culture itself in terms of biology:

»›Kultur‹ ist daher ein anthropo-biologischer Begriff, der Mensch von Natur ein Kulturwesen. Schon der Australier verfügt über etwa 200 Geräte und Techniken, mittels deren er sich in seiner trostlosen Umgebung behauptet. Kultur ist also in erster Annäherung der Inbegriff der Sachmittel und Vorstellungsmittel, der Sach- und Denktechniken, einschließlich der Institutionen, mittels deren eine bestimmte Gesellschaft ›sich hält‹, in zweiter Annäherung der Inbegriff aller darauf fundierten Folgeinstitutionen.« (Gehlen 1986: 80f)

With institutions Gehlen means e.g. family, but also laws, constitutions, social ranking, the arts etc. (i.e. some of the constituents of Hegel's concept of »geist«). The culture of humans becomes the »umwelt« of this strange animal, and within this world humans are adjusted and adapted exactly in the same manner as animals to their umwelt. And it is culture produced by humans as a necessary by-product of their specific form of activity that allows humans to survive. Culture then holds the place of umwelt, which allows as »world« the guidance of human action. This guidance is possible because of the existence of institutions substituting the rigid functional circuits of Uexküll's organism-environment-relationship. The institutions are those structures that guarantee the (biological!) survival of a deficient animal within a world that is not constituted as a natural Umwelt. Guiding the actions of individuals they guarantee the stability of this world, which can accidentally function as an Umwelt in the original sense of Uexküll. Accordingly, each development that threatens these institutions must be assessed as a direct attack on the viability of humans – such a development »back to nature« would result in a »naturalisation« of humans. In Gehlen's approach this contradicts the very *nature* of humans, being *culture* with its institutions that serve as devices of human survival. The resulting description leads to a very restrictive concept of society with obvious political consequences. In the context of this paper I will neither identify the authoritarian political consequences nor present a methodological criticism of the underlying naturalist argument.[1] In short, just to outline the argumentative strategy of this criticism, the starting point would be the analysis of the presuppositions of the animal-human-comparison, the methodological core of Gehlen's criteriological approach. One of the prerequisites of this comparison is the availability of a language of description. If we use biological knowledge here, the validity of this knowledge has to be supposed. And at least the evaluation of this validity itself must be independent from biological knowledge itself. To put it with Husserl:

»Sind, allgemein gesprochen, gewisse Rätsel der Naturwissenschaft prinzipiell immanent, so sind ihr selbstverständlich deren Lösungen nach Prämissen und Ergebnissen prinzipiell transzendent. Die Lösung eines jeden Problems, das der Naturwissenschaft als solcher anhaftet – also ihr durch und durch, von Anfang bis Ende abhaftet – von der Naturwissenschaft erwarten zu wollen, oder auch nur zu meinen, daß sie für die Lösung eines derartigen Rätsels irgendwelche Prämissen besteuern könne, das heißt sich in einem widersinnigen Zirkel bewegen.« (Husserl 1981: 20f)

Setting aside this objection here, I want to determine the role that technique plays in the description of humans as being cultural entities by nature. Gehlen derives the very form of technique from the underlying description of humans as deficient animals. Thus technique has three basic functions:

1. It substitutes the specialised organs which are found in proper animals.
2. It supports the weak biological constitution of human organs.
3. It excels by far the biological organs which can be found in the realm of animals.

Human beings as a biological species only survived within a hostile environment – because of the means they used in order to transform their environment.

»Die Welt der Technik ist also sozusagen der ›große Mensch‹: geistreich und trickreich, lebensfördernd und lebenszerstörend wie er selbst, mit demselben gebrochenen Verhältnis zur urwüchsigen Natur. Sie ist, wie der Mensch ›nature artificielle‹.« (Gehlen 1993: 149)

Technique becomes the essential character of human existence and by applying means and tools Humans *detoxify* their environment. But because they *toxify* their environment at the same time, they *depend* on their means- and tool-application. Culture originating in this process of the transformation of first nature then becomes »second nature«, the »nest which humans build into nature«. Technique as

1 This has been done already in another paper and it would exceed the scope of this paper (for further readings see Gutmann 2002a & b).

a character that guarantees the survival of human beings (as a biological species) allows Gehlen to define humans as cultural beings *qua* nature. Development of technique becomes initiated and guided by external forces (which may be conceptualised as analogs or homologs of the driving selection-forces of a specific type of an evolultion theory).

4. Mediation as a starting-point

In contrast to Gehlen, Cassirer proposes a mediation oriented approach of *human* being and *being* human. The new methodological starting-point beyond the limitations of criteriological substantialims is the realm of human individual activity as well as societal activities.

»Man's outstanding characteristic, his distinguishing mark, is not his metaphysical or physical nature – but his work. It is his work, it is the system of human activities, which defines and determines the circle of ›humanity‹. Language, myth, religion, art, science, history are the constituents, the various sectors of this circle.« (Cassirer 1972: 68)

Cassirer's early writing on *Substanzbegriff und Funktionsbegriff* leads him to the reconsideration of the substantialist treatment of (particularly) scientific, here mathematical, logical, chemical and physical objects as the function of a specific type of propositional speech and the underlying type of operations and actions. The results of this philosophy of sciences – dealing with the most developed forms of ideal-, formal- and empirical sciences of his time – are for Cassirer the entry-point for the philosophy of symbolic forms. What is presented in *Substanzbegriff und Funktionsbegriff* as the highest form of abstraction is to be reconsidered now as a type schematisation. The development of this schematisation, the reconstruction of its genesis is the aim of *Philosophy of Symbolic Forms*. As the concept of *function* allowed the reformulation of substance-ontology in terms of a pure methodology, the *Philosophy of Symbolic Forms* conceptualises the function of reason itself. The reconstruction of this function takes place in the realm of its respective systems of images, signs, schemata and symbols, applied in the respective modes of world-making. The »epistemological« Kantian project of critics of reason is transformed into comprehensive critics of culture tempting to understand all types of world-making as *modes* of generation and creation. The action of the subject cannot longer be reduced towards its function within the narrow limits of a theory of knowledge. Not only scientific objects but every possible object is to be reconsidered as the expression of human activity:

»Die Kritik der Vernunft wird damit zur Kritik der Kultur. Sie sucht zu verstehen und zu erweisen, wie aller Inhalt der Kultur, sofern er mehr als bloßer Einzelinhalt ist, sofern er in einem allgemeinen Formprinzip gegründet ist, eine ursprüngliche Tat des Geistes zur

Voraussetzung hat. Hierin erst findet die Grundthese des Idealismus ihre eigentliche und vollständige Bewährung. Solange die philosophische Betrachtung sich lediglich auf die Analyse der reinen Erkenntnisform bezieht und sich auf diese Aufgabe einschränkt, solange kann auch die Kraft der naiv-realistischen Weltansicht nicht völlig gebrochen werden. Der Gegenstand der Erkenntnis mag immerhin in ihr und durch ihr ursprüngliches Gesetz in irgendeiner Weise bestimmt und geformt werden – aber er muß nichtsdestoweniger, wie es scheint, auch außerhalb der Erkenntnis als ein selbständiges Etwas vorhanden und gegeben sein. Geht man dagegen nicht vom allgemeinen Weltbegriff, als vielmehr vom allgemeinen Kulturbegriff aus, so gewinnt damit die Frage alsbald eine veränderte Gestalt. Denn der Inhalt des Kulturbegriffs läßt sich von den Grundformen und Grundrichtungen des geistigen Produzierens nicht loslösen: das ›Sein‹ ist hier nirgends anders als im ›Tun‹ erfaßbar.« (Cassirer 1988: 11)

Following the concept of symbolic forms as the basis of a generic definition of human being as a developing entity, leads from the narrow limits of substantialism towards the wide and seemingly unrestricted area of *functional* characterisation of humans, referring to the specific type of their activities and actions:

»Language, art, myth, religion are no isolated, random creations. They are held together by a common bond. But this bond is not a vinculum substantiale, as it was conceived and described in scholastic thought; it is rather a vinculum functionale. It is the basic function of speech, of myth, of art, of religion that we must seek far behind their innumerable shapes and utterances, and that in the last analysis we must attempt to trace back to a common origin.« (Cassirer 1972: 68)

The resulting double-movement of *tracing back* the origin and *analysing* the expression of mediated human activity can be seen as a main leitmotif of Cassirer's culturalism. From this point of view the philosophy of symbolic forms becomes a Hegelian project – and as in the case of Hegel's developmentalism we should chose not a constitutive-theoretical but a *reconstructive* perspective. Cassirer considers this perspective – after a longer citation from Hegel's *Phenomenology of Spirit*:

»Schärfer kann es nicht ausgesprochen werden, daß das Ende, das ›Telos‹ des Geistes nicht erfaßt und nicht ausgesprochen werden kann, wenn man dasselbe als ein für sich bestehendes, wenn man es losgelöst und abgesondert von Anfang und Mitte nimmt. Die philosophische Reflexion setzt nicht in dieser Weise das Ende gegen Anfang und Mitte ab, sondern nimmt alle drei als integrierende Momente einer einheitlichen Gesamtbewegung. In diesem Grundprinzip der Betrachtung stimmt die ›Philosophie der symbolischen Formen‹ mit dem Hegelschen Ansatz überein; – sosehr sie in der Begründung wie in der Durchführung desselben andere Wege gehen muß. Auch sie will dem Individuum ›die Leiter reichen‹, die es von den primären Gestaltungen, wie sie sich in der Welt des ›unmittelbaren‹ Bewußtseins finden, zur Welt der ›reinen Erkenntnis‹ hinführt. Keine Sprosse dieser Leiter ist, sub specie der philosophischen Betrachtung, entbehrlich: jede darf und muß den Anspruch erheben, berücksichtigt, gewürdigt, ›gewußt‹ zu werden, wenn es sich darum handelt, die Erkenntnis nicht sowohl in ihrem Ergebnis, in ihrem bloßen Produkt, sondern in ihrem reinen Prozeß-Charakter, in der Art und Form des ›Procedere‹ selbst, zu verstehen.« (Cassirer 1990: VII)

The process of development should be understood in terms of a *reconstruction*. It is not the report of a *progression*, which inevitably and necessarily would have to result in the *Philosophy of Symbolic Forms* as its final and masterly accomplished implicit goal, which has become explicated by the history of philosophy itself.

5. The architecture of symbolic forms

Symbolic forms are paradigmatically introduced by Cassirer in reference to an extended version of Hegel's objective (and absolute) spirit. The symbolic forms show an intrinsic conceptual structure – expressed in the ambigious term of »energy«, namely as »ergon« as well as »energeia«:

»Unter einer ›symbolischen Form‹ soll jede Energie des Geistes verstanden werden, durch welche ein geistiger Bedeutungsgehalt an ein konkretes sinnliches Zeichen geknüpft und diesem Zeichen innerlich zugeeignet wird. In diesem Sinne tritt uns die Sprache, tritt uns die mythisch-religiöse Welt und die Kunst als je eine besondere symbolische Form entgegen. Denn in ihnen allen prägt sich das Grundphänomen aus, daß unser Bewußtsein sich nicht damit begnügt, den Eindruck des Äußeren zu empfangen, sondern daß es jeden Eindruck mit einer freien Tätigkeit des Ausdrucks verknüpft und durchdringt. Eine Welt selbstgeschaffener Zeichen und Bilder tritt dem, was wir die objektive Wirklichkeit der Dinge nennen, gegenüber und behauptet sich gegen sie in selbständiger Fülle und ursprünglicher Kraft.« (Cassirer 1988: 175f)

Symbolic forms are at the same time *forma formata* and *forma formans*. Translating the expression of »Bildung« they are forming, shaping agencies, structuring human action and activities. And, having their own peculiar structure, they are the formed products of human action and activities. This peculiarity becomes lucid when we refer to the three functions of each single symbolic form, namely expression, representation and conceptualisation, and meaning (pure meaning in the case of sciences). The active aspect of forming and shaping is expressed in the first line, the resulting »opera«, the products of this formation in the second.

Expression	→	*Representation*	→	*Notion*
↓		↓		↓
Language	→	*Image*	→	*Construction*

Language (and other types of expression), images and notions are not only products, they are themselves the means and tools of the forming-process itself. If we read the line from expression to notion in the sense of a classical constitutional theory of objectivity and knowledge (e.g. Husserl's phenomenological approach), then we will be urged to determine the emergent aspects of each single step of this line. The referents of expression, representation or notion existed independent of the means of expression, representation or cognition and were – so to speak – in a second step to be expressed, represented and conceptualised or apprehended. And it is exactly this option of reading, which Cassirer *excludes* by describing the function of a symbolic form in terms of a media:

»Die Wirklichkeit scheint für uns nicht anders, als in der Eigenart dieser Formen faßbar zu werden; aber darin liegt zugleich, daß sie sich in ihnen offenbart. Dieselben Grundfunktionen, die der Welt des Geistes ihre Bestimmtheit, ihre Prägung ihren Charakter geben, erscheinen andererseits als ebenso viele Brechungen, die das in sich einheitliche und einzigartige Sein erfährt, sobald es vom ›Subjekt‹ her aufgefaßt und angeeignet wird. Die Philosophie der symbolischen Formen ist unter diesem Gesichtspunkt gesehen, nichts anderes als der Versuch, für jede von ihnen gewissermaßen den bestimmten Brechungsindex anzugeben, der ihr spezifisch und eigentümlich zukommt. Sie will die besondere Natur der verschiedenen brechenden Medien erkennen; sie will jedes von ihnen nach seiner Beschaffenheit und nach den Gesetzen seiner Struktur durchschauen. Aber, wenngleich sie sich bewußt in dieses Zwischenreich, in dieses Reich der bloßen Mittelbarkeit begibt, so scheint doch die Philosophie als Ganzes, als Lehre von der Totalität des Seins, nicht in ihm verharren zu können. Immer von neuem regt sich vielmehr der Grundtrieb des Wissens: der Trieb, das verschleierte Bild von Saïs zu enthüllen und die Wahrheit nackt und hüllenlos vor sich zu sehen.« (Cassirer 1990: 3)

The intermediary realm, the realm of pure mediacy and mediation is the actual and privileged referent of philosophical reflection, within which the determination of »objects« and »subjects« as determined functions takes place within means-structured activity. This process of determination is understood as self-differentiation in the realm of pure mediacy. The term »medium« is used here in three meanings:

1. The respective media are the »between« of the subject-object-relation.
2. Medium is a physical metaphor referring to the refraction of a light-beam at the interface between two media (e.g. in the case of the air-glass-interface of a spectrum). The mode of refraction will depend on the physico-chemical quality of the respective media. The media interfere with the light-beam, i.e. we see the light *only insofar as it is refracted*, i.e. we see it only *mediated*. Analogically the apprehension of something as something takes place only qua symbols and signs; thoughts are »public entities« becoming observable insofar as they are *expressed* in terms of signs (of whatever kind).

3. This leads to the third meaning namely the function of media as »means« (and tools).

Cassirer determines human activity and action as mediated in all of these three meanings of the word. The specific kind of mediation then characterises the form of activity. Consequently, the specific type of knowledge (of world access) depends on the respective means which are applied; their impact and effect in the procedure of production and generation cannot be disregarded – we cannot abstract from them in order to achieve putative objects *per se*. The generation of objects is not a process of a secondary application of symbols and signs in order to schematise a pre-existing, with distinct objects already well-equipped world. The difference of subjects and the objects of their respective activities is generated within the symbolic systems themselves:

»Denn freilich bleiben wir auch hier in einer Welt der »Bilder« befangen – aber es handelt sich nicht um solche Bilder, die irgendeine an sich bestehende Welt der ›Sachen‹ wiedergeben, sondern um Bildwelten, deren Prinzip und Ursprung in einer autonomen Schöpfung des Geistes selbst zu suchen ist. Durch sie allein erblicken wir und in ihnen besitzen wir das, was wir die ›Wirklichkeit‹ nennen: denn die höchste objektive Wahrheit, die sich dem Geist erschließt, ist zuletzt die Form seines eigenen Tuns. In der Totalität seiner eigenen Leistungen und in ihrer Erkenntnis der spezifischen Regel, durch die jede von ihnen bestimmt wird, sowie in dem Bewußtsein des Zusammenhangs, der alle diese besonderen Regeln wieder zur Einheit einer Aufgabe und einer Lösung vereint: in alledem besitzt nunmehr der Geist die Anschauung seiner selbst und die der Wirklichkeit.« (Cassirer 1988: 48)

The term »image« (meant generally in the sense of verbal expression, scheme and construction, model or pure symbol) plays with the both meanings of »bild« in German. Namely as a product (a picture) of a generative process and as this process itself (»bilden« – generate). The process of »bildung« in this sense is an autonomous generative process, whereby the means and tools that constitute the respective medium become transformed during and by their application. This generative aspect is universal, insofar as it characterises all image-worlds – including scientific representation of our world-making activities and action. The scientific structuralisation of »world« has insofar no privileged status here – despite the very fact, that the most developed sciences build the actual *starting point* of the philosophy of symbolic forms. »Reality« as referent of the term »world« is the symbolic unity of all the different functional relationships that are constituted by these types of activities. But the symbolic forms are not only internally articulated with reference to the applied means of the generative and creative processes. They even show a specific functional arrangement to each other insofar as language has a peculiar function in relation to all other symbolic forms. Accordingly, we must reorganise the linear ordering of symbolic forms, as they are presented in reference to the title of the volumes, by relating myth and logos to language (and as we will see later on to technique):

Myth ↔ *Logos*
↑
Language/Technique

When we understand the term »myth« as an indicator for »life-forms« within communities (i.e. the original meaning of bios)[2], and »logos« as an indicator for the reflection of this life-form, we can integrate further symbolic forms such as the arts, religion etc. Language (and technique) serves in all these cases as a particular referential-system within which the respective life-forms is articulated and reflected. At the same time language itself becomes articulated and transformed by the respective common and communitarian praxes. From this point of view, the history of the respective symbolic forms becomes a process of the systematic self-differentiation and self-development of the means- and tools-relationships and their transformation.

symbolic form			*media*
Re presentation	↔	*Notion*	*Reflection*
	↑		
	Language		
	↕		*Expression /*
	Technique		*Constitution*

I cannot explicate the form of this reconstructive approach here – but we should keep in mind, that the Hegelian perspective, which Cassirer has chosen, results in a significant turn of the orientation of the *reconstruction* itself and its *presentation* in the form of the three book-titles. The reconstruction starts with the anticipation of a theory of knowledge and further with the results of the analysis of contemporary epistemology, logics and sciences. In the light of this anticipation – which we could call a »vorgriff« in the hermeneutic sense of the word – human activity and their transformation become reconsidered. The presentation of the results of this reconstructive project then starts with final stages of the reconstruction itself. I.e. despite the fact, that »language« is the title of the first issue, it is in fact the last referent of reconstruction. Language is fundamental, but we achieve the knowl-

2 At the same time, the term »myth« represents a specific type of thought, which characterised by an immanent tendency of identification and non-conceptual reflection.

edge about its structure and function only in reference to its differentiated and differentiating *use* in the context of the respective symbolic forms. Consequently, culture is not a character or trait of the species homo sapiens but a *generic* concept (comparable the notions of reflection in Kant's terminology), referring to a comprehensive reflection and reconstruction of the development of these respective relationships. The *Philosophy of Symbolic Forms* can be considered as a reconstructive program of continuing self-generation of human beings.

$$\overbrace{SF_1 \leftrightarrow SF_2 \leftrightarrow \ldots \quad SF_n}^{\text{philosophy of culture}}$$

↑	↑		↑
Arts	*Myth*		*Sciences*

Cassirer deals within the scope of the *Philosophy of Symbolic Forms* only incidentally with the problem of technique and the use of material means and tools. It is particularly in his later writing (on *Form and Technique*) were he becomes aware of the *systematic* relevance of this aspect of human practise, which resembles the symbolic structure of the medium language but nevertheless has its peculiar structure and impact of human world and self-formation and bildung.

6. Technique as the form of human action

Technique is usually assumed to be the opposite of nature. Even within social-constructivism nature receives frequently the status of »non-technical«. Technique can be conceptualised at least in two – contrary – ways. First we understand the term technique as a pure *title*, an epitome, indicating a general and summarising speech about different techniques such as glass-blowing, the composition of a madrigal, the pure-line breeding of horses or the melting of metal. In a second sense technique denotes the *way and method* by which humans constitute the relation to their surroundings. Technique thus defines the productive and reproductive structure of societies. Within societal relations, technique designates the very form of human action itself, structuralising the systematic relation between the individual and the society. For Cassirer »technique« resembles language insofar as it is at the same time and (on the level of individual (speech-)acts) *eodem actu* the subject-matter (the object) and the *form* of world-making. Technique, being *forma formata* and *forma formans,* is from this point of view neither a collection of material tools nor a kind of applied sciences; it is in an exact sense the *precondition* of both of them. To elaborate the fundamental relevance of technique in this approach it is necessary to reconstruct the categorical aspects of human action, conceptualised as means- and tools-related action. Cassirer starts his consideration with the statement, that objects are determined only insofar, as they are determined for a *purpose*:

»Der Gegenstand ist als Etwas bestimmt immer nur sofern er zu Etwas bestimmt ist. Darin liegt, daß es in der Welt des Werkzeuges niemals bloße Dingbeschaffenheiten, sondern daß es in ihr, um einen mathematischen Ausdruck zu brauchen, nur ein Ganzes von ›Vektorgrößen‹ gibt. Jedes Sein ist hier in sich bestimmt, aber es ist zugleich Ausdruck einer bestimmten Verrichtung, und in dieser Anschauung der Verrichtung geht dem Menschen ganz allgemein eine prinzipiell neue Blickrichtung, geht ihm die Auffassung einer ›objektiven Kausalität‹ auf.« (Cassirer 1985: 64)

Causality is a concept derived in the light of human action. The hermeneutical phrase of »something as something« is not exclusively located within language – but also within technique as a poietic form of human action. By dealing with something, handling something we *always already* determined objects *as* something in reference to the structure of this »dealing with« itself. Even »means« (mittel) – as well as all other objects – are thus *functionally* defined things. Humans – as entities that use means – can be defined as a »tool-making animal« (Cassirer 1985:51)[3]. Despite its similarity to biological descriptions, the term »animal« here does not signify a biologic definition of humankind. The specific form of action, which is a *proprium* of humans, denies such an interpretation, because it is the *form* of means-application, which provides the definiens of humans – namely as a »non-animals« (in the sense of »bestia« beasts here):

»Denn der Abstand zwischen jeglichem noch so ungefügem und unvollkommenen Werkzeug, dessen sich der Mensch bedient, und den höchsten Erzeugnissen und Errungenschaften technischen Schaffens mag in rein inhaltlicher Hinsicht noch so gewaltig erscheinen: er ist dennoch, wenn man lediglich das Prinzip des Handelns ins Auge faßt, nicht größer, sondern geringer als die Kluft, die die erste Erfindung und den ersten Gebrauch des rohesten Werkzeugs vom bloß tierischen Verhalten trennt.« (Cassirer 1985: 61)

The distinction between *means, educts* and *products* are *analytical* differentiations of the concrete generative procedures and not material distinction. Within work, the aspects of the process (educts, products, means, etc.) are articulated by constituting a relationship not only between the experiencing human and the concrete objects, but between concrete objects themselves. Experience is thus *concrete* and *determined* experience of something *as* something, confronting humans with the resistance and resilience of the objects of *their action* and *activities*[4]. We can

3 In contrast to our differentiation, Cassirer does not discern tools from means.

4 These »objective« aspects of human activity and action do not exist without reference to these activities themselves.

comprehend these *relations* by considering the fact, that the concrete objects themselves we deal with during production represent *relations*. The product represents not only the goal of the production – it is the realised and materialised end of the respective application of these means. And the means themselves are represented by a concrete object, which is transformed during its application. Within the process of work we transform not only the educts in accordance with the ends, we also transfer the means and in this sense we gain *two* differing products. In order to iterate the production, it is necessary to recover the means and this recovering is nothing else but a specific type of production for which again we will apply means. We indicate this process of the re-establishment of means by extending our terminology: means applied, in order to produce means, we will call *tools* (werkzeuge*)*. And insofar as means and tools serve for the reproduction of societies, i.e. of the conditions of the action and activities in which they originate, we refer to them as »media« (medien). Technique insofar as it is a medium of societal reproduction is a symbolic form.

7. Culture as a comprehensive relation

Understanding technique as a symbolic form, we have to reconsider now the consequences for the nature-culture difference from a developed (non-alienation-theoretical) standpoint. If technique is not merely a natural feature of the genus homo, even the nature-culture-difference cannot be thought any longer as being embedded within nature. Additionally the difference between nature and culture cannot be gained by referring to Aristotle's definition of nature as the realm of processes and objects that are shaped and transformed without human intervention. Neither nature (as first nature) nor culture (as second nature) can be found pre-existing to human action; they both are aspects of a fundamental world-relationship, which is constituted and articulated by humans technically:

> »Was die Instrumente der vollentwickelten Technik von den primitiven Werkzeugen trennt, ist eben dies, daß sie sich von dem Vorbild, das ihnen die Natur unmittelbar zu bieten vermag, freigemacht und gewissermaßen losgesagt haben. Erst auf Grund dieses ›Lossagens‹ tritt das, was sie selbst zu sagen und zu leisten haben, tritt ihr selbständiger Sinn und ihre autonome Funktion vollständig zutage.« (Cassirer 1985: 73)

This process of emancipation from the archetypical example of nature – which humans would have to follow if we based our consideration of the human-nature-relation upon the *naturalness* of technique – is itself not a process which starts *within* nature. It is an autonomous world-relationship in the sense, that the transformation of human-means-tools-media-relations takes place autonomously: the *reproduction* (identical as well as non-identical) of technical relations occur immanently without stimulating or guiding inputs from outside the relation:

»Als das Grundprinzip, das die gesamte Entwicklung des modernen Maschinenbaus beherrscht, hat man den Umstand bezeichnet, daß die Maschine nicht mehr die Handarbeit oder gar die Natur nachzuahmen sucht, sondern daß sie bestrebt ist, die Aufgabe mit ihren eigenen, von den natürlichen oft völlig verschiedenen Mitteln zu lösen. Mit diesem Prinzip (dem Grundprinzip technischen Handelns, MG) und seiner immer schärferen Durchführung hat die Technik erst ihre eigentliche Mündigkeit erlangt. Jetzt richtet sie eine neue Ordnung auf, die nicht in Anlehnung an die Natur, sondern nicht selten in bewußtem Gegensatz zu ihr gefunden wird. Die Entdeckung des neuen Werkzeugs stellt eine Umbildung, eine Revolution der bisherigen Wirkungsart, des Modus der Arbeit selbst, dar. So wurde, wie man betont hat, mit der Nähmaschine zugleich eine neue Nähweise, mit dem Walzwerk eine neue Schmiedeweise erfunden – und auch das Flugproblem konnte erst endgültig gelöst werden, als das technische Denken sich von dem Vorbild des Vogelfluges freimachte und das Prinzip des bewegten Flügels verließ [...].« (Cassirer 1985: 73f)

The relation between technique on the one hand and the relation between nature-culture on the other hand is only on the first glance a contradiction: nature is a specific qualification of the relation between humans and the technical form of their action. Nature and culture are *diaphora* and not *hetera*! Consequently, the development of the technical relation of means and ends is not a process, which leads from nature to culture but from culture (state1) to culture (state2). ***Within*** the transformation from culture (state1) to culture (state2) the index indicates that nature is an aspect of the former cultural constitution; the process of cultural development generates aspects, which we determine as natural aspects of the respective culture. And this nature is an aspect of the technical self-reproduction of the respective society (s. Gutmann 2003). The transformation of the »wise of working« results in the self-discrimination of those aspects that are maintained from the antecedent cultural-relations, from the older form of production. What was culture before becomes nature now, and what will be nature now can be assumed only in reference to the development of the form of production. Nature and culture are relations respectively. The relation between nature and culture then is embedded in a comprehensive relation – i.e. culture itself. Consequently the term culture occurs *twice*, namely on the one hand as a *relatum* of nature and on the other hand as the comprehensive (reflective) unifying *relation*, within which the *first* relation is embedded. And it is this comprehensive relation we deal with, when we assume that the humans-means-tool-media-relations are developing relations (s. Gutmann & Weingarten 2001). The internal transformation-process of technical development can be described as a relation which leads from nature(culture) towards culture(nature). Apprehending a determined status of the productive-reproductive-structure of a society as nature, insofar as it is the very starting-point of a transformation, we can denominate the new status which results from the transformation as culture – keeping in mind, that even the very nature, from which we started off was already *culture*. The status we start with the transformation can be called the realm of reality of (former) transformations. The resulting status is then the realm of possibility of this realisation. And it is a concrete possibility insofar as it represents a determined possibility *within* the starting-point of the transformation itself. The technical form of action leads beyond realm of the realised possibility:

»Dieses innere Wachstum erfolgt nicht einfach unter der ständigen Leitung, unter der Vorschrift und Vormundschaft des Wirklichen; sondern es verlangt, daß wir ständig vom ›Wirklichen‹ in ein Reich des »Möglichen« zurückgehen und das Wirkliche selbst unter dem Bilde des Möglichen erblicken. Die Gewinnung dieses Blick- und Richtpunkts bedeutet, in rein theoretischer Hinsicht, vielleicht die größte und denkwürdigste Leistung der Technik. Mitten im Umkreis des Notwendigen stehend und in der Anschauung des Notwendigen verharrend, entdeckt sie einen Umkreis freier Möglichkeiten. Diesen haftet keinerlei Unbestimmtheit an, sondern sie treten dem Denken als etwas durchaus Objektives entgegen. Die Technik fragt nicht in erster Linie nach dem, was ist, sondern nach dem, was sein kann. Aber dieses ›Können‹ selbst bezeichnet keine bloße Annahme oder Mutmaßung, sondern es drückt sich in ihm eine assertorische Behauptung und eine assertorische Gewißheit aus – eine Gewißheit, deren letzte Beglaubigung freilich nicht in bloßen Urteilen, sondern im Herausstellen und Produzieren bestimmter Gebilde zu suchen ist.« (Cassirer 1985: 81)

The *concreteness* of possibility, which is realised and possible by the concreteness of action itself, constitutes a determined relation between goals and means – the means themselves originate within the respective form of production and reproduction of and within a respective society. The purposes, which are to be realised by applying means and tools, are in the same sense concrete as the form of action itself. Purposes are only (but *necessarily*) seemingly subjective decisions or settings of acting individuals. Insofar, as purposes are *analytical* aspects of the realised form of (societal) production and reproduction, they become *discovered* at and within the realm of the technically organised form of human action itself. Unquestionable it is the individual, which acts, decides and realises purposes – insofar goals *are* as subjective as the tools and means, which are applied in order to achieve the purposes. But as aspects of the societal production they are objective i.e. the relation between purposes and means follows a specific rationality that cannot be reduced to the decision of the individuals. This abstraction then, which starts in the realm of realised purposes and results into the realisation of not yet realised possibilities is always also an anticipation of the »might-be« of reality. It could be misunderstood as a process, which starts with a seemingly »given« *unmediated* status (i.e. nature in the usual definition) and results into the realm of *mediated* products and actions. This misunderstanding comes into being only, if we neglect the constitutive reference of the (societal) realised reality of purpose-tools relations and finally leads to classical alienation-stories as Simmel's *Tragedy of Culture* might show paradigmatically. In this reading the starting-point of the realisation of concrete possibilities degenerates towards a seemingly pre- and extra-conceptual nature, and the products of the transformation process comes to be exactly the type of technique, which usually is supposed to be the counterpart to and contradiction of nature itself. Technique then seems to be the contra-natural agent *per se*. This differentiation between an *unmediated* nature and a *mediated* realm of technique holds only, if we identify the nature with the very origin of the unnatural and mediated technique itself. Following the *Philosophy of Symbolic Forms*, the form of their action defines humans as technical entities. Consequently, even the characterisation of humans as *natural* entities must be redefined as a characterisation of human nature as nature(culture), which becomes realised within his respective culture(nature). Liberation or emancipation from nature does not imply necessity of liberation from technique. In very contrast humans must be conceptualised as entities which realise themselves in their work – understood as a reproductive societal action. This »reproduction« is of a completely different structure than »biological« phenomena. Cassirer determines this difference, by emphasising the »Larmakian« Aspect of human reproduction by means of their »work«:

»Die Variationen, die sich im Kreise der Pflanzen- und Tierwelt in einzelnen Exemplaren vollziehen, bleiben biologisch belanglos; sie tauchen auf, um wieder zu versinken. Wollne wir diesen Sachverhalt in der Sprache der Weismannschen Vererbungstheorie ausdrücken – wobei wir die Frage nach der empirischen Richtigkeit und Beweisbarkeit dieser Theorie hier natürlich dahingestellt sein lassen –, so können wir sagen, daß diese Veränderungen nur das Soma, nicht aber das ›Keimplasma‹ betreffen, daß sie demgemäß an der Oberfläche bleiben und nicht in jene Tiefenschicht hinabwirken, von der die Entwicklung der Gattung abhängt. In den Kulturphänomenen aber ist diese biologische Schranke beseitigt. Der Mensch hat den ›symbolischen Formen‹, die das eigentümliche seines Wesens und seines Könnens sind, gewissermaßen die Lösung einer Aufgabe vollzogen, die die organische Natur als solche nicht zu lösen vermochte. Der ›Geist‹ hat geleistet, was dem ›Leben‹ versagt blieb. Hier ist das Werden und Wirken des einzelnen in ganz anderer, tief eingreifender Weise mit dem Ganzen verknüpft. Was die Individuen fühlen, wollen und denken, bleibt nicht in ihnen selbst verschlossen; es objektiviert sich im Werk. Und diese Werke der Sprache, der Dichtung, der bildenden Kunst, der Religionen werden zu den ›Monumenten‹, zu den Erinnerungs- und Gedächtniszeichen der Menschheit.« (Cassirer 1994: 126)

The relation between the individual and the society, within which they live their »symbolising« life, is constituted and reproduced by work. And in reference to work, reflecting the specific structure of the form of action and of the products, generated by this process, the individuals become »individualised« by – at the same time – *reproducing* the *conditions* of their work:

»Man hat mit Recht hervorgehoben, daß es vielleicht keinen einzelnen Akt des Sprechens gibt, der nicht irgendwie ›die‹ Sprache beeinflußte. Aus unzähligen solchen Akten, die in gleicher Richtung wirken, können sich bedeutsame Änderungen des Sprachgebrauchs, können sich lautliche Verschiebungen oder formale Wandlungen ergeben. Das liegt daran, daß die Menschheit sich in ihrer Sprache, ihrer Kunst, in allen ihren Kulturformen gewissermaßen einen neuen Körper geschaffen hat, der allen gemeinsam zugehört. Der Einzelmensch als solcher kann individuelle Fertigkeiten, die er sich im Laufe des Lebens erworben, freilich nicht fortpflanzen. Sie haften am physischen ›Soma‹, das nicht vererbbar ist. Aber was er in seinem Werk aus herausstellt, was sprachlich ausgedrückt, was bildlich oder plastisch dargestellt ist, das ist der Sprache oder der Kunst ›einverleibt‹ und dauert durch sie fort. Dieser Prozeß ist es, der die bloße Umbildung, die sich im Kreise des organischen Werdens vollzieht, von der Bildung der Menschheit unterscheidet.« (Cassirer 1994: 127)

The »Lamarkian« mode of human reproduction, the specific form of activity, namely »work«, transcends the pure (biological) reproduction – a process, which Cassirer considers to be a re-iteration of former states of biological development. But because of its connection to the very form of human activity, the reproduction of humanity within the circle of media, described as symbolic forms, this reproduction must be conceptualised as a collective activity. Consequently, individuals are not *tokens* of a *type* (as in the field of biological re-production insofar as a single human entity is a member of the species *homo sapiens*) but the necessary and irreducible agents by and through which the process of reproduction takes place.

8. Conclusion

Work then is the constitution of mediated self-relationships, reflectively articulated in terms of medial societal reproduction of the conditions of individual action. From this point of view the transformation of technique is not the result of external motivation but a necessary by-product of the immanent structure of human activity as well as human action. Mediation does – at least from a methodological point of view – not imply alienation, but »objectivation« *sensu verbis* – a difference that we emphasise with Cassirer (and with Marx – opposing some prominent Marxists' Marx-interpretation) by discerning *work* from *labour*. Humans are developing entities – and referring to the autonomous creativity of the transformation of the form of human activity and action they are self-developing and conceptualising entities. The authentic task of human development is to *be* human and at the same time to increasingly *becoming* human.

9. Reference

Cassirer, E. (1972). *An Essay on Man*. New Haven, London: Yale University Press.

Cassirer, E. (1985). Form und Technik. In E. W. Orth & J. M. Krois (eds.), *Symbol, Technik, Sprache* (pp.39-90). Hamburg: Meiner.

Cassirer, E. (1988). *Philosophie der symbolischen Formen. Bd. 1 Die Sprache*. Darmstadt: Wissenschaftliche Buchgesellschaft.

Cassirer, E. (1987). *Philosophie der symbolischen Formen. Bd. 2 Das Mythische Denken*. Darmstadt: Wissenschaftliche Buchgesellschaft.

Cassirer, E. (1990). *Philosophie der symbolischen Formen. Bd. 3 Phänomenologie der Erkenntnis*. Darmstadt: Wissenschaftliche Buchgesellschaft.

Cassirer, E (1994). Die »Tragödie der Kultur«. In *Zur Logik der Kulturwissenschaften. Fünf Studien* (pp.103-107). Darmstadt: Wissenschaftliche Buchgesellschaft.

Gehlen, A. (1986). *Der Mensch. Seine Natur und seine Stellung in der Welt*. Wiesbaden: Aula.

Gehlen, A. (1993). Der Mensch und die Technik. In: *Anthropologische und sozialpsychologische Untersuchungen* (pp.147-162). Hamburg: Rowohlt.

Gutmann, M. (2002a). Die »Sonderstellung« des Menschen. Zum Tier-Mensch-Vergleich. In M. Weingarten, M. Gutmann & E.-M. Engels (eds.), *Jahrbuch für Geschichte und Theorie der Biologie. 8/2001.*

Gutmann, M. & Weingarten, M. (2001). *Die Bedeutung von Metaphern für die biologische Theoriebildung. DZPh, 49 (4)*: 549-566.

Gutmann, M. (2002b). Human Cultures' Natures. In A. Grunwald, M. Gutmann & E.-M. Neumann-Held (eds.), *On Human Nature. Antropology: Biological and Philosophical Foundation* (pp.190-240). Berlin, Heidelberg, New York: Springer.

Gutmann, M. (2003). Technik-Gestaltung oder Selbst-Bildung des Menschen? Systematische Perspektiven einer medialen Anthropologie. In A. Grunwald (eds.), *Technikgestaltung* (pp.39-71). Berlin, Heidelberg, New York: Springer.

Husserl, E. (1981). *Philosophie als strenge Wissenschaft*. Frankfurt: Klostermann.

Scheler, M. (1988). Probleme, Methode, Einteilung I und II. In M. Scheler, *Schriften aus dem Nachlaß. Bd. III. Philosophische Anthropologie* (pp.16-23). Bonn.

Sandra B. Rosenthal

Cultural Pluralism and the Issue of Relativism: The Significance of Pragmatic Perspectivism

The uprootedness of experience from its ontological embeddedness in a natural world is at the core of much contemporary thinking which, like pragmatism, aims to reject foundationalism or objectivism in all its forms, positions which all hold, in varying ways, that there is a bedrock basis on which to build an edifice of knowledge, something objective which justifies rational arguments concerning what is the single best position, the single position that conveys the objective truth of the matter at hand as it exists independently of our various contextually set inquiries. There can be no non-perspectival framework within which differences (social, moral, scientific, etc.) can be evaluated and resolved. These positions may, like pragmatism, focus on the pluralistic, contextualistic ways of dealing with life, on the role of novelty and diversity, on a turn away from abstract reason to imagination, feeling and practice, and on the need to solve the concrete problems of political, social, and moral life. However pragmatism, in rejecting foundationalism or objectivism does not embrace the alternative of relativism or its equivalent dressed up in new linguistic garb.

This refusal to embrace either of these traditional alternatives cannot be understood as an eclectic synthesizing of both. As Mead warns, in a statement echoed in various ways throughout the writings of the classical American pragmatists and applicable to virtually each the traditional alternatives offered by the assumptions of past thinking, »There is an old quarrel [...] which can never be healed as long as either sets out to tell the whole story of reality. *Nor is it possible to divide the narrative between them.*«[1] Rather, pragmatic philosophy, through its focus on experience as experimental and organism-environment interaction rethinks the nature of foundations, standing the tradition on its head, so to speak. And what emerges from this rethinking is a reconstructed realism housing a perspectival pluralism which avoids the perspectival closure of relativism, a pluralism of perspectives which open onto a common reality that demands commitment. The ensuing discussion will turn the pragmatic understanding of the nature of experience as experimental and organism-environment interaction as these lead to its perspectival pluralism, a position which can also aptly be called perspectival realism.

While pragmatism is concerned with the findings of science and its import for concrete human existence, its *systematic* focus on science is not on the con-

1 G.H. Mead, *The Philosophy of the Present,* ed. Arthur Murphy (La Salle, Ill: open court, 1959), 98.

tents of science but rather on science as *method* or as lived through human activity, on what the scientist *does* to gain knowledge.[2] Pragmatism views knowledge as continuous with science not in terms of scientific contents but scientific method, a method which in itself implies no particular type of content. In turning to scientific or experimental inquiry what pragmatism finds is that the very first stage of scientific inquiry requires human creativity. We are not mere passive spectators gathering ready made data, but rather we bring creative theories which enter into the very character and organization of the data grasped. Secondly, there is directed or goal oriented activity dictated by the theory. Finally, the test for truth is in terms of consequences: does the theory work in integrating the relevant experience? Valid conceptualizations are not something passively attained, either by the contemplation of absolutes or by the passive accumulation of data, but by activity shot through with the theory that guides it. This role of purposive activity in thought and the resultant appeal to relevance and selective emphasis which must ultimately be justified by workability are key pragmatic tenets. Such creativity involved in scientific method thus implies a radical rejection of the »passive-spectator« view of knowledge and an introduction of the active, creative agent who, through meanings, helps structure the objects of knowledge, and who cannot be separated from the world in which such objects emerge.[3]

The pragmatic focus on the human biological organism and organism-environment adaptation is intertwined with this understanding of experience as experimental. The human being is within nature. Neither human activity in general nor human knowledge can be separated from the fact that this being is a natural organism dependent upon a natural environment, but for all the pragmatists, human behavior is irreducibly meaningful, and this behavior of the human organism in interaction with its natural environment is the foundation of the noetic unity by which humans are bound to their world. Within the context of organic activity and behavioral environment there emerge irreducible meanings which allow the universe to come to conscious awareness in significant ways,[4] a universe

2 This stress on pure method is not intended to deny that pragmatism is influenced in its philosophical claims by the findings of various sciences. Indeed, it pays careful attention to these findings. However, pragmatic philosophy's inextricable linkage to the model of scientific method as pure method is one thing. Its attention to various findings of various sciences achieved by the general method is something quite different. These two issues should not be conflated, and it is the *method* of science which provides the key to pragmatism.

3 See for example, Dewey, *The Quest for Certainty*, vol.4 (1984), *The Later Works*, ed. Jo Ann Boydston (Carbondale and Edwardsville: University of Southern Illinois Press, 1981-1991), pp.163-165.

4 Thus, both Dewey and Mead stress that meanings can be expressed both in terms of the ongoing conduct of the biological organism immersed in a natural universe and in terms of the phenomenological description of the appearance of what is meant.

rich with ontologically real value-laden qualities that span the gamut of the richness of human existence in its fullness, qualities that themselves emerge in the interactive contexts of humans with the universe in which they are enmeshed. Value qualities are contextually emergent facts, and so- called brute facts are value laden through the contexts in which they emerge. There is no fact-value distinction, and value claims, like factual claims, arise through the dynamics of experimental method.

From the backdrop of the non-spectator understanding of human experience, humans and their environment – organic and inorganic, take on an inherently relational aspect. The properties attributed to the environment belong to it in the context of that interaction, and it is within such an interactional context that experience and its qualities function; what we have is interaction as an indivisible whole. In this way, the human organism and the nature within which it is located are both rich with the qualities and values of our everyday experience. With the rejection of the spectator theory of knowledge comes the rejection of the correspondence theory of truth and, instead, a view of reality as richer than, or overflowing, our conceptual demarcations. Diverse perspectives grasp the richness of reality in different ways, but must be judged in terms of their ability to expand and harmonize interactive contexts.

As indicated above, one of the most distinctive and most crucial aspects of pragmatism is its understanding of experience as a rich ongoing interactional or transactional unity between organism and environment, and only within the context of meanings which incorporate such an interactional unity does what is given emerge for conscious awareness. Such a transactional unity is more than a postulate of abstract thought for it has experiential dimensions. The interactive ontological unity of organism-environment transaction is reflected in the phenomenologically grasped features of experience. That which intrudes itself inexplicably into experience is not bare datum, but rather evidences itself as the over-againstness of a thick reality there for my activity. Thus Lewis asserts that independent factuality »does not need to be assumed nor to be proved, but only to be acknowledged«,[5] while Dewey observes that experience »reaches down into nature; it has depth.«[6] This description of the ontological dimension of experience is well evinced in Mead's claim that, in becoming an object, something has the character of »actually or potentially acting upon the organism from within itself.«

Dewey, *The Quest for Certainty*, p.142; »The Experimental Theory of Knowledge«, *The Middle Works*, ed. Jo Ann Boydston (Carbondale and Edwardsville: Southern Illinois University Press, 1976-1983), vol. 3, pp. 114-115. G. H. Mead, *The Philosophy of the Act*, (Chicago: University of Chicago Press, 1938), pp.115-116.

5 C. I. Lewis, *Mind and the World Order*, (New York: Dover Publications, 1929), Appendix D, pp. 425-426.

6 Dewey, *Experience and Nature*, The Later Works, vol. 1, 1981, pp.12-13.

He calls this character that of having an inside.[7] Such acting upon the organism cannot be understood as passive resistance, but as active resistance, resistance to our organic activity. Peirce captures this ontological dimension of experience in his understanding of the Dynamical Object, which is »the Reality which by some means contrives to determine the Sign to its Representation.« [8] Signs engage the interpreter with a dynamic reality through habits of action as living meanings. In this way habit creates the immediate object under the constraints of the dynamical object which is its ultimate referent, and provides the vital, living link between signs and the universe.

The interactional unity contains a two directional openness: the primordial openness of the character of experience itself opens in one direction toward the features of the human modes of grasping the independently real, and in the other direction towards the features of the independently real, for the character of experience emerges from an interaction of these two poles and thus incorporates characteristics of each, though it mirrors neither exactly. In the interactional unity which constitutes our worldly experience, both poles are thus manifest: the independently-there otherness onto which worldly experience opens, and the structure of the human way of being within whose purposive activity worldly experience emerges.

The pervasive textures of experience, which are exemplified in every experience, are at the same time indications of the pervasive textures of the independent universe which, in every experience, gives itself for our responses and which provides the touchstone for the workability of our meanings. As Peirce so well summarizes, though »everything which is present to us is a phenomenal manifestation of ourselves« this »does not prevent its being a phenomenon of something without us, just a rainbow is at once manifestation of the sun and the rain.«[9] For all the pragmatists, the flux of life as it concretely occurs contains already a phenomenological dimension of human thrown-outness onto the universe through a vital intentionality constitutive of the nature of experience as experimental. Thus, the being of humans in the natural universe and the knowing by humans of the natural universe are inseparably connected within the structure of experience and its pervasive textures, which include the features of continuity, temporal flow, novelty and vagueness.

In this way, there is an elusive resistance at the basis of meaning selection which must be acknowledged in our creative development of meaning systems

---

7 Mead, *The Philosophy of the Present*, ed. Arthur Murphy (La Salle, Illinois: Open Court, 1959), p. 137.

8 Charles Peirce, *Collected Papers*, Vols. I-VI ed. Charles Hartshorne and Paul Weiss(Cambridge: Belknap Press of Harvard University, 1931-1935); Vols. VII and VIII ed. Arthur Burks (Cambridge: Harvard University Press, 1958), 4.536; See also 8.314 Hereafter cited using only conventional two-part notation

9 Peirce, 5.283.

and choices among them. Moreover, the very textures of experience indicate that this resistance cannot be understood in terms of discrete, structured realities as the furniture of the universe which we merely find, and the finding of which requires that we in some way escape our interpretations and the structures they provide. Rather, this resisting element provides a general compulsiveness which constrains the way networks of beliefs interrelate, and may at times lead to changes, sometimes radical changes, in our understanding of the world which our beliefs – both perceptual and more reflective, incorporate.

What we experience, what we know, then, is reducible neither to what is antecedently there nor to a social construction. There is no sharp distinction between the natural and the social in the sense that one can situate particular objects exclusively within one or the other. The contextualism of pragmatic philosophy is rooted in a naturalism which both gives rise to interpretive activity and is the test of its adequacy. Our interpretive activity emerges within and embodies organic activity and is grounded in a world not exclusively of our own making. At the very heart of the temporal stretch of human behavior as anticipatory is a creativity, expressive of the experimental nature of experience, that is at once unified with a natural universe but that renders its grasp in terms of any absolute grounding impossible. As such, human awareness is at once theoretical, practical, and richly embedded within a thick, resisting nature. This rich epistemic-ontological unity at the heart of experience, rather than any falsely reified interpretive content emerging from it, provides the foundational level for ongoing human activity, both as a way of being and a way of knowing.

The passage from temporality as the basis of meaningful experience to the temporality of the natural world is operative in all the pragmatists. It is found in Lewis' claim that »The absolutely given is a specious present fading into the past and growing into the future with no genuine boundaries. The breaking of this up […] marks already the activity of an interested mind.«[10] Or, as Mead states in similar fashion, »At the future edge of experience, things pass, their characters change and they go to pieces.«[11] The role of human constitutive activity in transforming a processive, »independently there« natural universe into structured things unified in terms of their function within our environment is succinctly indicated in Dewey's claim that »structure is constancy of means, of things used for consequences, not of things taken by themselves absolutely.«[12] Further, the »isolation of structure from the changes whose stable ordering it is, renders it mysterious – something that is metaphysical in the popular sense of the word, a kind of ghostly queerness.«[13]

10 Lewis, Mind and the World Order, p.58.
11 Mead, Philosophy of the Act, p.345
12 Dewey, Experience and Nature, pp.64-65.
13 Ibid, p.65.

The two directional openness of experience carries temporality from one pole to the other, from a phenomenology of worldly experience toward a process nature. The temporal structure that belongs to our interpretive processes belongs as well to the universe within which they emerge. Human habits of response, which are for the pragmatist the living embodiment of meaning, are precisely »naturally thick« dynamic tendencies or processes structuring emerging activities in the context of alternative possibilities for ongoing actualization. Thus, when James asks, »How far into the rest of nature may we have to go in order to get entirely beyond« the overflow of experience,[14] his answer is clear. One may »go into the heart of nature«, one may grasp the most pervasive textures of its most characteristic features and one will not get beyond its overflow. Humans are natural beings in interaction with a natural universe. And at the heart of nature is process. Conversely, a temporal universe reinforces the pragmatic understanding of knowledge, for as James observes, »when the whole universe seems only [...] to be still incomplete (else why its ceaseless changing?) why, of all things, should knowing be exempt?«[15]

Within the dynamics of creativity and constraint, the search for fully determinate, the fully fixed, the fully discrete yields to the basic pragmatic intuition of the continuity and indeterminacy which pervade a radically temporal universe in the fullness of its space-time concreteness. Thus, Peirce and James alike stress the role of infinitesimals in ridding us of the notions of discreteness and determinacy, be it notions of experiential bits, ontological bits, or temporal bits.[16] As Dewey stresses, the indeterminate, problematic situation is objectively indeterminate and problematic, independently of consciousness.[17] In a similar vein, Peirce, James, and Lewis alike deny that the principles of non-contradiction and excluded middle apply to reality apart from the organizing mind.[18] As Peirce aptly encapsulates the character of this processive reality, it »swims in indeterminacy.«[19]

---

14 James, *A Pluralistic Universe*, (1977), *The Works of William James*, p.129.

15 James, *Essays in Radical Empiricism* (1976), The Works of William James, p.37.

16 James, *A Pluralistic Universe*, 153-154. Peirce, 6.109, 6.111, 6.87, 5.282, 6.138. For an integration of these and the immediately following references in terms of the above issue see my *Time, Continuity, and Indeterminacy: A pragmatic Engagement with Contemporary Perspectives* (Albany: State University of New York Press, 2000.), Chapters 8 and 9.

17 *The Quest for Certainty*, p.194 The Later Works, Vol.4, 1984

18 James, *A Pluralistic Universe*, p.117.; C. I. Lewis, C. I. Lewis, »A Pragmatic Conception of the A Priori«, *Collected Papers of Clarence Irving Lewis*, ed. John Goheen and John Mothershead,Jr.(Stanford: Stanford University Press, 1970), p. 232; Peirce asserts that the general is that to which the law of excluded middle does not apply, while the vague is that to which the principle of non-contradiction does not apply (5.448). He then explicitly identifies continuity with generality. For the way continu-

Neither intelligibility nor truth requires either the ontologically discrete or the ontologically determinate. Neither the ceaselessly »becoming other« of reality nor its inherent indeterminacy leads to unintelligibility. The postmodern tendency to so relate the two stems from the refusal to separate intelligibility from discreteness and fixity. The reality of the continuity of becoming other and the indeterminacy this brings with it provides for rational discourse and ongoing inquiry which is rooted in and provides perspectival knowledge about reality, so long as knowledge is not understood as a direct, uninterpreted seizure of what immediately »is«, and truth is not understood as conformity or correspondence to the fixed discretes of a fully determinate reality.

Underlying the supposedly necessary choice between the groundlessness of Derridian play or Rortyian conversation on the one hand and the grasp of reality in its »pristine purity« on the other is the assumption that without a »place« for the fully determinate, the groundless alternative wins out, an assumption that flourishes within frameworks that ignore the fundamental, creative, interactive unity at the heart of lived experience which is central to the spirit of pragmatic philosophy. Pragmatic naturalism demands realism, but demands as well that it be reconstructed to rid itself of all vestiges of and trappings surrounding the spectator theory of knowledge and the concomitant correspondence theory of truth and fully structured reality of traditional realism. We do not *think to* a reality to which language or conceptual structures correspond, but rather we *live through* a reality with which we are intertwined, and the intertwining with which constitutes experience. Our primal interactive embeddedness in the world is something which can never be adequately objectified. Within the interactive context of creativity and constraint human experience is analogous to reality in that our activities are continuous with, and emergent levels within, the reality which we attempt to characterize by the interpretive nets we cast upon it; and the indeterminately rich, continuous nature of a temporal universe emerges as facts and objects within the interpretive context of organism-environment interaction.

Truth is relative to a context of interpretation, then, not because truth is relative, but because without an interpretive context the concept of truth is meaningless. Truth is not an absolute grasp, a correspondence with an external reality, but neither is it relative. It is perspectival. We create the perspective, but whether or not it allows us to grasp in workable ways that which enters into experience is dependent not on our creativity but on the resistant features of that which enters our perspectival net and provides the touchstone for the workability of our interpretations. Truth as workability is understood in terms of answering. Peirce claims that a true thought is one which *answers*, which leads to thoughts in harmony with na-

---

ity pervades all of reality, see my *Charles Peirce's Pragmatic Pluralism* (Albany: State University of New York Press, 19)

19 Peirce, 1.171-172

ture[20] The relation of »answering« is ultimately two directional. Reality answers our questions, and determines the workability of our meaning structures, but what answers it gives are partially dependent on what questions we ask, and what meaning structures work are partially dependent upon the structures we bring. As Peirce stresses, »nothing else than a fact possibly can be a ›witness‹ or ›testimony‹«,[21] and facts are not »a slice of the Universe«[22] but are always relative to the framework of a discriminating mind. Yet the »witness of a fact« is the real, »since it is truly in that which occurs.«[23] A true belief is a tool that fits – not the fitting of a copy corresponding to an original, but the fitting of a key opening a lock.[24]

True beliefs allow us to engage reality in workable ways. As Lewis captures the import of this interactional unity: »It may be that between a sufficiently critical idealism and a sufficiently critical realism there are no issues save false issues which arise from the insidious fallacies of a copy theory of knowledge.«[25] Dewey's own frustration at being pushed into traditional alternatives by his critics is captured in one of his letters to James, in which he stresses that unless ideas take account and function in the transformation of independent existence his instrumental theory of knowledge is self-contradictory. As he summarizes, »I have repeated ad nauseam that there are existences prior to and subsequent to cognitive states and purposes, and that the whole meaning of the latter is the way they intervene in the control and revaluation of the independent existence.«[26] Indeed, throughout his logical considerations Dewey presents a running attack on what he calls analytic, presentative, and epistemological realisms as well as on their traditional idealistic or relativistic alternatives. His objection to all of these are variations of one theme, his objection to the »ubiquity of the knowledge relation«, which involves the confusion between mediated and non-mediated knowledge.[27] As Peirce well expresses the significance of noetic creativity within the pragmatic position, it does not force us into »ontological ignorance.«[28] The indefinitely rich concreteness of a process universe is revealable in various ways through various meaning structures, and is universalizable and »intelligible« through the network

---

20 *Microfilm Edition of the Peirce Papers* (Houghton Library, Harvard University), MS 934, p. 24.

21 Ibid, MS 647, p.26

22 Ibid, MS 647, p.8

23 Ibid, MS 647, p.9

24 James uses this precise analogy.

25 Lewis, *Mind and the World Order*, p. 194.

26 Quoted in Herbert Schneider, *A History of American Philosophy*, 2nd ed., New York: Columbia University Press, 1963, p.473.

27 See especially »Brief Studies in Realism«, *The Middle Works*, 6, pp.103-122.

28 *Writings of Charles Peirce, Vol.1*, ed. Max Fisch (Bloomington: Indiana University Press, 1982), p.489. Italics in text.

of such structures, though »in itself« it contains no inherently intelligible order. However, as Dewey carefully point out, this »does not mean that nature has lost intelligibility. It rather signifies that we are in position to realize that the term intelligible is to be understood literally [...]. Nature is capable of being understood [...]. The devotion we show to the ideal of intelligence determines the extent« to which the universe »is congenial to mind.«[29]

Our perceptual environment, which grounds the emergence of facts and objects and provides the foundation for other, more abstract or more imaginative environments, is existentially one with the spatio-temporal unfolding of an indeterminate reality. It is, metaphysically, that independently real. Yet, our various environments are dependent upon the meaning systems or interpretive contexts which grasp in a way in which the full concreteness of spatio-temporal reality is not, for they are perspectives of the indefinitely rich reality which has been »fixed« or »carved out« by systems of meanings. Knowledge is abstractive and selective. Our everyday environment, though concrete, is nonetheless selective in the sense that it is the concrete content denoted by a system of meanings, a system that is one way in which the indeterminate concreteness of reality can be delineated or »fixed.« A system, once chosen, limits the alternatives possible within it, but alternative systems may be possible. The indefinite richness of a processive universe is there. Where the conceptual »cuts« are imposed is, in part, our decision. Any environment is delineated by a system of facts, but facts are not independent of the selective knowledge process, for facts are abstracted portions of interacting continuities.

Throughout many levels, truth is both made and found. The so-called tensions between truth as made and truth as found, between truth as changing and truth as fixed, result from focusing on diverse dimensions operative within the intertwining of human interpretive activity and the temporal unfolding of a processive universe. We create the interpretive frameworks within which beliefs can emerge and be found true or false and within which investigation can tend toward agreement. The creative intelligence involved in radical changes and shifts of interpretive frameworks is influenced by socio-cultural conditions, but is ultimately founded not in a relativistic, perspectivally closed historicism, but in an ontologically grounded, perspectivally open temporalism. The criterion for adequately cutting into the indefinitely rich array of possibilities of experience offered by the dynamics of an indeterminately rich concrete universe is workability, but workability can be established only relative to some meaningful network by which experience is »caught«.

Here it may be objected that the view of knowledge as perspectivally and temporally rooted involves relativism and historicism. However, such objections again sever experience from its creative, interactive unity with, and openness

29 Dewey, The Quest for Certainty, p.215.

upon, that which is independently there. As previously indicated, the unity denies the arbitrariness of antifoundationalism, antirealism, relativism, a historicism of present happenstance, the demise of metaphysics. The temporally founded creativity denies the absoluteness of foundationalism, realism, objectivism, the absolute grasp. Instead of the stultifying self-enclosement of a relativism in terms of arbitrary conceptual schemes, this pragmatic view houses an open perspectivalism in which perspectives open onto the common concrete ground of their possibility. Instead of an historicism of present happenstance, it involves a temporalism in which historical rootedness is at once rootedness in a thick, resisting, natural universe, and in which the rootedness of perspective emerges within the context of a past that presents itself in the richness of the potentialities and possibilities of a processive present oriented toward a novel and indefinite future. Valid knowledge claims are fallibilistic, perspectival, and temporal, but nonetheless grounded in a thick reality.

As long as pragmatic doctrines are understood within, or developed in terms of, one of the family related sets of the very alternatives it has rejected, then though specific aspects of its position may be further developed for specialized purposes, the significance and uniqueness of its systematic vision is lost.

Pragmatism attempts neither to freely create nor to free itself from commitments, but rather to reveal the way in which there a primal commitedness or rootedness at the very heart of the experience that grounds such alternative attempts. It attempts to draw one toward an awareness of the interactive openness, at the heart of experience, of humans and the natural universe in which they are embedded, and in so doing provide the path for freeing thinking from premature ontological assertions, from illicit reifications, and from a tradition of philosophy which, in its search for supposed foundations, lost the illusive but pervasive existential foundations of its search. Pragmatism, in illuminating the creative interactive unity at the heart of experience, develops a position which eludes the false alternatives and misplaced dichotomies which still haunt philosophy today. If, as pragmatism holds, the pulse of human existence at its very core is, both existentially and epistemically, creatively and perspectivally intertwined with, and thus attuned to, an indeterminately rich processive universe which reveals itself in various ways both within and among various levels and modes of human activity, then attunement to this sense of human existence can yield at once both a more demanding and more tolerant master than any of the diverse second level articulations to which it gives rise. Pragmatic perspectival realism gives philosophical legitimacy to this prethematic sense that is born of our essential interactive unity with a thick dynamic cosmic process which we must creatively engage in fruitful ways.

When a community is operating within a common system of meanings on any one issue, then investigation can tend toward an ideal limit of convergence. But, when different segments of interpreters experience different facts because of different sets of meaning structures for cutting into the indefinitely rich continuity of possibilities of ordering, then such convergence cannot occur. The criterion for adequately cutting is workability, but workability can be established only relative to some meaningful network by which experience is »caught«. Thus there may be a plurality of interpretations among varying groups of interpreters on any topic. For, each group, identifiable by varying nets or perspective for the catching of experience, are variously structuring some contours of an environment. But, even the lines of demarcation of distinct groups of interpreters are difficult to discern, for such differing networks are embodied in differing attitudes of response and may be present when disagreeing interpreters think their differences can be resolved merely »by collecting the facts.« In this way, the essential pluralism is often hidden from view in the misplaced drive toward a common conclusion based on »the evidence«.

Such pluralism must ultimately be dealt with in terms of a generalized stance of agreement concerning what standards are to be applied in making decisions among »incommensurable« frameworks for delineating facts. Such standards may be difficult to elucidate, but as implicitly operative they can be elicited for clarification. However, perspectives may emerge which are not only »incommensurable« with another conceptual net for the catching of experience through the determination of what kind of facts exist in the world, but which also incorporate standards and criteria and solutional goals, or kinds of problems important to resolve, which are »incommensurable« with those of another perspective. Thus, there are not only different facts, but different methods, standards, and criteria for determining which system of facts should be accepted.

The function of »persuasion« comes into play here. Persuasion, however, does not involve a contrast between the rational and the non-rational, but rather requires a new understanding of the nature of rationality. Pragmatism implicitly reveals the way in which the rational cannot be confined to what can be explicitly formulated in a series of propositions, for facts and their propositional formulations emerge from the backdrop of a horizon of meaning which by its very nature cannot be brought to such formulation. As Peirce stresses, the irrationality of humans consists in »an exaggerated loyalty to their own principles«[30] rather than willingness to change in the light of the dynamics of scientific method. This method incorporates at all levels of its functioning the vague sense of workability and, as holistic in nature, is not reducible to rigid rules of procedure. Yet incommensurable perspectives, whether at the level of common sense or science, though in a sense structuring differing »worlds«, cannot, by their very nature as opening onto a natural universe with which we must successfully interact, be closed to rational discussion. In the ongoing course of experience some arguments

30 6.181

or reasons gain vitality while others fall by the wayside. Though neither are proved right or wrong, we »get over« some, but yield to the force of others. Such a »getting over« or reinforcement is based on rational discussion, guided by a vague, elusive, but real sense of the inescapable criteria of workability.

The adjustment of perspectives through rational reconstruction requires not an imposition from »on high« of abstract principles but a deepening to a more fundamental level of human rapport. While experience arises from specific, concrete contexts shaped by a particular tradition, this is not mere inculcation, for the deepening process offers the openness for breaking through and grasping different contexts. Ongoing dialogue and debate about experimental reconstruction of problematic situations, and about resultant new norms and ideals which develop as working hypotheses out of such concrete situations, must ultimately be rooted in the creative utilization of an attunement to the valuings of humans and their ongoing flourishing, or there is nothing for the debate to be about. Reconstruction of concrete situations in their richness as involving authentic growth thus ultimately requires both a deepening attunement to the pulse of human existence and the development of creative intelligence. In this ongoing process, differences are not to be eliminated or melted down, for these differences provide the necessary materials by which both humans and societies alike can continue to grow.

In this way, perspectival pluralism allows for a pluralism of valid frameworks while yet allowing for their openness onto both the »other« or different perspectives and a thick, independent universe to which they are answerable. And thus the position avoids the extremes of either relativistic irresponsibility or dogmatic commitment or imposition, replacing both with the importance of ongoing inter-perspectival dialogue which allow for the advancement of knowledge and the ongoing enrichment of human existence. It calls for commitment to one's perspective as it proves to advance these goals, but yet openness to other perspectives which may, in their own way, be accomplishing the same goals. Knowledge as cumulative and knowledge as changing do not lie in opposition. Rather, knowledge as changing is also knowledge as cumulative, for any novel perspective emerges from a cumulative process or history which yields enrichment of intelligibility both of the old and of the new. But, to demand of such a cumulative process that it tends toward a final unchanging truth is to misunderstand the nature of the indeterminately rich natural universe, the nature of noetic activity, and the nature of the interactive contexts within which both are unified.

Julio Raúl Méndez

Logic and Culture

Translated by Vincent Capuano sj

1. Universality and particularity in logic

The experience of making trips abroad and human communication has always made clear *the diversity of languages* within the universality of language as a human act. The surprise and the confusion that this experience produces has an explication in the bible story of the tower of Babel. The differences that separate men one from another and plunge them into confusion is presented as a divine punishment for human pride.

Throughout history the search for a way to overcome this situation has taken many forms. One of the forms that requires much sacrifice is the learning of foreign languages that permit dialogue and common action. The learning of a foreign language involves a very human commitment to meeting the other. The opposite and more violent way to overcome language barriers is the imposition of one language over another as a refection of triumphal superiority. A third way, many time attempted and never successful, is the project of inventing a universal language that would be common for everybody.

These efforts respond to *the universal desire to communicate*. Man naturally not only desires to know but also to communicate with other men. For this reason the story of the tower of Babel is seen as a story of punishment. The punishment consists in the mutual lack of understanding that the diversity of languages represents. This supposes of course the assumption that if the linguistic problem is solved communication is produced. This assumption implies another that seems obvious: that human thought is universally the same, that ideas are common to all, and for that reason if a common language could be found the desire to communicate would be satisfied.

The cultural history and cultural anthropology have studied the phenomenon of *cultural diversity*. These disciplines also begin from the premise that it is possible to understand other cultures and that the problem is found in the codes of expression, it is assumed that human thought is universally the same. The premise of *formal logic* is that mental processes have an absolute character, that is to say they are independent from factors that could render them relative. It concerns itself with establishing laws of thinking that are universally valid. The important logician I. M. Bochenski affirms that throughout history in the various problems that he has studied, in both Western and Eastern literature, formal logic is one. The same problems always appear, and the same solutions are a ways found (see *Formale Logik*, 1956; introduction).

Science, with its theoretical epistemological rigor, as well as international politics and international law rest on premise that all men think in the same manner, therefore the question is to identify a common starting point and from there proceed rationally. That premise would lead us to believe that the key is having all the *information* necessary to have a discussion. Discussions make sense in so far as it is possible to resolve the differences either by means of irrefutable facts (*contra facta non fit argumentum*), or by means of evidence produced by reason. The later is formal evidence and as such in a debate one tries to find the logical faults in the opponents argument.

Aristotle clearly saw that logic is not a science but an instrument (»organon«). He pointed out the value of formal logic in the argumentative, dialogical phase of human thought. In the aristotelic scheme the best way to construct solid knowledge is by means of eliminating errors in the discussion. However in the experience of global human relations, especially in international politics and international law and in intercultural dialogue, make clear that often discussions do not advance past a certain point. The result is the temptation for the stronger party to impose a solution, using force in someway to suppress the adversary or his controversial projects and proposals. If we can avoid falling into this temptation, in front of the impasse in the discussion the question may arise: What do these people think? Why can't we just agree on what seems so evident? Maybe formal logic is not so absolute?

2. Not only the formal

When Aristotle wrote *The Topics* he clearly saw that at the beginning and during the course of the argumentation there are more than just empty formal principles. Frequently logicians dismiss this work. Even the pragmatic rhetorician Cicero found the casuistic style of *The Topics* a challenge, because it meant entering into a vast number of experiences in particular times and places that probably could not be reconstructed and were far from universal or at least demanded preparatory work for those who did not have them.

Aristotle distinguishes the task of the philosopher from the task of the dialectician. The philosopher investigates only for himself, he is concerned with the reality of things that establish whether thoughts are true and the reality is known. On the other hand, the dialectician needs also to order the topics and formulate questions because his work leads to the discussion (*The Topics*, VIII, 155b 11-15.) The origin of the book *The Topics* is an Athenian society habituated to public debate. It is a valuable resource for us living in a context of globalized debate. *The Topics* is not dismissive of formal logic. In fact in the book one discovers empty formal structures that are ways to predicate (*Topics* I, 101b 15 ss). Therefore, it deals with what can be predicated and with analogy (*Topics* I, 106a ss). But also the character of the thesis and the problems is discovered.

There are problems that require argumentation, others that require a correction (e.g. »that parents should not loved«), others that require a sensation (e.g. »whether snow is white«) (*Topics* I 105a 4ss). But also »all that seems to be a given in all of the cases, or in the majority of cases should also be taken into account as a principle and admitted as a hypothesis« (*Topics* I 105b 10). This is similar to how the ideas and hypotheses of the wisest or of philosophers are (provisionally) accepted as valid »as long as they are not contrary to observed facts« (*Topics* I, 105a 35ss). Just as in a legislative assembly it is the custom to present bills for consideration and if they seem better than the laws actually in effect they are accepted. Thus in the (scientific or philosophical) debate the hypotheses can be challenged and modified according to formal laws (*Topics* VI 151b 4 ss). That means the recuperation of the vertical superiority of the formal topics over the horizontal topics of the majority opinion or of the scientific authority. The universality of logic is maintained, but the multiplicity has been recognized.

Discounting the cases when one of the parties does not practice goodwill and intentionally denies reason and makes discussion useless (*Topics* VIII, 164b 8 ss) the multiplicity must be considered as a valid although a divergent form of organizing information to serve as a starting point constructing an hypothesis as well as in testing it. This is *the multiplicity of ways of thinking* that is necessary to keep in mind in order to understand some of the roadblocks of discussion and to remove them. The recognition of this multiplicity will save us from the monist and hegemonic pretensions interpreting history of Francis Fukuyama (*The End of the History and the Last Man,* 1992). This formal multiplicity also challenges the pretensions of Carl G. Hempel (*The Function of General Laws in History*, 1942) who held that history is explained by the same type of laws that govern natural sciences. According to his theory the events and historical processes are able to be foreseen. According to Hempel there exists a *principle of rationality* according to which men normally act rationally. By this principle, given the situation *S* the subject *A* acts rationally if and only if he produces an action of type *B*. If placed in situation *S* the subject *A* does not do *B*, it is because in this case he is not acting rationally. For Hempel the principle of rationality admits an exception, when the man decides not to act rationally.

But this principle supposes that there is only one universal rationality. The previously mentioned misunderstanding that produces questions like: *What are these people thinking? And how could they do that?* occurs on both sides. Both parties consider the position of the other as irrational and that the other party decided not to observe the principle of rationality. Thus the other side can seem to have its reason clouded by their emotions, or be perverse, or be unbalanced, or not to take in account the facts about the starting point of the argument. For Karl Popper (*Of Clouds and Clocks: An Approach to the Problem of Rationality and the Freedom of Man*, 1966) it is better to formulate the principle of rationality in this way: Men act rationally according to the situation *as they see it.* Thus it is not so easy to label a conduct »irrational«. There is neither fatalism nor axiomatic foresight in history. Popper insists in the in the particularity of individuals and their original contributions to history. We should also consider this originality in terms of *particular cultural subjects*. That A does not necessarily produce B means that S is not necessarily the same for all those A. That every subject acts rationally according to his view of the situation, means that *each subject reasons according to those principles and experiences from which he starts*. This variant puts to one side the cases of emotional confusion, unbalance and perversion. This is the variant of *multiple horizontal forms of thinking.* The recognition of this multiplicity makes it possible to respond to the questions: What do these people think? What does that guy think? The response is to ask: What does that people see? From what context does that man begin? Asking these questions is helpful because it opens oneself horizontally to human otherness and disposes oneself to see more what *the other sees*. It may be because one discovers and incorporates new viewpoints and guiding principles of thought or it may be because one critically rediscovers one's own viewpoints and principles in the confrontation with the diversity.

The perception of formal horizontal multiplicity by an individual can be understood as a perception that does not close itself in simple information but rather discovers *how the information is received and processed.* The fact that the same information delivers different content to different people argues against the idea that the richness of the object of knowledge is readily disposable to a subject. The subjective reception of the known object by the intellect conditions future acts of reception by the formation of *habits of knowledge* that are formal modes of interpreting the object. When these habits are shared within a community they generate scientific, philosophic and cultural *traditions*. Further, it is necessary to recognize the role of the *interaction between knowledge and affectivity* in these habitual and traditional ways of thinking.

Paul Ricoeur (*The Metaphorical Process as Cognition, Imagination and Feeling*, 1980; *Le temps et la narration*, 1987) has pointed out the existence of affective schemes that in the moment of filtering content from raw information selects according to affective preference. As a result of this favorable treatment the full richness of the preferred content is developed. Thomas Aquinas (*Summa Theologica* II-II q. 45 *et alia*) made clear the role of the *cogitative,* an internal sense that grasps the value of the object in relation to the subject for its *connaturality*, generating the horizontal multiplicity that we have been talking about. This framework permits us to recognize the vertical and horizontal articulation in the forms or categories used in the thinking process. From this perspective we want to approach the case of Latin American thought as an example of a cultural subject with its own *tradition* and *connaturality* in the plural universe of human thought.

3. Latin American thought

It has always been the characteristic and constitutive condition of philosophy (and of science) its *academicality*, as universal communication of human thought in diachronic and synchronic axis. In this dialogue not only is truth sought in a shared way, but there is a shared self-consciousness of its own thought with its own identity, its own limits and its own contributions to universal human thought. For historical reasons and for its intrinsic vigor *Western philosophy* has been disseminated in the whole world. This is true of Latin America. Western philosophy acts as a fermenting agent that stimulates the development of philosophy as such and is the standard against which regional philosophies distinguish themselves and form their self-conscious identities. This too is true of Latin American Philosophy. Resisting the temptation of hegemony, we propose to offer a report on a fundamental characteristic of *Latin American thought*, as a specific act of the superior faculties of the mind with self defined cultural features.

Before beginning our argument it is worth while clarifying that what we call *Latin American thought* is based in the practice of philosophy done in an environment larger than the departments of philosophy and centers of investigation of universities. Without dissolving the continuity with Western philosophy we must recognize that the aesthetic expressions of Latin American thought are rooted in popular culture. Exercising the Latin American self-consciousness one discovers that Latin American thought is *estimative*, that's to say that it recognizes as its proper object not just the truth but *the truth and the good* as inseparably united. This is a complex phenomenon that only a more profound analysis can penetrate. What the Latin mind collects as data is presented as a *content of reality* that for its very *intensity of being* produces in the Latin American man *an attitude of recognition and movement toward or rejection of the object.*

The two activities the Western thought separated analytically as *logos* and *eros* are presented in Latin American thought concomitantly as one complex act. Without a doubt an analysis psycho-logical by the European school is able to suggest the distinction with some advantage without demanding a strong separation, but for Latin American thought this always remains a difficult exercise. This is the characteristic of the *estimative logic* as a mental structure that corresponds to the regional mentality and permeates the distinct cultural expressions: there is no pure *logos,* there is no *logos* without *eros*. Because in and from the very fabric of the logos springs the *eros*, the act of openness and recognition of the reality is in itself a bonding act. Because of this the context that surrounds the Latin American man is perceived as his landscape and homeland, other men are perceived as brothers, and in everything the presence of the Absolute is discovered.

This triple bond places the Latin American man in the middle of an initial and spontaneous harmony. It is not that the land has the meaning of homeland because there is no preliminary instance of simple »land« that latter acquires the content of »homeland«, rather the land *is* homeland. The connection or bond between *logos* and *eros* is not another moment, *there are no neutral contents*. We can clarify by saying that this phenomenon is what those classic philosophers called *the identity of transcendentals*: being, the good, the truth and the beautiful. What does not appear in the Latin American Mind is the later cleavage between being and the good, or being and the beautiful: a cleavage that is introduced by the mediation of the subjectivity. Reducing the reality to »*essence*« has produced its de-signification, its estimative neutrality, because of the loss of its original intensity. This is the origin of the »*plainness*« of essence totally indifferent and malleable in the hands of subjectivity that European philosophy has developed especially since the start of modernity. The designified essences are not in themselves connective. It is clear that the bonding character of reality presupposes that the density that generates the bonds is *original* and not imposed by the subject. In regards to the idea that bonds are imposed by the subject, it would seem then that the only articulation possible is of the subject with himself. On the other hand, the bondage that is produced in the subject as an effect by the presence of the real is the unitive efficiency of the real-consistent it is the inclusion in the oneness of being, the good, the truth and the beautiful.

While the essencialist reduction dissolves the differences of the real in *the pure logic of coherence* that makes possible because it is thinkable, the estimative logic receives the differences of what is real as that which is found relevant and not simply found manageable. Here we can add another feature that defines the Latin American thought that we have called *estimative logic*. The density of the real, its goodness that is displayed as value is something *discovered*: and for that reason attracts and defines the bonds by means of acceptance of what is real. More than an elaboration or a cultural mediation, it is an experience of an *immediacy* of communion with the reality that is manifested. For that reason in estimative logic the reality is presented as *given*. Here sound with all its force the voice of those philosophers of epistemology that wanted to begin with the *data*, but later backed off and introduced the rule of subjectivity. Without this later move, and even less the move of those epistemological models that are conceived the as pure mental constructs, for Latin American thought the *starting point*, *the process and the end point of knowledge are considered as a communion with the real in all its density*. Communion is often expressed in *multiple locutions* because of inadequacy of language to express the real. This communion with the ontological density of the real is expressed by means of the metaphor. Here the metaphor is not just a literary convention nor is it self-conscious, rather it is the royal road of analogical thinking moving from the known to the unknown in a manner different from dialogical thinking. By means of different metaphors thought becomes *more logical*.

What modern Western thought has viewed as a break and mediation in reason Latin American thought views, only as mediation and not as a break. The metaphor arises from the community and is used as an ascending spiral of human communion with the real. The language repeats that which is always most richly given. The distance that marks the environment of the subject is not in the terrain of knowledge but of language. To say that the reality is *given* implies that it is *freely given*, it is something that comes from something else without a specified reason. Latin American metaphysical thought understands the real as something presented as dense and with a good foundation, i.e. with its own consistency but as produced by something else. The origin of reality is not the so called »*principle of sufficient reason*« of western metaphysics.

Contrary to the attitude of Western metaphysics that processes the real according to the demands of reason, looking for or imposing attributes and satisfactory conditions for the subjective universe of the ideal, the metaphysics of the estimative logic discovers in the density of the reality as presented a pure gift. What is real does not appear questioned nor questionable; rather than to speak of a *problem* it is more apt to speak of a *mystery*. Because what is real is presented as something that cannot lead to what is foreign to the real. The only thing that the reality as a *given* can lead to is the *giver*. In as much as the real is coming to us in partial measures it alludes to the Total Absolute of what is coming. Therefore what we could call the »*metaphysical question*« is not a question of why there is something and not nothing, in absolute terms, but the question is about the itinerary of the given presence of reality from its origin in the Giver. From this perspective, we can say that the Latin American metaphysical thought does not treat the problems of the beginnings of reason but the mysteries of the foundation of Love. In this very treatment the greatest bond or link is extended and affirmed, that is the bond that unites man with the Absolute by means of the always unitive dynamism of reality, and all the more unitive the more denser and original it is.

In this brief report on Latin American thought the where the contradistinctions appear it cannot be left unrecognized the great contribution of *critical philosophy* gestated in European modernity. The question is the following: Is it necessary for Latin American philosophy to assume the philosophy that was born in Europe? I think that it is not posible to ignore; as we have pointed out, the universal academicity of thought. But it is important to keep in mind that in this academic *dialogue*, as a search for the truth, one must be faithful to the dynamism of one's own logos. In this sense the acceptance of the goods of Western philosophy does not constitute an indiscriminate acceptance of all its assumptions and historical baggage as if they were the structural attainments that make up all human thought. It is necessary in order for the dialogue to be fruitful, to critically consider the Western philosophical horizon within the multiple human horizons. The first observation is that the assumptions of modern Western philosophy imply abandoning the original experience of the subject that encounters the real. While Western philosophy assumes that this encounter with the real is something the subject does, the Latin mind view the encounter as an encounter with one's self and finds oneself co-implicated with the world and communicates with it. The Western philosophical notion of subjectivity seen from the Latin American point of view is less an exaltation of the subject than the emptying of the subject. The *destruction of the human subject* occurs on account of the destruction of the bonds that make and sustain being. The objective dissolution of the bonds with the earth (the home), other men, and the Absolute because of the uncontrolled primacy of subjectivity is expressed in ecological destruction and disaster, in individualism, in anonymity and in nihilistic secularism.

4. The new dialogue

In the context of a world linked by communications, the philosophic worries and concerns have become more shared, as in the paradigmatic case of *cultural dialogue*. To further intercultural dialogue the message from Latin America, for Europe awash in references to postmodern nihilism, is a call to self examination and consideration of the original experience of learning. In this ineludible experience the presence of the reality (one's own and the surrounding) is confirmed, and not as something neutral to which one must add sense, but rather as something *given* coming uninterruptedly with a sense that moves attracting and pushing forward. This is the original experience that is the source of thought according to the estimative logic of Latin America. In dialogue with the logic of subjectivity, of sufficient reason, and of the nihilism of »weak thought«, the Latin American estimative logic is clearly seen not as modern, nor as post-modern but as *post-contemporary* in the current of universal thought. This Latin American thought is not based on some founding thought, some big idea that is sure of it self and constructs a self-contained system without bonds to the outside, nor is it based on the loss of all reference in the disorientation of the weakness of thought. It is however founded on a thought that is *consolidated by the collection of experiences of a reality that is continually coming to be*, Latin American thought is conscious of the future and of the possibility of a consistent and fruitful dialogue.

The possibility of dialogue is given by this first and primary *access and acceptance* of what is real. In effect, from the immanence of the subject the closed and aggressive languages and cultures are projected, vehicles of militant truths or of those petty tyrants of nihilist egoisms. From the *acceptance and openness* to the very basic reality, as real human language expressed in diverse tongues, it is possible to indicate the dialogue in a womb of common belonging. Here Latin

American thought lifts up the fundamental role of *body*. Defining man as »*ru-miallpa kamashka*« as »*land that walks*« those wise men amautas of the Tahuatisuyo, define man in a connection and continuity with the world. From this viewpoint the closed immanence, or the absence and impossibility of referent seems to be a violent systematic abandoning of oneself, it seems unpractical because of the original experience of thought.

Far from the closed immanence and the absence or impossibility of references, the first linguistic proposal, the first step of dialogue is assured by the *gesture* as the first tongue of human universal communication. Before a word is spoken, the body expresses its corporal continuity with the universe. Starting from gestures it is possible to consolidate the word and launch the dialogue. A dialogue that for its very original continuity will turn *not only* on the truths but also on the concomitant values or estimative significance. These values are generated in man because of the fabric of connections with the reality. In midst of the remains and in the desert of the post-modern crisis that has affected the whole planet, the Latin American estimative thought that we have presented faces the future with confidence and optimism.

Heinrich Beck

The Relation of European Thought to the ›Logos‹ and ›Logic‹. A Possible Contribution to Cultural World Integration?

The modern secular culture primarily is the result of world wide extension and influence of the European culture. Therefore, in order to determine the constructive and destructive power of the modern secular culture for shaping a dynamic world peace in encounter with traditional Asiatic and African cultures, an analysis of positive and negative characteristics of the European culture seems to be necessary. These characteristics are to be comprehended by means of their historical manifestations, especially of the development of European philosophy from antiquity and middle ages to modernity, which we have to look over in the following exposition under this aspect.

In the first part, we will elaborate the primordial positive disposition and capacity of the European spirit. This consists, as I will demonstrate, in the development of λογοσ and logic; European culture, from its basic onto-anthropological identity and tendency, is a rational culture. This fundamentally means a particular faculty of an objectifying and distancing consciousness of being, which makes possible a critical understanding and transcending of the past and an active projection and creation of the future. This rational ability gave birth to the sciences, which have to analyse and divide the original unity of experienced reality into its components and partial functions, and it produced modern techniques, which have to synthesise and recompose the parts to new ingenious unities. Hence it follows an especial progressivity of European mind and culture. This consciousness confronting and dividing reality further included the evolution of individual rights of the human person, as well as the construction of rational orders of society and economy. In these human values the possible contribution of the European culture to world integration is grounded.

But simultaneously this particular capacity of the λογοσ and of logical structuring of empirical reality seems to have been partially perverted into negative attitudes: in alienation, exploitation and destruction. Pointing out these negative attitudes is the intention of the second part of this exposition. Here historical phenomena like rationalism, empirism, positivism occur indicating the permanent danger and tendency of the European spirit to fall into a subjectocentric nihilism. It is to be understood as a partial privation and perversion of the originally positive faculty and disposition just mentioned, and signifies a deep crisis of the European culture and – in its enlargement in the modern secular world civilisation – a threat for mankind's survival and therefore a strong provocation. The task of overcoming this crisis demands a creative encounter with Asiatic and African cultural traditions which exactly embody those human values which could balance out the one-sidedness of the European access to reality.

1. Representation of the λογοσ as pimordial capacity and destiny of the European culture, as a possible contribution to world integration

a) Looking upon the historical development of the European mentality in its philosophical conceptualisation, we see the idea of the λογοσ as the leading motive of thinking since the earliest times. In antiquity, as it seems, the pre-socratic thinker Heraclitus[1] was the first who called the λογοσ the supreme and inmost principle of reality and the law of all processes and events, combining and determining the differences and contrarities of being to an all-embracing floating unity, as a παλιντροποσ ηαρμονιαε, and in Pythagoras[2] this λογοσ assumed more mathematical-harmonical and psychical features. Later on, with Sokrates[3], the λογοσ in the play of questioning dia-logues and dia-lectics was recognised as the methodical principle of finding out the truth; and according to his disciple Plato[4]

---

1 Concerning the general conception of the *λογοσ* in Greek philosophy cf. M. Henze, *Die Lehre vom Logos in der griechischen Philosophie*. Repr. of the ed. Oldenburg 1872, Aalen 1984; W. Nestle, *Vom Mythos zum Logos. Die Selbstentfaltung des griechischen Denkens von Homer bis auf die Sophistik und Sokrates*, Stuttgart 1942; B. Snell, *Die Entdeckung des Geistes. Studien zur Entstehung des europäischen Denkens bei den Griechen*, Hamburg 1955; W. Kelber, *Die Logoslehre, von Heraklit bis Origenes*, Stuttgart 1976; M. Bartling, *Der Logosbegriff bei Heraklit und seine Beziehung zur Kosmologie*, Göppingen 1985; especially to Heraclitus cf. K. Deichgräber, *Rhythmische Elemente im Logos des Heraklit*, Wiesbaden 1963; E. Kurtz, *Interpretationen zu den Logos-Fragmenten Heraklits*, Hildesheim 1971; W.H. Pleger, *Der Logos der Dinge. Eine Studie zu Heraklit*, Frankf./M. 1987.

2 Cf. W. Burkert, *Weisheit und Wissenschaft. Studien zu Pythagoras, Philolaos und Platon*, Nürnberg, 1962; B.L. van der Waerden, *Die Pythagoreer. Religiöse Bruderschaft und Schule der Wissenschaft*, Zürich-München 1979; D.J. O'Meara, *Pythagoras Revived. Mathematics and Philosophy in Late Antiguity*, Oxford 1989.

3 Cf. H. Kuhn, *Sokrates. Versuch über den Ursprung der Metaphysik*, München 1948; B. Waldenfels, *Das sokratische Fragen. Aporie, Elenchos, Anamnesis*, Meisenheim 1961. – We can also mention here that in Platonic dialogues Socrates is the person which demands from his partners »to give the reason«, that means literally: »to give the logos« (λογοσ διδοναι as in *Menon*, 81a or in *Protagoras*, 336d). Socrates himself says that the essential aim of his life is »to follow the logos« (*Kriton* 46b: πειδωσδαι τω λογω).

4 Cf. P. Friedländer, *Platon. Vol I-III*, Berlin-New York 1964-75; A. Graeser, *Platons Ideenlehre. Sprache, Logik und Metaphysik*, Stuttgart 1975; W.D. Ross. *Plato's theory of ideas*, Westport (Conn.) 1976; see also B. Witte, *Der εικως λόγος in Platos ›Timaios‹. Beitrag zur Wissenschaftsmethode und Erkenntnistheorie des späten Plato.*

all physical reality is transparent to its meta-physical λογοσ, it is to an order of through-shining archetypes or hypostatic ›ideas‹, as the good and the love or truth, beauty, equality, harmony and justice; and at least, Aristotle[5] put these transcendent principles of sense and cognoscibility into the matter of the world, as the immanent forms of the physical beings and happenings. As to be seen, for the ancient Greeks the whole world was ordered homogeneously by harmonical mathematical principles and reigned by the λογοσ working out the chaos to the cosmos. But, because the material substratum to a certain extent resists the λογοσ, he does appear in the visible world only in a limited manner, and order can't overcome the chaos perfectly. This metaphysical opposition and dualism in the constitution of the world's being also is the reason for an ultimate failing of all ethical efforts and for a deeply tragical of fate. Therefore, human education was understood as the task to elaborate, represent, imitate and actualise the λογοσ and a λογοσ-corresponding order of being: theoretically in the rational consciousness, practically in the ethical will and character, and poietically in the constructing of external culture. This European conception of cosmic λογοσ, embracing all nature and mankind and grounding world order, may be found in a similar way also in other cultures and certainly opens a basic perspective for future world integration.

b) In the second period of the historical development of the European culture, the so called Middle Ages, under the influence of Jewish and Christian revelation the cosmocentric image of being changed to a theocentric one. That means, in the centre of being it is not the logic of an anonymous divine energy that works, but the one and omnipotent personal God, who creates the world through the λογοσ, his personal word, by which he calls all things into being. Now, the λογοσ is no longer understood as a part of the world, as its immanent forming and structuring force, but as a personal divine reality. According to Christian philosophers such as Saint Augustine[6] or Thomas Aquinas[7] God in Himself realises an interpersonal

---

In: Archiv für Gesch. der Philos. 46 (1964) 1-16; K. Bärthlein, Der oρδος λόγος und das ethische Prinzip in den Platonischen Schriften. Ibid.46 (1964) 129-173.

5 Cf. J. Stallmach, *Dynamis und Energeia. Untersuchungen am Werk des Aristoteles zur Problemgeschichte von Möglichkeit und Wirklichkeit*, Meisenheim 1959; H. Seidl, *Beiträge zu Aristoteles' Erkenntnislehre und Metaphysik*, Würzburg-Amsterdam 1984; H. Schmitz, *Die Ideenlehre des Aristoteles. Vol.1.2*, Bonn 1985; M. Furth, *Substance, Form, Psyche. An Aristotelian Metaphysics*, Cambridge 1988.

6 Cf. M. Schmaus, *Die psychologische Trinitätslehre des hl. Augustinus*, Münster 1927, repr. ibid. 1967; F.M. Sladeczek, *Die Selbsterkenntnis als Grundlage der Philosophie nach dem hl. Augustinus*. In: Scholastik 5 (1930) 329-356; V. Warnach, *Erleuchtung und Einsprechung bei Aurelius Augustinus*. In: Augustinus Magister. Vol.1, Paris 1954, p.429-449; R. Berlinger, *Augustins dialogische Metaphysik*, Frankf./M. 1961; J. Mader, *Die logische Struktur des personalen Denkens. Aus der Methode der Gotte-*

life; His act of being consists in a trinitarian dialog: By intellectual self-penetration God perceives His own infinite essence and expresses and pronounces it in the λογοσ, who therefore is named the co-essential ›Son of God‹; He perfectly represents Him and corresponds to Him. The co-acting of self-pronouncing and of responding culminates in the origination and aspiration of the Holy Spirit, by which both accept each other in perfect love and unity. In this unlimited divine dialog, the world as a limited being in space and time participates. Thus God the creator occurs as the father both of His consubstantial Son, the Divine λογοσ, and of all His creation which is pronounced through the same λογοσ – in the love of Holy Spirit; and the world, especially the human person, is invited to integrate itself into the λογοσ and His correspondence to God, that is in His responding and answering son-partnership to God. In this horizon, the evolution and history of the world appears as nothing less than an increasing or decreasing conformity to the reality of the λογοσ, that means: History is the response and responsible answer to the call of the creator, or also its denial.

It implies a mystery of Christian belief, that in the history of his fatherly partnership with the world, God has sent his Son as an incarnated brotherly being with the humankind, and that He was crucified; hence the cross is understood as a sign for the disturbed order of being and for the suffering, as a consequence of the denial against creative divine λογοσ and love, and simultaneously as a permanent offer to reconciliation and freedom.

Philosophically, thereby two important aspects of the λογοσ have been elaborated:

- λογοσ means personal dialog and creative encounter, and all human being from its absolute divine fundament is disposed and directed to dialog and interpersonality; in this λογοσ-participating similitude to the Divine, especially an irreplaceable dignity of every human person is rooted, and this is the fundament of its individual rights and its social and cosmic obligations as dimensions of a dialogical and responsible being. This value, articulated in a peculiar way in the Christian middle ages, means an indispensible supposition and contribution for world integration.

---

serkenntnis bei Aurelius Augustinus, Wien 1965; O. du Roy, *L'intelligence de la foi en la Trinité selon saint Augustin*, Paris 1966.

7 Cf. A. Malet, *Personne et amour dans la théologie trinitaire de saint Thomas*, Paris 1956; E. Bailleux, *Le personnalisme de saint Thomas en théologie trinitaire*. In: Rev. thomiste 61 (1961) 25-42; H. Beck, *Der Akt-Charakter des Seins. Eine spekulative Weiterführung der Seinslehre Thomas v. Aquins aus einer Anregung durch das dialektische Prinzip Hegels*, 2Fft/M. 2003; K. Kremer, *Die neuplatonische Seinslehre und ihre Wirkung auf Thomas v. Aquin*, Leiden 1966; F. Inciarte, *Forma Formarun. Strukturmomente der thomistischen Seinslehre im Rückgriff auf Aristoteles*, Freiburg-München 1970.

- But λογοσ and all λογοσ-participating order in reality also is violated and is deeply suffering; therefore the aim of history seems to be liberation and freedom through the relation to the λογοσ, by His personal assimilation and subjectification. Thus, in the line of λογοσ-accentuated the European culture development after the cosmocentric world view of the Antiquity and the theocentric of the Middle Ages, now in a third period, modernity, a more anthropocentric version is initiated.

c) In modernity, the cultural and intellectual evolution of the European-occidental world appears as a spiritual movement of liberation; now occidental philosophy understands its fundamental intentions as ›philosophy of freedom and liberation‹.

This setting out towards freedom and liberty first announced itself in a new relation to nature and gained from in the modern sciences and techniques. In Antiquity and the middle ages human reason was considered as the capacity to perceive the λογοσ, the intelligible content of the sensorily given reality and to express it in rational concepts; the logical order of human reason had to correspond to the preceding order immanent in nature. In modernity, however, a new task has been attributed to human reason, the task of taking the empirical reality logically into its potency, of forming it as a disposable material according to man's subjective intentions – whether according to innate ideas, as in Descartes[8], or according to apriori forms, as in Kant[9], or according to interests of the society, as in positivism or neo-positivism[10]. Man intended to grasp reality rationally by ›logical‹ con-

---

8 Cf. R. Descartes, *Discours de la méthode pour bien conduire sa raison et chercher la verité dans les sciences*, Paris 1986; idem, *Meditationes de prima philosophia*, Hamburg 1977; further F. O. Rose, *Die Lehre von den eingeborenen Ideen bei Descartes und Locke. Ein Beitrag zur Geschichte des apriori*, Bern 1901; W. Schulz, *Die Aufhebung der Metaphysik Descartes' in den konstruktiven Systemen der Neuzeit*. In: Schulz, Der Gott der neuzeitlichen Metaphysik, Pfullingen 1957, p. 58-87; C.F. von Weizsäcker, *Descartes und die neuzeitliche Naturwissenschaft*, Hamburg 1958; W. Röd, *Descartes. Die innere Genesis des cartesianischen Systems*, München-Basel 1964; Ch. Link, *Subjektivität und Wahrheit. Die Grundlagen der neuzeitlichen Metaphysik durch Descartes*, Stuttgart 1978.

9 I. Kant, *Kritik der reinen Vernunft*, Riga 1981, 2nd ed. 1987 *(passim)*; further F. Kaulbach, *Die Dialektik von Vernunft und Natur bei Kant*. In: Wiener Jahrb. für Philos. 10 (1977) 51-72; W. Teichner, *Kants Transzendentalphilosophie. Grundriss*, Freiburg-München 1978; K. Gloy, *Das Verhältnis der ›Kritik der reinen Vernunft‹ zu den ›Metaphysischen Anfangsgründen der Naturwissenschaft‹, demonstriert am Substanzbegriff*. In: Philosophia naturalis 21 (1984) 32-53; H. Schmitz, *Was wollte Kant?* Bonn 1989.

10 Cf. H. Beck, *Der wissenschaftstheoretische Positivismus*. In: Beck, *Natürliche Theologie. Grundriß philosophischer Gotteserkenntnis*, München-Salzburg [2]1988, p. 244-262; a lot of corresponding publications you can find ibid., p. 382-392.

cepts, and to dominate it theoretically by science. In this way he could subject it also practically and dispose of it by technics. He confronted himself with nature, opposed it as a ›determined object‹ and imposed himself on it as the ›determining and free subject‹. By means of the ›objectifying of nature‹ the ›subjectifying‹ of man should be mediated; the ›constitution of nature as a determined object‹ served the ›self-constitution of man as a dominating and free subject‹.

Especially the quantifying character of the modern exact natural sciences can be understood by this tendency of reason to freedom. Because, if the concrete qualities of the object of the sensorial experience lose significance and importance for the abstracting view of the natural sciences, and only the quantitative-mathematical aspects of reality formulatable in general laws are observed, then the human spirit gains distance from concrete nature and makes itself free from it. So, the paradigm of a ›reduction of quality to quantity‹ serves as an instrument for an intellectual taking in possession of reality, as Hobbes[11] says, and thus for mediating freedom.

A similar phenomenon to that in the natural sciences, especially in physics, chemistry, and biology can be observed in the modern development of psychology, whose prototype is the so called psycho-analysis, initiated by Freud[12]. By an objectifying cognition of the unconscious psychic complexes which determine human life, and by dissolving them into their elementary functional components, man intends to subtract himself from their narrowing hindering and so to liberate himself. By means of psycho-analytical dissolution and destruction of opposite and undesired structures and by free psycho-synthetical construction of desired structures man will be the free creator of the psychic structure of his life.

In modern history of the Occident an analogous process is equally realisable in the human co-existence; it is in structuring society, in economy and in politics. Here the concept of individual rights, tolerance, and solidarity was more elaborated – work of a dividing and distancing, but also unifying and ordering λογοσ, perhaps with an accent on distancing and liberating. Furthermore, the so called ›capitalistic liberalism‹ is conceivable as an expression of an unlimited aspiration of the individual towards freedom vis-à-vis the whole society; in the subsequent phenomenon of a ›collectivistic socialism‹ there operates a will to liberation of the

11 Cf. B. Gert, *Hobbes and psychological egoism*. In: Journ. of the hist. of ideas 28 (1967) 503-520; H. Fiebig, *Erkenntnis und technische Erzeugung. Hobbes' operationale Philosophie der Wissenschaft*, Meisenheim 1973.

12 Cf. S. Freud, *Studienausgabe. Vol I-X*, Frankf./M. 1982 [Vol. I: Vorlesungen zur Einführung in die Psychoanalyse; Vol. II: Traumdeutung; Vol. III: Psychologie des Unbewussten]; spezial explications in: H. Beck/A. Rieber, *Anthropologie und Ethik der Sexualität. Zur ideologischen Auseinandersetzung um körperliche Liebe*, München-Salzburg 1982, p. 46-63; see also E. Fromm, *S. Freuds Psychoanalyse. Größe und Grenzen*, Stuttgart 1979.

lower classes or also of the whole humankind from the predominating and repressive higher classes of society.

As notable figures, who searched to interpret philosophically and to favour historically this direction of social development, primarily Kant, Hegel and Marx are to be mentioned. Kant[13] proclaimed the free and strongly transcendentally valid self-determination as that state which solely corresponds to the dignity of man as the autonomous subject of morality. Hegel[14] saw in the liberating and victorious anti-thesis of the third social class, the citizens, to the first and second class, the clerics and the nobles, as manifested in the French revolution, a progress of the ›spirit of world‹ and the ›λογοσ of being‹; this Hegelian ›λογοσ‹ with his three dialectical steps of self-realisation identifies the world-history with the trinitarian structure of the Deity in the Christian middle ages, and so he understands the social progress to more freedom as a step of an absolute divine logic. Marx[15] saw – in a dialectical continuation of Hegel – in the desired victory of the fourth society-class, the proletariat of the physical labourers, in a socialistic world-revolution the last and definitive step towards freedom in the all-embracing ›equality‹ and ›fraternity‹ of the whole humankind. This progress to an always more unlimited freedom should in reality mediate itself by means of a rational analysis of the historical structures and complexes in their single causal factors – with the intention to dominate and manipulate them psycho- and sociotechnically, for instance by application of mediums of communication and propaganda, in order thus to create social structures of more humanity.

d) To sum up: What is the prevalent feature of the European-Occidental culture and mentality, as it has shown itself in its self-explication in the course of history? It seems to be an especial relation to λογοσ, logic and rationality. In the first epoch, the more cosmocentrically thinking Greek antiquity, the λογοσ seemed included in the cosmos, as its innermost fundamental part and forming principle; and so, as human values were generated: an intellectual sensibility for cosmic or-

---

13 Cf. I. Kant, *Kritik der praktischen Vernunft*, Riga 1788 *(passim)*; idem, *Schriften zur Geschichtsphilosophie*. Ed. by M. Riedel, Stuttgart 1974.

14 Cf. G.W. Hegel, *Vorlesungen über die Philosophie der Geschichte*, Frankf./M. 1973, espec. p. 491-540; further explications in: M. Riedel, *Fortschritt und Dialektik in Hegels Geschichtsphilosophie*. In: Neue Rundschau 80 (1969) 476-491; E. Coreth, *Die Geschichte als Vermittlung bei Hegel*. In: Philosoph. Jahrb. 78 (1971) 98-110; D. Brauer, *Dialektik der Zeit. Untersuchungen zu Hegels Metaphysik der Weltgeschichte*, Stuttgart 1982.

15 Cf. K. Marx/Fr. Engels, *Ausgewählte Werke*, Moskau 1983 [p. 26-28: Thesen zu Feuerbach; p. 29-63: Manifest der Kommunistischen Partei]; in other respects H. Kesting, *Zur Geschichtsphilosophie von Karl Marx*. In: Archiv für Rechts- und Sozialphilos. 43 (1957) 545-554; L. Kolakowski, *Marx' anti-utopische Utopie*. In: Merkur 28 (1974) 616-627.

der and harmony, and its representation, imitation, and continuation both in the theoretical rational consciousness and in the practial, ethical, and external culture. In the second period, the more theocentrically oriented Christian middle ages, the λογοσ transcended the world and faced it as the word of the all-mighty divine creator, who has even spoken it into his creation up to its personal incarnation Jesus Christ; by association with Him and participation in Him, the possibility was offered to mankind to in-sist and engage in the world from the basis of its absolute and free divine fundament, and so, new values-dimensions were opened such as free personal partnership on the basis of an unsubstitutable God-representation of human person and responsibility. In the third and ultimate era, modernity, with its anthropocentric turn and orientation, the λογοσ is appropriated from its divine transcendence and in a certain way identified with human rationality and human history. In modernity the Occidental spirit conceives itself in evolution and realisation in the tendency towards freedom, exceeding and transcending every status that it already has reached and rejecting it again: gaining distance from it theoretically by means of ›acts of a rational objectification‹, and dominating it practically by ›real acts of techniques‹; so this spirit searches for its progress towards a greater freedom in all regions of physical nature and the psychic structure of the individual and the society.

It may occur that in the differentiation and cooperation of the geographically and culturally distinct sectors of Europe this process is accentuated differently. In the northern part, it is the Anglo-Saxon culture which also has expanded to North-America, a more abstract logico-analytical theory of science and the search for an economic appropriation of the world prevails – and in this sense here we have a progressive culture. In a certain contrast to this, in the southern part, it is the Roman culture which also is extended to South- and Latin-America, a concrete intuitive and esthetical access to the λογοσ is prevalent, as seen in a typical development of arts and religion – and in this sense here the expressive dimension of culture is accentuated[16]. Situated in the centre of Europe, Germany participates in both regions and therefore seems particularly called to their ideological confrontation and creative conciliation as realised in great German scientists, inventors, artists, philosophers and innovators of religions who have influenced world history. So, the cultural identity of Europe, according to the explicating and differentiating character of the λογοσ itself is not a monotonous, but a polyphonic one; it does not express uniformity, but analogy.

---

16 Cf. E. Spranger, *Lebensformen. Geisteswissenschaftliche Psychologie und Ethik der Persönlichkeit*, München-Hamburg 1965; S.T. Alisjabana, *Values as integrating forces in personality, society and culture*, Kuala Lumpur ^{2}1986; idem, *Socio-cultural creativity in the converting and restructuring process of the new emerging world*, Jakarta 1983.

2. The crisis of the European culture in modernity and overcoming it through a world cultural encounter

The peculiar ability of European spirit for λογοσ and logical structure of reality, as described above, which basically means a creative capacity for culture and a positive disposition for integral human being, especially in modern and present times seems to have been partially perverted to a negative state, and so it has thrown all humankind into a deep survival crisis. One can't deny that domination and freedom, gained by means of science and techniques, on the basis of nominalism, rationalism and positivism have led to a removal, alienation and estrangement of the theoretical consciousness from the structures of sense of reality – and consequently to a practical attitude of hybris, it is of exploitation, destruction and unlimited manipulation.

According to the early modern nominalistic philosopher Occam[17], our rational concepts have not to perceive and represent a preceding sense or immanent λογοσ of being, but to grasp the empirical reality and to bring it under the ordering intention and potency of human subjective consciousness; according to its rationalistic continuation in Kant[18] the rationally forming intentions were to be understood as expressions of the so called ›transcendental subject‹ or of the whole humankind as such; then positivism[19] substituted the strongly universal and transhistorical Kantian ›transcendental subject‹ with the multiple concrete human societies and their partial and variable interests, which now were considered to be the ultimate sense-giving instances and authorities. Hence nature was no longer comprehended as a subject of its own being and sense, but still more as an object for man, who intends nothing else but only himself as an unlimitedly free subject. Nature was regarded as a pure medium and instrument for human self-realisation; it was not apprehended and respected as ›value of sense in itself‹, but merely as ›value of use and utility for man‹. It is in the end an effect of this mentality and attitude, that we are nowadays threatened by the danger of a destruction of life through contamination of the air with poisonous emissions, by unintended secondary effects of radioactivity and through certain evolution of gene-techniques which escapes human responsibility; and further in the future it cannot be ruled out that there will be a disturbance of the cosmic equilibrium by atomic energy, which is at no time absolutely controllable. A provocation of history becomes manifest, touching the possibility of survival for mankind from its physical basis.

17 Cf. W. of Ockham, *Philosophical writings*. Ed. by Ph. Boehner, Edinburgh 1957; idem, *Texte zur Theorie der Erkenntnis und der Wissenschaft*. Ed. by R. Imbach, Stuttgart 1987.

18 See above the footnotes 9 and 13.

19 See above the footnote 10.

A similarly lugubrious view is given by modern evolution in the regions of the psychic, the social and the political. It seems that the relations of the sexes and the generations are falling more and more into neurotic forms and the economic and intercultural activities of the peoples are most heavily disturbed by lacking mutual respect and confidence. Where are reason and freedom going to?

It is evident, that occidental history of freedom manifests itself not only as a rational movement of opening, representing and confronting reality, but also partially perverts itself in sense-failing estrangement and destruction; confer in this context Sartre's[20] conception of freedom as rejection of all obligating claims of the beings, and Heidegger's[21] interpretation of the occidental ›Seinsgeschick‹ as an ›eclipse of being‹ in the line of Nietzsche's[22] prophecy of nihilism. The fall into a subjectocentric nihilism attacking the ontical fundament of the human subject and of his freedom is threatening. It is true that recently a new ethics is demanded, for instance in the realms of bio-chemical genetic manipulation and socio-economic activities; but one must ask if here an adequate conception of ›ethics‹ is commonly included: if ›ethics‹ is intended as an attitude of ›respect for the being because of itself‹ and not only another form of ›techniques‹, namely a mere techniques of survival.

So is seems concretely proved under different aspects that the peculiar capacity of European spirit to distance and objectify reality – which is the fundament of free self-determination and projecting the future, and which signifies an originally positive quality – has to a great extent become perverted to removal and estrangement from reality; occidental rationality has fallen into a rationalistic attitude, not sufficiently opened and susceptible for the voice of being; the Occidental λογοσ in its concrete habit means – if one might interpret it in a Christian perspective – a particular participation in the crucified λογοσ. What the Occidental λογοσ is missing in its actual state of alienation is the corresponding re-ference, the adequate re-obligation and re-implication to the original sense of being. Nowadays the European culture seems unilaterally more progressive by looking at the physical matter to dominate it rationally as a mere medium for economic prosperity,

20 Cf. E. Schadel, *Sartres Dialektik von Sein und Freiheit. Existentialistische Absurditätserfahrung als Konsequenz positivistischen Wirklichkeitsverständnisses.* In: Theologie und Philosophie 62 (1987) 196-215; H. Beck, *Sartre: Nihilistischer Existentialismus.* In: Beck, *Ekin-sistenz: Positionen und Transformationen der Existenzphilosophie*, Frankf./M.-Bern-New York-Paris 1989, p. 71-100.

21 Cf. M. Heidegger, *Zur Seinsfrage*, Frankf./M. 1956; idem, *Nietzsche. I-II*, Pfullingen 1961; idem, *Was ist Metaphysik?* Frankf./M. [12]1981; G. Siewerth, *Das Schicksal der Metaphysik von Thomas zu Heidegger*, Einsiedeln 1959.

22 Cf. K. Löwith. *Nietzsches Philosophie der ewigen Wiederkehr des Gleichen*, Stuttgart 1956; E. Heftrich, *Nietzsches Philosophie. Identität von Welt und Nichts*, Frankf./M. 1952; D. Arendt, *Nihilismus. Die Anfänge von Jacobi bis Nietzsche*, Köln 1970; E. Fink. *Nietzsches Philosophie*, Berlin-Köln-Mainz [3]1973.

than expressive by representing and mediating an intuitively perceived metaphysical sense in spiritual concordance and love; in short: it seems more mental and ›logical‹ than spiritual.

Therefore, as the way to a more integral and free humanity, there suggests itself a creative encounter with other cultures, which in their basic onto-anthropological disposition are accentuated more spiritually, that means with cultures of the Asiatic Orient and of Africa. And it seems, that in the ultimate and most recent development of the European modern and secular culture, in the so called »postmodernity«[23], under the influence of Asiatic and African spiritual impulses, there is opened a new sensibility for the metaphysical expressivity of the physical world, and initiated cosmic consciousness, transparent to the totality of being. But the first signs of breaking up to a New Age of mankind seem to a great extent to be rather confused, and more distinctness would be required, through a rationality which has regained its intuitive fundament and, on this basis, its metaphysical competence. Then there is hope that the abstracting and analysing rational reflection which dissects reality in its parts would be accompanied and balanced by an emotional devotion which rebinds the separated parts and acknowledges the whole. Thus the full and integral act of being in its triadic structure will be realised: in its basic first step, the initial in-sisting and reposing of the being in itself; the second step, the recognising and opening ex-sistence or outwards-movement and confrontation; and the third and ultimate step, the re-specting and loving inwards-movement and re-insistence, by which the being expressively accepts itself and the others and perfects its unity and identity.

A creative encounter of the modern secular world civilisation which mainly originated in Europe, and traditional Asiatic and African cultures, forced and favorized by the present survival-provocation of Being of all humankind, could initiate in the scientific technological civilisation a critical self-consciousness: both of the positive human values, elaborated in the history of European culture since antiquity and middle ages as we have described it, and of its own unilateralities, limits and deficits. Out of this could arise a practical impulse to actualise and develop the positive qualities and to accept and gradually overcome the negative ones – in mutual dialog and completion. Motivation and inspiration for change and evolution of habits come from the experience that we can complete one another and so reach our own fuller identity. Perhaps the present sufferings of man-

23 Cf. J.F. Lyotard. *Grundlagenkrise*. In: Neue Hefte für Philos. 26 (1986) 1-33; R.G. Renner, *Die postmoderne Konstellation. Theorie, Text und Kunst im Ausgang der Moderne*, Freiburg 1988; W. Welsch (ed.), *Wege aus der Moderne. Schlüsseltexte der Postmoderne-Diskussion*, Weinheim 1988; idem, *Unsere postmoderne Moderne*, ibid. [3]1991; J. Roberts, *Postmodernism, Politics and Art*, Manchester 1990; G. Vattimo, *Das Ende der Moderne*, Stuttgart 1990.

kind are to be understood as the pains on the way to an essentially new kind of human being, expressing more integration, humanity and freedom.

Concluding Remark

Cf. the further elaboration of these perspectives in: Heinrich Beck, Gisela Schmirber (ed.), *Creative Peace through Encounter of World Cultures* (Germ.: Frankf./M, Berlin, Bern, New York, Paris, Wien 1995; Engl.: Delhi 1996; Span.: Maracaibo 1996, Chin.: Peking 1998), and there esp. the contribution of H. Beck, *World peace as dynamic unity of cultural contrarieties. The onto-hermeneutic basis for an understanding of the structure of the culture of mankind as a perspective for a dialectic-triadic conception of reality*, and the contribution of Fritz Wallner, *Intercultural identity in relation to variability and its possible contribution to peace*. – In reference to the discussion of the author's with Fritz Wallner's point of view cf. Heinrich Beck, *Metaphysische Implikationen im Konstruktiven Realismus*, in: F. Wallner, B. Agnese (ed.), *Konstruktion und Verfremdung. Von der Wirklichkeit zur Realität*, Wien 1999.

Martin J. Jandl

The Non-Intellectual View of Language in the Works of Humboldt and Wittgenstein: Language as Speaking

1. De-transcendentalising and the intellectual view of language

I understand philosophy of language as a kind of philosophical reflection that focuses on language structuring traditional issues of philosophy newly from this viewpoint. Like any dating, it is difficult to date the ›linguistic turn‹, but it takes place when ›speaking‹ is no longer conceived as the mere expression of universal thoughts, and reasoning is no longer the mere grasping of natural facts to be scientifically formulated in words, numbers, or symbols, but when reasoning and speaking is conceived as a process of linguistic understanding between the reasoning of two or more individuals (see Borsche 1996, p.11). In this conception philosophy of language there is another conception of reasoning and being, of truth and knowledge that are not longer situated in the modern difference of subject and object, but that are now situated in the tension field of different subjects who are formed in this process as reasonable individuals, and out of this field of intersubjective tension emerges what is philosophically called ›world‹. Focusing on language means to abolish the conception of world as a sum of objects presupposed and founding the process of knowledge; it means to emphasise intersubjective processes creating ›our‹ world. Thus it is tempting to date the linguistic turn on September of 1800 because of a line written by Wilhelm Humboldt to Friedrich Schiller: »Language is [...] the means by which humans form simultaneously themselves and the world, or rather by which humans become conscious that they cut off a world from themselves. [*Die Sprache ist daher, wenn nicht überhaupt, doch wenigstens sinnlich das Mittel, durch welches der Mensch zugleich sich selbst und die Welt bildet, oder vielmehr seiner dadurch bewußt wird, daß er eine Welt von sich abschneidet.*]« (Humboldt 1981b, p.196)

When Habermas (1999b, p.186) states that the most interesting movements of philosophy in the last two centuries are the endeavours to de-transcendentalise the recognising subject bringing Kant's transcendental subject back into lifeworld contexts and situating reason that runs through these lifeworld contexts in social space and within historical time; and when Habermas names as the most important protagonists of this movement of de-transcendentalisation Humboldt, Peirce, Dilthey, Cassirer, Heidegger and Wittgenstein who all in their special way conceive language, practice or life form as symbolic medium of reason, then it becomes obvious that the linguistic turn is a turn away from transcendental philosophy.

However, Habermas' point of view is controversial. Rorty (1987, pp.283) scents in philosophy of language the continuation of Kant's project of philosophy of knowledge applying different means. He assumes the source of philosophy of language as a kind of philosophy of knowledge that tries to uphold Kant's picture of philosophy as a discipline that provides scientific research with an unhistorical system of concepts. Rorty (1987, pp.284ff) names for instance Russell, Carnap and Lewis who conceives beside receptivity of sensuality and instead of spontaneity of reason the subjective contribution to the object constitution in form of meaning of its parts. But, sure, Rorty's philosophy is based on a kind of philosophy of language that situates on the place of the transcendental subject a linguistic composed reasoning.

To understand the difference between Habermas' and Rorty's view, Rorty's suspicion and the de-transcendentalising push of philosophy of language I suggest a further terminological distinction that differentiates not only between transcendental and non-transcendental philosophy, but that differentiates one more time the de-transcendentalisation that emerges philosophy of language. This terminological differentiation was introduced by Sybille Krämer (2001) who distinguishes philosophy of language (in the 20th century – what is not the point in issue here) in ›intellectual‹ and ›non-intellectual‹ philosophy of language. In this chapter I will focus on the intellectual philosophy of language, and in the following chapters I will sketch out the features of the non-intellectual philosophy of language by discussing briefly Humboldt's and Wittgenstein's view of language.

Krämer (2001, p.95) names as protagonists of an intellectual understanding of language Saussure, Chomsky, Searle, and Habermas. Saussure and Chomsky focus on the structure dimension of language dealing with the question ›What is language?‹. Words or sentences are structures (Saussure does not use the term ›structure‹, as far as I see) composed of linguistic tokens that are identifiable and analysable independently of the concrete context of application. In the works of Searle and Habermas the pragmatic dimension of language is in the foreground dealing with the question ›What for do we use language?‹. In the pragmatic dimension utterances as a communicative action come to the fore of reflection that is specifyable only in relation to the speaker's intention and within communicative contexts. Beside the contrasts of structure orientated and pragmatic orientated positions with subject concerned contrasts there are shared presuppositions. The core of these presuppositions is the two-worlds-model of language, or a two-worlds-ontology (see Krämer 2001, p.95).

A characteristic feature of the intellectual view of language is, firstly, the separation of language in two regions – the region of pure language or communication and the region of every-time speaking. According to this view language disposes of an element that founds unity and closure in form of grammatical, semantic or pragmatic rules and by its application, actualisation and concretisation speaking emerges. Language and speaking are related like pattern and its realisation, like type and its instantiation in space and time. Thus language and speaking belong to different ontological registers (see Krämer 2001, p.96). Not this distinction as such is crucial but – and this is the second characteristic feature of the intellectual view of language – its conception as hierarchy. Saussure differentiates between ›langue‹ and ›parole‹ what he grasps as a difference of system and execution or between substance and accidence. Chomsky introduces the difference between ›competence‹ and ›performance‹ or ›i-language‹ (›internalised language‹) and ›e-language‹ (›externalised language‹) what he interprets as language and its epi-phenomenon. Searle and Habermas formulate the same understanding on the side of linguistic pragmatics: The propositional-performative double structure of speech act, the typology of speech acts that comprises a specified set of speech act classes (completed by Habermas' typology of validity claims) lead to a system of pragmatic universals, and every event of speaking is only analysable as a actualisation of this system to count as speaking filling its purpose of communication (see Krämer 2001, p.96). Thus the two-worlds-ontology and the logic-genealogic priority of language in relation to speaking are the characteristic features of the logos-orientated or intellectual view of language.

The intellectual view of language influenced philosophy strongly. It made language autonomous, and its autonomy leads to de-transcendentalisation. Language is no longer defined as a representation means of the not linguistically given and its privileged purpose as representation of thoughts is abolished. And this is the feat of the two-worlds-model of language. The new autarky of language is not only guilty in the scope of thoughts, but in all scopes. To quote Krämer in original: »*In dem bis in die Moderne hinein wirksamen repräsentationalen Sprachkonzept, mit seiner Referenztheorie der Bedeutung und seiner Auszeichnung des Behauptungssatzes, gilt die Sprache als Abbild, Medium oder Organ einer der Sprache selbst vorgängigen Ordnung, die bevorzugt interpretiert wird als eine Ordnung des Denkens. Eine Leistung des Zwei-Welten-Modells besteht darin, diesem repräsentationalen Sprachkonzept die Nachfolge aufzukündigen, insofern Form, Ordnung, System und Regel durch Sprache nicht bloß zur Darstellung kommen, sondern jetzt in der Sprache selbst lokalisiert werden und durch sie auch alleine begründbar sind. Die Sprache wird zur Springquelle von Form, Systematizität und Regel, und das macht sie autonom; die Sprache stellt Strukturen nicht dar, sondern wird selbst zur strukturgebenden Instanz.*« (Krämer 2001, p.97)

The intellectual view of language pushes pure reason from its pedestal, but it maintains transcendental-philosophical argumentation patterns. The intellectual view of language detaches language from its solitary function to represent the inner world of thoughts, but it establishes a relation within language that is analogous to the relation of language and reason (see Krämer 2001, p.97). And this is the relation between language and speaking as the hierarchical relation between pure language and every time speaking. If language is conceived as a higher scope that is separated from every time speaking and so takes the place of pure reason,

Rorty's suspicion is justified that philosophy of language is the continuation of transcendental philosophy with different means – even though that the very fact of philosophy of language is equal with de-transcendentalisation.

Further, Krämer analyses that there is an intellectual fallacy in the intellectual view of language. Krämer emphasises that this fallacy is not a mistake or a flaw in reasoning confessing that she appreciates the intellectual force of authors like Habermas or Chomsky. The intellectual fallacy is not a simple confusion of model and reality. It is true that Taylor (1995) diagnoses exactly this intellectual confusion of model and reality in philosophy of language, but against this diagnosis Krämer states: »When Chomsky conceives natural languages just not as languages in the sense of a universal grammar, and when Habermas accepts by his distinction of communication and discourse that actual communication just doesn't takes place like an ideal speaking situation, then the intellectual strategy is more subtle than the simple confusion of ideal and reality suggests. [*Wenn Chomsky die natürlichen Sprachen gerade nicht als Sprachen im Sinne einer Universalgrammatik versteht und wenn Habermas durch seine Unterscheidung von Kommunikation und Diskurs anerkennt, daß wirkliche Kommunikation nicht wie eine ideale Sprechsituation sich vollzieht, dann ist die intellektualistische Strategie subtiler, als es die bloße Verwechslung von Ideal und Realität nahelegt.*]« (Krämer 2001, p.104) It is due to the two-worlds-ontology to overcome this confusion. And thus the problem is not the two-worlds-ontology itself, but the additional postulate of a logical-genealogical priority of the language level to the speaking level. This gets a metamorphosis of every time speaking going and mutates it to a representation of language or communication respectively. »The intellectual fallacy is not to coin a concept or a model of language and to provide this noumenal creation with the index of reality and finally to consider the every time speaking as the reality of pure language. There is no simple mix up of model and reality, but rather reality is transformed in a representation of the model to the disadvantage of reality. The fallacy is to view the reality of speaking as if it were a representation, or more pointedly: a instantiation of language. With it the border of language/non-language is imported in speaking. Then it is a characteristic feature of speaking vis-à-vis of language to mingle linguistic and extra-linguistic components. Because of this mixture speaking is vis-à-vis of language incomplete, deficient, and distorted; it is less form than deformation. And it is thus the task of theory to employ the concept of language as an instrument to purify speaking. [*Der ›intellektualistische Fehlschluß‹ besteht also nicht darin, einen Begriff oder ein Modell von Sprache zu bilden, dieses ›noumenale Gebilde‹ dann mit einem Realitätsindex zu versehen und schließlich das jedesmalige Sprechen für die Wirklichkeit der reinen Sprache selbst zu halten. Es wird nicht einfach Modell und Wirklichkeit verwechselt, vielmehr wird die Wirklichkeit verwandelt in eine Repräsentation des Modells, was stets zuungunsten der Wirklichkeit ausfallen wird. Der Fehlschluß besteht also darin, daß die Wirklichkeit des Sprechens so angesehen wird, als ob sie Repräsentation, genauer: eine Instantiierung der Sprache sei. Damit wird in das Sprechen selbst die Grenze zwischen Sprache/Nicht-Sprache eingeführt: Es ist dann die Eigenart des Sprechens gegenüber ›der‹ Sprache, Sprachliches und Außersprachliches zu vermischen. Kraft dieser Mixtur ist das Sprechen gegenüber der reinen Sprache prinzipiell etwas Unvollständiges, Mangelhaftes, Defizitäres, Verzerrtes: weniger Form denn Deformation. Und es ist die Aufgabe der Theorie, den Begriff der Sprache zum Instrument einer Purifizierung auf der Seite des Sprechens einzusetzen.*]« (Krämer 2001, p.105)

The non-intellectual view of language doesn't make the difference between a language level and a speaking level. There is no attempt to purify language from extralinguistic components. The contrary is the case. I will demonstrate the non-intellectual view of language by discussing Humboldt and Wittgenstein.

2. Notes on Humboldt's linguistic-sensual world constitution

Wilhelm von Humboldt (1767-1835) is a political man who travelled around the whole globe (sometimes together with his famous brother Alexander), and his philosophy reflects the variety manifested in different human worlds he became acquainted with. Humboldt's philosophy is an anthropological reflection that fathoms the forms in which the human mind unfolds itself. In this anthropological reflection language is not one matter beside others, but Humboldt declares language as the core matter of his philosophy. According to Humboldt, language is the form of human mind (see Cesare 1996, p.278). Reason and being get their place from the viewpoint of language because they are constituted by language. Sure, Humboldt's work is voluminous, thus I restrict my lecture to his writing on philosophy of language, especially to *Über die Verschiedenheit des menschlichen Sprachbaues (About the Difference of Human Language Construction)*.

Humboldt refuses to conceive language as a mere means of communication because of an instrumentalistic misunderstanding of language: »To conceive language as an instrument means on the one hand to reduce it to a set of conventional signs without any force to form the world, to reduce it to signs that humans use to refer to a given world more or less exactly; and it means on the other hand to understand language as something that is not in its core human, to conceive it as an aid humans apply to cope with an external need, the need of communication. [*Die Sprache als Instrument zu betrachten, bedeutet auf der einen Seite, daß man sie auf eine Menge konventioneller Zeichen ohne jede weltgestaltende Kraft reduziert, Zeichen, mittels deren der Mensch mehr oder weniger genau auf eine vorgegebene Welt verweist, und auf der anderen Seite, daß man sie sich als etwas dem Menschen Äußerliches denkt, ein Hilfsmittel, das einem äußeren Bedürfnis abhelfen soll, dem Bedürfnis nach sozialer Kommunikation.*]« (Cesare 1996, p.278)

Hence Humboldt employs the metaphor of organ understood in the Kantian sense as a part of a living organism. Language as an ›inner organ‹ of humans is to attribute originally and naturally to humans; language arises from an inner ›instinct‹ of humans and it is not possible to explain that fact further. According to Humboldt humans are natural beings that are originally united with the world within human live. It is the act of reflection that bursts open this unity, and in this act of reflection humans determine themselves as subjects and things of the world as objects simultaneously. Hence language becomes what – to quote the letter to Schiller once more – »the means by which humans form simultaneously themselves and the world, or rather by which humans become conscious that they cut off a world from themselves.« (Humboldt 1981b, p.196) Humans are humans only through language and humans conceive the world as world only if it is constituted linguistically (see Cesare 1996, p.279).

Humboldt is a romantic philosopher, and thus it is necessary to remember his famous words formulating the emergence of language: »The touch of world and man is the electric shock which bursts language, but not only in its emergence, but permanently as long as humans will think and speak. The manifold of the world and the depth of the soul are the sources out of which language scoops. [*Die Berührung der Welt mit dem Menschen ist der elektrische Schlag, aus welchem die Sprache hervorspringt, nicht bloss in ihrem Entstehen, sondern immerfort, so wie Menschen denken und reden. Die Mannigfaltigkeit der Welt und die Tiefe der menschlichen Brust sind die beiden Punkte, aus welchen die Sprache schöpft.*]« (Humboldt 1981a, p.252) Humboldt's philosophy is a linguistic foundation of knowledge. Without words there are no concepts and furthermore no objects because objects obtain objective determination only conceptually. Thus Humboldt conceives the way out of dullness in which subject and object are not separated up to knowledge in two steps, and language as the organ of the mind is constitutive for both of them – first in its cognitive function and then in its communicative function, to formulate Humboldt's two steps in the words of Habermas (1999a).

To sketch Humboldt's first step, we can start with Humboldt's idea that language is the forming organ of thoughts and that intellectual activity and language are an inseparable unity; it isn't even possible to view the first one as the producing and the second one as the product: »*Die intellectuelle Thätigkeit und die Sprache sind daher Eins und unzertrennlich voneinander; man kann nicht einmal schlechthin die erstere als das Erzeugende, die andre als das Erzeugte ansehen.*« (Humboldt 1981a, p.191) Like Kant who conceives mind and sensuality as equally original (›*gleichursprünglich*‹) in their object constituting synthesis, Humboldt doesn't view the fixing of the idea (›Vorstellung‹) by sound (or more exactly: by word) as additional or as something that follows the emergence of ideas (›Vorstellungen‹). The fixing of ideas (›Vorstellungen‹) is only possible by sound and hence both are equally original – according to Humboldt notions (›Vorstellungen‹) find their primary objective form as concepts in the interplay of intellectual activity and linguistic sensuality. Humboldt gives up the Kantian concept of sensuality that is focused on time and space in favour of the sensuality of sound. In Humboldt's philosophy the primacy of the eye is abolished. »The essence of reasoning is to reflect, that means to distinguish the thinking person and the thought. To reflect the mind must stand still in his progressive activity for a moment and combine the just thought in a unit confronting this newly formed unit as an object to itself. [...] The essence of reasoning is to make sections in its own course; by it to form whole units using portion of its activity; and to confront these formations individually each one with the others and in sum as objects to itself as the recognising subject. Even pure reasoning can't happen without the universal form of our sensuality because with it we can conceive and grip it. [...] Thus language starts immediately and simultaneously with the first act of reflection, and when human awakes from the dullness of desire (›Begierde‹) in which the subject devours the object to self-consciousness there is the word – the first impulse that gives human to himself to stand still, to look around and to orient. [*Das Wesen des Denkens besteht im Reflectiren, d.h. im Unterscheiden des Denkenden von dem Gedachten. Um zu reflectiren, muss der Geist in seiner fortschreitenden Thätigkeit einen Augenblick still stehn, das eben Vorgestellte in eine Einheit fassen, und auf diese Weise, als Gegenstand, sich selbst entgegenstellen. [...] Das Wesen des Denkens besteht also darin Abschnitte in seinem eignen Gange zu machen; dadurch aus gewissen Portionen seiner Thätigkeit Ganze zu bilden; und diese Bildungen einzeln sich selbst unter einander, alle zusammen aber, als Objecte, dem denkenden Subjecte entgegenzusetzen. Kein Denken, auch das reinste nicht, kann anders, als mit Hülfe der allgemeinen Form unsrer Sinnlichkeit geschehen; nur in ihnen können wir es auffassen und gleichsam festhalten. [...] Die Sprache beginnt daher unmittelbar und sogleich mit dem ersten Act der Reflexion, und so wie der Mensch aus der Dumpfheit der Begierde, in welcher das Subject das Object verschlingt, zum Selbstbewusstseyn erwacht, so ist auch das Wort da – gleichsam der erste Anstoss, den sich der Mensch selbst giebt, plötzlich still zu stehen, sich umzusehen und zu orientiren.*]« (Humboldt 1981c, S.97f) The sound fixes the idea (›Vorstellung‹) and contrasts it with the intellectual activity that creates it. Without the sound, without a sensual husk the idea wouldn't find a place in the intelligible subject, but it would disappear without a trace (see Cesare 1996, p.280). Humboldt keeps the old, but famous insight of theory of knowledge that there is not knowledge without differentiation by the sensual activity of linguistic articulation. »*Das Denken ist eine geistige Handlung, wird aber durch sein Bedürfnis nach Sprache ein Antrieb zu einer körperlichen.*« (Humboldt 1981a, p.195)

To summarise the first step of the linguistic world constitution according to Humboldt: To become a concept the idea (›Vorstellung‹) must become an object to the subject who is the instance of the idea forming intellectual activity, and this process of objectification is linguistic in nature. In the sensual form of the word the idea (›Vorstellung‹) obtains its objective existence. At this point the second step sets in that Habermas names the communicative step (the first step is the cognitive one). In Humboldt's work the communicative function of language is inseparably interwoven with the cognitive function. If the idea (›Vorstellung‹) is fixed by linguistic sensualisation and is contrasted as object to the subject (that means the idea is externalised), the concept won't be achieved. According to Humboldt concepts are not the result of a mere subjective process. Hence Humboldt walks not one inch on the Kantian way of philosophising claiming that all subjects constitute the same objects because of the same transcendental equipment and by it reach a unified world view without intersubjective communication. Rather the process of objectification and of concept formation is accomplished when the ›I‹ perceives its own ideas (›Vorstellungen‹) objectified out of itself. And that is only possible in another imagining and reasoning human being.

Without this second step banking on the communicative function of language and letting the cognitive function taking effect, the idea connected with the word (that's exactly the result of the first step) would be nothing more than a dream vision or a mere appearance. According to Humboldt speaking is a necessary condition for reasoning of a single person even in total seclusion. Humans understand themselves only if they try whether other persons understand their words. These definitions literally quoted: »*Ohne daher irgend auf die Mittheilung zwischen Menschen und Menschen zu sehn, ist das Sprechen ein nothwendige Bedingung des Denkens des Einzelnen in abgeschlossener Einsamkeit. In der Erscheinung entwickelt sich jedoch die Sprache nur gesellschaftlich, und der Mensch versteht sich selbst nur, indem er die Verstehbarkeit seiner Worte an Andren versuchend geprüft hat.*« (Humboldt 1981a, S.196) Thus it is obvious when Humboldt states: »The concept gets its determination and clarity only by radiating back from another force of reason. [*Der Begriff erreicht seine Bestimmtheit und Klarheit erst durch das Zurückstrahlen aus einer fremden Denkkraft. Er wird [...] erzeugt, indem er sich aus der bewegten Masse des Vorstellens losreisst, und dem Subject gegenüber zum Object wird. Es genügt jedoch nicht, dass diese Spaltung in dem Subjecte allein vorgeht, die Objectivität ist erst vollendet, wenn der Vorstellende den Gedanken wirklich ausser sich erblickt, was nur in einem andren, gleich ihm vorstellenden und denkenden Wesen möglich ist. Zwischen Denkkraft und Denkkraft aber ist die einzige Vermittlerin die Sprache, und so entsteht auch hier ihre Nothwendigkeit zur Vollendung des Gedankens.*]« (Humboldt 1981a, S.201) And that is the reason why language is necessary requirement for the first creation of thoughts and for the ongoing education of the human mind: »*So ist die Sprache ein nothwendiges Erforderniss zur ersten Erzeugung des Gedanken, und zur fortschreitenden Ausbildung des Geistes.*« (Humboldt 1981a, S.217)

The dialogue between I and You takes place in a perspective opened by language, in a linguistically formed world. The nature of language admits that the world is a world in between (›Zwischenwelt‹), that means that objectivity of concepts never will take the value of something absolute firm or something of universal and invariable validity (see Cesare 1996, p.283). In addition every actually spoken word sounds and requires the whole language (see Humboldt GS IV, p.15). »In general it is the nature of language to be glued to all given, bodily, singular and contingent things and to transport them to an idealistic, mental, universal and necessary region giving to them a form that reminds of its origin. [*Es ist überhaupt die Natur der Sprache, sich an alles Vorhandene, Körperliche, Einzelne, Zufällige zu heften, aber dasselbe in ein idealistisches, geistiges, allgemeines, nothwendiges Gebiet hinüberzuspielen, und ihm darin eine an seinen Ursprung erinnernde Gestaltung zu leihen.*]« (Humboldt 1981a, S.158)

The synthetic activity of the imagination (›Einbildungskraft‹) transforms the masses of singular and separated appearances into an inseparated unity and an organised whole (see GS II; pp.128ff) by grasping the inner coherence that connects one object with the other and with the whole – by analogy (see GS III, p.295). The totality of the analogies grasped of the appearance's reality (›Erscheinungswirklichkeit‹) leads to a world view. In his later works Humboldt replaces the term ›analogy‹ by the term ›form‹ to explain the dynamic feature of language. According to Humboldt the formal striving of language is form giving. This formal striving of language is realised differently in different languages, and language as a forming activity follows a form – the form of a historic language. Humboldt compares the form of the language with a path that the activity must follow to work. What Humboldt calls form of language is the way a language realises its individual striving for form or the individual urge by which a nation enforces thought and feeling – »*die Form der Sprache ist der durchaus individuelle Drang, vermittels dessen eine Nation dem Gedanken und der Empfindung Geltung in der Sprache verschafft*« (GS VII, p.47). To follow a path means in this context: to form according to special principles. Language is both the form principle and the result of this principle. Or, in other words, language has a form and is a form (see Cesare 1996, p.284).

From this determination of language rises immediately as a consequence: »The human being doesn't speak, because he wants to speak in this way, but because he must speak in this way. *[Der Mensch spricht nicht, weil er so sprechen will, sondern weil er so sprechen muss.*] (Humboldt 1981a, p.162) That language forms the human thought also means: »The human being is not born as a pure intellectual being who vests completed thoughts with sounds, but as a sounding creature out of whose sound emerges all great, pure and intellectual according to a wonderful nature. [*Der Mensch kommt nicht nach Art eines reinen Geistes in die Welt, der den fertigen Gedanken nur mit Tönen umkleidet, sondern als ein tönendes Erdengeschöpf, aus dessen Tönen sich aber, nach ihrer wundervollen Natur, durch ein in ihrem scheinbar zufälligen Gewirr ruhendes System alles Grosse, Reine und Geistige entwickelt.*]« (Humboldt 1981a, p.154) Humboldt (1981a, p.163) emphasises that it is necessary to distinguish the dead form of language that is represented in the sum of existing words and systems of analogies from the language that is living in the reasoning, feeling and acting human. The dynamic of language also opens possibilities of going beyond the fixed forms by the creative act of speaking. The possible change of form makes the dynamic relation between a special historic language form and the single speech acts clear (see Cesare 1996, p.284). This dynamic reflects the tension of universality and individuality, and Humboldt pleads for the creative force of the individual.

Now the non-intellectual view of language in Humboldt's work is emerging. It becomes even more obvious if we consider that there is no empty phrase for the dynamic feature of language – what Cesare (1996, p.284) calls a characteristic feature of Humboldt's work. There is one exception, and that's Humboldt's definition of language as ›*ενεργεια*‹ in contrast to ›*εργον*‹: »*Die Sprache, in ihrem wirklichen Wesen aufgefasst, ist etwas beständig und in jedem Augenblicke Vorübergehendes. [...] Sie selbst ist kein Werk (*εργον*), sondern eine Tätigkeit (*ενεργεια*). Ihre wahre Definition kann daher nur eine genetische seyn.*« (GS VII, p.45f) In this definition Humboldt tries to conceive the true essence of language that is recognisable at the transition between language to speaking. According to Cesare (1996, p.285) it is inevitable that Humboldt's attempt to define language leads to the definition of every time speaking. Thus the concept of ενεργεια initiates a view of language as an active process of producing and as a development; it also stresses the priority of the act in favour of the potency what is an expression of superiority. Hence the individual linguistically creative activity that arises from speech possibly modifies the manner of linguistic procedure. And therefore founds speech language and not conversely. »Language produces itself out of speaking. [*Aus dem Sprechen erzeugt sich die Sprache.*]« (GS VI, p.180) Pointedly formulated, Humboldt is an exponent of the non-intellectual view of language.

So that Humbodt rejects the monologue model of knowledge claiming that the relatedness of subject to object is crucial. Humboldt replaces this monologue model of knowledge by a dialogue model of knowledge claiming that the relatedness of subject to subject founds object constitution and thus knowledge. By intervening in its dialogue form and in its institutionalised form language mediates between human and world, and the more the concepts of subject and object must be defined differently. Humboldt's ›I‹ is not Fichte's absolute ›I‹ that is confronted with the ›non-I‹, but a concrete historical individual who unfolds himself/herself in the dialogue with the ›You‹. In this dialogue the objectifying estrangement of the subject takes place by which the matter of appearances is formed and simultaneously the internalisation of the objective world by the subject is initialised. This process is linguistic and thus can only happen within language between subjects. Thus the linguistic process is not only the subject-object relation constituting *ποιεσισ*, but more and mainly a *πραξισ* realised between subject and subject (see Cesare 1996, p.281).

Humboldt transfers knowledge from the intelligible transcendental subject to the concrete human by language, or more exactly: by every time speaking. He notes: »Language belongs to humans and has not other source than his essence [...]. But if language identifies with humans in this way, then it will do so not only with humans in a general and metaphysical sense, but with the actually existing and living human who is constituted by the manifold of local and historical circumstances [...]. By this language becomes an external force for the single human and for a single nation, but always in a way that even the strangest sound announces an inner kinship. [*Die Sprache gehört aber dem Menschen selbst an, sie hat und kennt keine andere Quelle, als sein Wesen, wenn man sagt, dass sie auf ihn wirkt, sagt man nur, dass er sich in ihr nach und nach in immer steigendem Umfang und immer wechselnder Mannigfaltigkeit bewusst wird. Wenn sich aber die Sprache so mit dem Menschen identificirt, so thut sie dies nicht bloss mit dem Menschen, allgemein und metaphysisch gedacht, sondern mit dem wirklich vorhandenen, lebendigen, durch alle die vielfachen örtlichen und geschichtlichen Verhältnisse der Irdischheit enge bedingten, nicht mit dem einzelnen, nicht mit der Nation allein, zu der er sich rechnet, nicht mit der jedesmaligen Generation, sondern mit allen Völkern und allen gewesenen Geschlechtern, die, wie fern und mittelbar die Verknüpfungen gewesen seyn mögen, mit ihm in Sprachberührung gestanden haben. Dadurch wird die Sprache dem einzelnen Menschen und der einzelnen Nation auch zu einer äusserlichen Macht, aber so, dass auch aus dem fremdesten Laut ihm innige Verwandtschaft entgegenklingt.*]« (Humboldt 1981a, S.155)

3. Wittgenstein's theory of language games: De-discoursifying of language

Referring to Humboldt's philosophy I argued that language as a sensual activity governs human reasoning as the means of differentiation within the intellectual activity. Furthermore Humboldt formulates with his definition of language as *ενεργεια* a view of language that Krämer calls non-intellectual that refuses the primacy of language in favour of every time speaking. Sure, this thought traces back to the romantic idea that the universal form moulds the individual matter. Nevertheless it is striking that Humboldt pleads for a non-intellectual view of language that refuses the common distinction of the λογοσ.

Let's make a jump of 130 years to the theory of language games formulated by Ludwig Wittgenstein in the famous *Philosophical Investigations*. Following Krämer (2001, p.115) it is necessary to emphasise that understanding Wittgenstein's view of language requires to grasp the deep and fundamental difference between his conception of linguistic activity and the linguistic-pragmatic conception of language. We get on to this difference if we ask why Wittgenstein's language game may not be identified with speech acts. The difference between language games and speech acts is rooted in the latent iconicity that is a characteristic feature of Wittgenstein's language games and so in a kind of de-discoursifying or (in German) ›*Entdiskursivierung*‹ (see Krämer 2001, p.115). ›Language game‹ or (again in German) ›Sprachspiel‹ is the core concept in Wittgenstein's philosophy.

Wittgenstein does not relate language game to the essence of language. Language game doesn't aim at the final units that are not further analysable and that found the manifold of linguistic events as the universal order. Rather ›language game‹ is not a clearly outlined notion that is relevant for a theory of meaning because Wittgenstein doesn't try to explain how language works. In Wittgenstein's work we shouldn't expect to find a comprehensive theory of language (see Majetschak 1996, p.366), and that becomes obvious especially when this seems to be the case: when Wittgenstein defines the meaning of meaning. This famous definition reads: »The usage of a word in a language is its meaning. [*Der Gebrauch des Wortes in der Sprache ist seine Bedeutung*.] (Wittgenstein 1989a, p.262/§43; also see Wittgenstein 1989b, p.20f). But Wittgenstein shows proof that there is no homogeneous phenomenon of meaning that would be the subject matter of a semantic theory. Even though many interpretations of this usage-as-meaning-theory claim that Wittgenstein formulates a new theory on this issue, Wittgenstein rather discharges definitively every kind of meaning theory by explaining how the term ›meaning‹ itself used in a wide variety of usages in natural language is used normally (see Majetschak 1996, p.378).

Mindful of Wittgenstein's differentiation of ›celebration of language‹ and ›work of language‹, ›language game‹ belongs to the work mode of language if it is not an absurdity emerging when language runs dry. This absurdity is avoided when ›language game‹ is not conceived as a means of explanation, but rather as a means of language description. Thus ›language game‹ is a means of description to achieve survey, ›*ein Übersicht schaffendes Mittel der Darstellung*‹ (see Wittgenstein 1989a, p.304/§130). Language game is thus a scale: Language is not a language game, but we compare language with language games. And as a result we don't order language by this comparison, but our knowledge of language (see Krämer 2001, p.117). The category of language game has an epistemic function -- language game is a medium of description, not the described matter itself. To construct a language game is just a linguistic phenomenon (see Krämer 2001, p.117).

But what is the interesting feature of games so that Wittgenstein assesses them like no other phenomenon as an analogy of language? The answer maybe the manifold of games that is repugnant to the philosophical striving for universality. In the *Blue Book* Wittgenstein notes that we are inclined to suppose that there must be a common feature of all games justifying the application of universal term ›game‹ in respect to all games. But games establish a family, and the members of this family share common features. »We see a complex net of similarities that spread over and cross. [...] Like these similar features of a family spread over and cross: growth, features, colour of eyes, pace, temperament etc., etc. – And I will say: Games establish a family. And like this, for example, the different kinds of numbers establish a family. [*Wir sehen ein kompliziertes Netz von Ähnlichkeiten, die einander übergreifen und kreuzen. Ähnlichkeiten im Großen und Kleinen. [...] so übergreifen und kreuzen sich die verschiedenen Ähnlichkeiten, die zwischen den Gliedern einer Familie bestehen: Wuchs, Gesichtszüge, Augenfarbe, Gang, Temperament, etc., etc. – Und ich werde sagen: Spiele bilden eine Familie. Und ebenso bilden z.B. die Zahlenarten eine Familie.*]« (Wittgenstein 1989a, S.278/§66f) To speak about family similarities is a philosophical renunciation (see Wittgenstein 1989b, p.37ff). It is the renunciation of the assumption of universal features shared by all members of a family (see Krämer 2001, p.118). The thread of family similarities doesn't consist of fibres running through the whole thread, but many fibres spread over (see Wittgenstein 1989a, p.278/§67).

Wittgenstein formulates the analogy between games and language: »Instead of stating what the common feature of all what we call language is I claim that there is nothing what is common of all these appearances that is the reason for the fact that we use the same word for all of them –; but these appearances are related in many different ways. And because of this kinship we call them all ›languages‹. [*Statt etwas anzugeben, was allem, was wir Sprache nennen, gemeinsam ist, sage ich, es ist diesen Erscheinungen gar nicht Eines gemeinsam, weswegen wir für alle das gleiche Wort verwenden –, sondern sie sind mit einander in vielen verschiedenen Weisen verwandt. Und dieser Verwandtschaft wegen, nennen wir sie alle ›Sprachen‹.*]« (Wittgenstein 1989a, S.277f/§66) The philosophical striving for universality that discovers in the different objects a common feature that is a part of these objects and that designates these common features with a concept is discharged by the doctrine of family similarities. From this point of view Humboldt's first step becomes clearer: The fixation of an idea (›Vorstellung‹) is not an abstraction of a feature to be found in the objects: Form or family similarity is not primarily founded by the objects.

The question emerges how communication works. How is it possible to communicate about things when there are no universals that are to be abstracted out of objects falling then under common concepts? Wittgenstein answers this with his idea of life form, ›*Lebensform*‹. To speak about games is only possible if there is the activity of playing. With it the activity aspect and the embeddedness of language games in a life form shift to the centre of reflection. Wittgenstein notes: »The term ›language game‹ emphasises that speaking a language is a part of an activity or of a life form. [*Das Wort ›Sprachspiel‹ soll hier hervorheben, daß das Sprechen einer Sprache Teil ist einer Tätigkeit, oder einer Lebensform.*]« (Wittgenstein 1989a, p.250/§23) This quotation is not interesting because of the trivial fact that Wittgenstein conceives speaking as an activity, but because he conceives speaking as a part of an activity. That will become obvious if we continue the lecture of this passage: »The word ›language game‹ shall emphasise that speaking a language is part of an activity or of a life form. Make the manifold of language games clear by these, and other, examples: giving orders, and acting according to orders/describing an object [...]/producing an object according to a description/report on a course/making supposes about a course/formulating a hypothesis and verifying/[...]/begging/thanking/swearing/greeting/praying. It is interesting to compare the manifold of the linguistic tools and its use, the manifold of words and sentence forms with what logicians said about the construction of language. [*Das Wort ›Sprachspiel‹ soll hier hervorheben, daß das Sprechen der Sprache ein Teil ist einer Tätigkeit, oder einer Lebensform. Führe dir die Mannigfaltigkeit der Sprachspiele an diesen Beispielen, und anderen, vor Augen: Befehlen, und nach Befehlen handeln/Beschreiben eines Gegenstands nach dem Ansehen, oder nach Messungen/Herstellen eines Gegenstands nach einer Beschreibung (Zeichnung)/Berichten eines Hergangs/Über den Hergang Vermutungen anstellen/Eine Hypothese aufstellen und prüfen/Darstellen der Ergebnisse eines Experiments durch Tabellen und Diagramme/Eine Geschichte erfinden; und lesen/Theater spielen/Reigen singen/Rätsel raten/Einen Witz machen; erzählen/Ein angewandtes Rechenexempel lösen/Aus einer Sprache in die andere übersetzen/Bitten, Danken, Fluchen, Grüßen, Beten./ Es ist interessant, die Mannigfaltigkeit der Werkzeuge der Sprache und ihrer Verwendungsweisen, die Mannigfaltigkeit der Wort- und Satzarten, mit dem zu vergleichen, was Logiker über den Bau der Sprache gesagt haben. (Und auch der Verfasser der Logisch-Philosophischen Abhandlung.)*« (Wittgenstein 1989a, S.250/§23)

»I will call the whole: of the language and of the activities with that language is interwoven a ›language game‹. [*Ich werde auch das Ganze: der Sprache und der Tätigkeiten, mit denen sie verwoben ist, das ›Sprachspiel‹ nennen.*]« (Wittgenstein 1989a, p.241/§7) Linguistic usage is not just a doing, but embedded in a doing. Hence language games are interwoven with nonlinguistic actions constitutionally (see Krämer 2001, p.119). This interwovenness of language with actions is a very important definition of language games, and without grasping this definition it is impossible to understand neither Wittgenstein's famous private language argument (see Wittgenstein 1989a, §§243-315) or the no less famous sentence: »If a lion was able to speak, we couldn't understand it. [*Wenn ein Löwe sprechen könnte, wir könnten ihn nicht verstehen.*]« (Wittgenstein 1989a, p.568)

Wittgenstein's concept of action isn't to interpret emphatically, but totally prosaic. That becomes obvious in Wittgenstein's special liking for technical analogies that are the metaphor reservoir for Wittgenstein's philosophy of language – the signal box analogously to which language starts actions, the tools in the tool kit analogously to which words work, the instrument analogously to which the usage of a sentence is understandable. All these metaphors testify a special liking for plain actions (see Krämer 2001, p.119). Beside this latent instrumentalism Krämer diagnoses a further feature of the activity view of language games the non-reflexivity in Wittgenstein's philosophy. Wittgenstein isn't interested in speaking as an intentional, well-considered action, but he focuses on speaking as a cultural practice of a community, as inveterate ways of actions that became self-evident and natural. Accordingly learning a language is not explaining, but training: »The child uses such primitive forms in the phase of language acquisition. The teaching of a language is not to explain, but to train. [*Solche primitiven Formen der Sprache verwendet das Kind, wenn es sprechen lernt. Das Lehren der Sprache ist hier kein Erklären, sondern ein Abrichten.*]« (Wittgenstein 1989a, p.239/§5)

Wittgenstein who mercilessly exposes his existence to reasoning formulates a view of language that manages almost without reason. The theory of language games refuses the distinction of λογοσ – reflection and cognition themselves are special language games that are not over or above other language games, but beside them and one of them. Wittgenstein detaches linguistic communication from the role of being reasonable by its anchoring in life forms. That doesn't mean that there is no certainty in language games! On the contrary language games are bound to life forms that found a pre-reflexive and elementary certainty. Without this kind of certainty founded by life forms humans couldn't act, and the language game of doubting starts from this every day certainty. (It would be possible to doubt if there were nothing certain – and doubt requires certainty as a prerequisite). From an epistemological viewpoint life forms are the border of all foundations expressed in the words: ›That's the way I act.‹ (see Krämer 2001, p.120f.)

4. Philosophy as a survey providing description (›übersichtliche Darstellung‹)

According to Wittgenstein the most of philosophical problems emerge if language runs dry (see Wittgenstein 1989a, §132), if language ›celebrates‹ (see Wittgenstein 1989a, §38). It is the task of philosophy as therapy to reveal the usage and misuse of language and to open insights in the ›work of our language‹ (Wittgenstein 1989a, §109). Philosophical grammar achieves this task. E.g., if someone talks about the prejudice of ›crystal purity of logic‹ or about ›misunderstood role of an ideal‹, language will celebrate, and likewise if he talks about ›non-spatial and non-timely objects‹ in contrary to ›spatial and timely phenomena of language‹. The celebration of language is hence defined: »To predicate something about an object what is founded in its description. [*Man prädiziert von der Sache, was in der Darstellungsweise liegt.*]« (Wittgenstein 1989a, p.296/§104) Language will celebrate exactly if an idealisation achieved by means of language that is a feature of the description means is transferred to the described thing and if we hence ›live in the idea‹ that the ideal must be found in reality (Wittgenstein 1989a,

§101). It is not to run idealisations down, but to prevent a misuse of ideals that will be given if ideals are transferred into objects. »The ideal is immovable in our thoughts. You can't make a step out of it. The ideal is like glasses on our nose, and what we look at we see through it. We don't think of taking off the glasses. [*Das Ideal, in unseren Gedanken, sitzt unverrückbar fest. Du kannst nicht aus ihm heraustreten. [...] Die Idee sitzt gleichsam als Brille auf unserer Nase, und was wir ansehen, sehen wir durch sie. Wir kommen nicht auf den Gedanken, sie abzunehmen.*]« (Wittgenstein 1989a, §103)

Philosophy as reflection of the work of language assigns idealisation to an appropriate usage what will be the case if its postulates don't threaten to become idle: »The more exactly we look at the actual language the stronger becomes the conflict between language and our postulates. (Crystal purity of logic isn't a fact; it is a postulate.) The conflict becomes unbearable; the postulate threatens now to become idle. – We got on icy grounds where the frictions lack, where the conditions are, so to speak, ideal, but where we therefore are not able to go. We want to go; then we need friction. Back to the rough ground! [*Je genauer wir die tatsächliche Sprache betrachten, desto stärker wird der Widerstreit zwischen ihr und unseren Forderungen. (Die Kristallreinheit der Logik hatte sich mir ja nicht ergeben; sondern sie war eine Forderung.) Der Widerstreit wird unerträglich; die Forderung droht nun, zu etwas Leerem zu werden. – Wir sind aufs Glatteis geraten, wo die Reibung fehlt, also die Bedingungen in gewissem Sinne ideal sind, aber wir eben deshalb auch nicht gehen können. Wir wollen gehen; dann brauchen wir die Reibung. Zurück auf den Boden!*]« (Wittgenstein 1989a, S.297/§107) By looking at the phenomena we can go the way back to the rough ground. Krämer (2001, p.113) calls this way of looking at phenomena ›morphological procedure‹. The morphological procedure is directed to phenomena without the presupposition that phenomena conceal the essence behind their surface. »Philosophy just places everything and neither explains or concludes. – Because everything lies there openly there is nothing to explain. We are not interested in what is concealed. [*Die Philosophie stellt eben bloß alles hin, und erklärt und folgert nichts. – Da alles offen daliegt, ist auch nichts zu erklären. Denn, was etwa verborgen ist, interessiert uns nicht.*]« (Wittgenstein 1989a, p.303/§126) Although matters lie open, we don't see them because their everyday ordinarity veils them. »The most important aspects of things are concealed by simplicity and everyday existence. [*Die für uns wichtigsten Aspekte der Dinge sind durch ihre Einfachheit und Alltäglichkeit verborgen.*]« (Wittgenstein 1989a, p.304/§129) It is true that philosophy neither explains nor concludes, but now philosophy has nevertheless a task: Philosophy yields a ›survey providing description‹. »The concept of the survey providing description is fundamental for us. It designates our form of representation – the kind we see objects. [*Der Begriff der übersichtlichen Darstellung ist für uns von grundlegender Bedeutung. Er bezeichnet unsere Darstellungsform, die Art, wie wir die Dinge sehen.*]« (Wittgenstein 1989a, p.302/§122) The survey providing description makes coherence visible by grouping phenomena in a row and draws by this a ›face‹ or a ›gestalt‹. In this formulation coherence just means ›point of view‹. And phenomena can be grouped in a manifold of coherences or, in other words, they can be viewed from many perspectives.

At this point of argumentation Krämer (2001, p.114) sees the paradigm coming into play. The paradigm is a phenomenon characterised by the fact that it serves as a scale. There are two kinds of ›being a scale‹: Firstly because the other phenomena are grouped according to their similarity or dissimilarity with the model; or, secondly, because the paradigm serves as model of measuring the other phenomena. Which morphological coherence will exist between the phenomena depends on the selection of the one phenomenon that is never to compare, but always the means of comparison. Hence humans don't just find a coherence, but humans create coherences. The difference between a means of description and the described object is in the perspective of the morphological procedure equivalent with the difference between a paradigm and the phenomena grouped according to the paradigm. This difference is practically established and isn't a feature that is to be found in the objects (for example by abstraction).

The morphological procedure makes coherences obvious. In the *Tractatus logico-philosophicus* Wittgenstein yet claims that the function of a proposition is to carry the truth value and hence to be a picture of reality. This picture applied to reality as a scale (see Wittgenstein 1960, p.17/2.1512) contains the relation between world and language that can be showed, but never verbally expressed. Wittgenstein holds on to this claim that it is possible to show forms, but that it is not possible to express forms in his late work. Hence language functions like a picture. The morphological procedure of survey giving description makes coherences visible and that's why this procedure has an ›iconic dimension‹ (see Krämer 2001, p.115). This is exactly the reason why Wittgenstein prefers description and rejects explanation. In difference to explanation the description is not restricted to the modality of discourse, but its features are strongly iconic. Creating a survey giving description is a practice of making visible (see Krämer 2001, p.115).

5. Plural world views and the gain of necessary communication

Hence philosophy makes coherences visible. The survey giving description (the philosophical grammar), however, is itself a language game and language games are not pictures of the world. That was argued above. But now the question rises: Persons who share a common life form expressed in different language games can communicate without any problems. The commonly shared life form as a cultural matrix is the explanation for the mutual understanding. But what about two or more persons who don't share a common life form founding language games? What if persons communicate who don't live in the same world? And according to the non-intellectual view of language that is not only a metaphor. Different languages constitute in fact different worlds.

No doubt, Humboldt answers this question. As I noticed, Humboldt was a political man, and he was interested in the ways of communication without the arrogance that was and is the usual way of thinking and behaviour when Europeans meet indigenous people. Like Wittgenstein who conceives language games in plural language develops its knowledge constituting activity according to Humboldt not as a universal language, but as a special, individualised language. Language appears in the variety of individual forms. When Humboldt states that human reasoning and mind are determined by language, he claims that the special, individualised form of the language a certain person calls his/her mother tongue determines his/her reasoning and mind. The acceptance of the different languages as the historical conditions of human mind is Humboldt's ›Copernican turn‹ (see Cesare 1996, p.282).

This Copernican turn becomes obvious in two quotes. In the first quote Humboldt firstly refuses the view that language (in singular) is applied to the world or, in other words, Humboldt refuses the instrumentalistic view of language. Humboldt argues his refusal by life world embeddedness. »The idea that different languages just mark the same mass of objects and concepts that are independent of the languages with different words is natural to the human understanding of language, and before someone won't reflect about language, he won't refuse this view. [...]. According to this view the difference of languages is just a difference of sounds, and it is treated as a means to achieve objects. [*Die Vorstellung, dass die verschiednen Sprachen nur dieselbe Masse der unabhängig von ihnen vorhandenen Gegenstände und Begriffe mit andren Worten bezeichnen und diese nach andren Gesetzen, die aber, ausser ihrem Einfluss auf das Verständnis, keine weitere Wichtigkeit besitzen, an einander reihen, ist, ehe er tiefer über die Sprache nachdenkt, dem Menschen zu natürlich, als dass er sich leicht davon losmachen könnte. [...] Immer in Objecten lebend, webend und handelnd, bringt er die Subjectivitaet zu wenig in Anschlag, und gelangt schwer zu dem Begriff einer durch die Natur selbstgegebenen Objectiven in ihm beimischenden, und es, nicht zufällig, launisch oder willkürlich, sondern nach innern Gesetzen so umgestaltenden, dass das scheinbare Object selbst nur zu subejctiver, und doch mit vollem Recht auf Allgemeingültigkeit Anspruch machender Auffassung wird. Die Verschiedenheit der Sprachen ist ihm nur eine Verschiedenheit von Schällen, die er, gerichtet auf Sachen, bloss als Mittel behandelt, zu diesen zu gelangen.*]« (Humboldt 1981a, p.153) Humboldt places at the language in singular the plurality of historical, current and future languages: »The linguistic share of ideas is not just metaphysical founding the existence of the concept. Language has effect on the kind of its forming and coins it. In this way a language gives to the mass of ideas a coherent form. Hence language determines the way of combining ideas what radiates back to humans. [*Der Antheil der Sprache an den Vorstellungen ist nicht bloss ein metaphysischer, das Daseyn des Begriffs bedingender; sie wirkt auch auf die Art seiner Gestaltung und drückt ihm ihr Gepräge auf. Indem, bei aller objectiven Verschiedenheit in ihm, sie immer in dem ihr eignen Charakter auf ihn wirkt, giebt sie der ganzen Masse der Vorstellungen eine mit ihr zusammenhängende gleichmässige Gestaltung. Sie steht ebenso der Fügung des Gedankens in innerlicher oder äusserlicher Rede vor, und bestimmt dadurch auch die Verknüpfungsweise der Ideen, die wieder auf den Menschen nach allen Richtungen zurückwirkt.*]« (Humboldt 1981a, p.154)

The difference of languages is not only and not primarily a difference of sounds and signs, but primarily a difference of world views. World is formed only with and in language, and hence world is given only in different languages. Thus there is not one world, but there is a manifold of worlds according to the manifold of perspectives opened by languages. There is no sense to ask what the world itself is. Humboldt assesses the unreducable variety of languages and the resulting manifold of world views positively. »*Weltansicht aber ist die Sprache nicht bloss, weil sie, da jeder Begriff soll durch sie erfasst werden können, dem Umfange der Welt gleichkommen muss, sondern auch deswegen, weil erst die Verwandlung, die sie mit den Gegenständen vornimmt, den Geist zur Einsicht des von dem Begriff der Welt unzertrennlichen Zusammenhanges fähig macht. Denn erst indem sie den Eindruck der Wirklichkeit auf die Sinne und die Empfindung in das, als Organ des Denkens eigen vorbereitete Gebiet der articulirten Töne hinüberführt, wird die Verknüpfung der Gegenstände mit den klaren und reinen Ideen möglich, in welchen der Weltzusammenhang ans Licht tritt. Der Mensch lebt auch hauptsächlich mit den Gegenständen, so wie sie ihm die Sprache zuführt, und da Empfinden und Handlen in ihm von seinen Vorstellungen abhängt, sogar ausschliesslich so. Durch denselben Act, vermöge welches der Mensch die Sprache aus sich heraus spinnt, spinnt er sich in dieselbe ein, und jede Sprache zieht um die Nation, welcher sie angehört, einen Kreis, aus dem es nur insofern hinauszugehen möglich ist, als man zugleich in den Kreis einer andren Sprache hinübertritt. Die Erlernung einer fremden Sprache sollte daher die Gewinnung eines neuen Standpunktes in der bisherigen Weltansicht seyn, da jede das ganze Gewebe der Begriffe und Vorstellungsweise eine Theils der Menschheit enthält. Da man aber in eine fremde Sprache immer mehr oder weniger seine eigne Welt-, ja sogar seine eigne Sprachansicht hinüberträgt, so wird dieser Erfolg nie rein und vollständig empfunden.*« (Humboldt 1981a, S.225)

The emphasis of the manifold of world views delivers Humboldt to the reproach of relativism. I prefer to claim that Humboldt is not a proponent of relativism, but of relativity (what is assessed more positively in the philosophic community). Humboldt views humans on the one hand embedded in the world before the first linguistic act (but without cognition because object and subject are identical in dump desire), and on the other hand he maintains the idea of the world as the focus of the lingusitically determined world views. This is obvious when Humboldt claims that language works like a prism (GS III, p.167 ff) – Humboldt conceives difference as a difference of unity. The most striking evidence is that he speaks about language that shows itself in different languages and also about the unity of human beings.

Habermas (1999a, p.74f) states that the response in second person singular (the response of the ›you‹) unfolds not only the social-integrative power of agreement, but the critical-proving power of contradiction as well: We learn about the world by learning from each other. And it is due to Humboldt to emphasise the response of the ›you‹ cognitively important. What is to say, according to Habermas, that its definition marks the crossing of the cognitive and the communicative function of language in Humboldt's œuvre. Humboldt isn't interested in the claims of truth (›Wahrheitsansprüche‹), but in the moral implications of the exchange of competing world views and cultures: If the horizon of the own world view is widened, the own value orientation will be relativated. Humboldt claims an inner coherence between understanding and communication and that there is a cognitive dynamic working within the practice of communication contributing to a decentralisation of the own world views and to universalistic perspectives in morals.

The variety of world views opened by the variety of languages gains power that can't be ensured by the transcendental subject. Furthermore it won't be appropriate to conceive the concept constitution by spontaneity of the mind in mutual interaction with receptivity of the sensuality; the appropriate way of conceiving the process of concept constitution is to reflect on the linguistically given cultural influences on our mind and to bear in mind that the human mind must transcendent its own horizon of necessity to understand itself. Humans won't understand their mind by going into itself, by following the procedure of the *Criticism of Pure Reason* because this is not possible. Humans will be able to understand their own views only if they decentralise their perspectives by applying different world views. This way of de-transcendentalising doesn't hide in a particularism (and thus isn't a relativism in a bad manner), but it views relativity as a positive chance; by the way, it is a core postulate of Constructive Realism and should be reflected in the reflection of psychology.

Two further quotes make this line of thinking even clearer. »It is not possible to receive language like something physically completed. The receiver must cast it in a form having ready for it, what is usually called understanding. Either he forces the strange form in the form of his own language or he manages to transfer himself into the view of the other person's language who is at home in it requiring a vivid knowledge of the other language. The enlightening knowledge of difference resulting from this transfer requires the simultaneous consciousness of both languages. This requires furthermore having reached a higher viewpoint to which both linguistically different viewpoints are subordinated. [...] The possibility of reaching such a higher viewpoint is not constituted by different languages, but by being human. Thus humans understand each other without problems even if language doesn't offer a way of understanding to bridge the gap. [*Sprache kann auch nicht, gleichsam wie etwas Körperliches, fertig erfasst werden; der Empfangende muss sie in die Form giessen, die er, für sie bereitet, hält, und das ist es, was man verstehen nennt. Nun zwängt er entweder die fremde in die Form der seinigen hinüber, oder versetzt sich, mit recht voller und lebendiger Kenntnis jener ausgerüstet, ganz in die Ansicht dessen, dem sie einheimisch ist. Die lichtvolle Erkenntnis der Verschiedenheit erfordert etwas Drittes, nämlich ungeschwächt gleichzeitiges Bewusstseyn der eignen und fremden Sprachform. Dies aber setzt in seiner Klarheit voraus, dass man zu dem höheren Standpunkt, dem beide untergeordnet sind, gelangt sey, und erwacht auch dunkel erst recht da, wo scheinbar gänzliche Verschiedenheit es auf den ersten Anblick gleich unmöglich macht, das Fremde sich, und sich dem Fremden zu assimiliren. Das Gemeinsame liegt auch noch weit mehr im Menschen, als in den Sprachen selbst. Daher versteht der Mensch den Menschen leicht auch da, wo, genau untersucht, die Sprache keine Brücke des Verständnisses bietet.*« (Humboldt 1981, p.156)

In this quote I would like to stress the definition of the higher viewpoint that is important. Leaving one's own language and taking part of another language isn't exactly what leads to knowledge. Knowledge is only achieved if the simultaneous consciousness of both linguistically determined viewpoints are compared. Hence Humboldt (1981a, p.161) states: »Language combines even if it isolates, and the wrap of the most individual expression encloses the possibility of universal understanding. [*(Die) Sprache (verbindet auch), indem sie vereinzelt, und in die Hülle des individuellsten Ausdrucks die Möglichkeit allgemeinen Verständnisses einschliesst.*«

Reference

Cesare, Donatella Di (1996). Wilhelm von Humboldt (1767-1835). In T. Borsche (Hrsg.), *Klassiker der Sprachphilosophie. Von Platon bis Noam Chomsky* (S.275-290). München: C.H. Beck.

Borsche Tilman (1996). Einleitung. In T. Borsche (Hrsg.), *Klassiker der Sprachphilosophie. Von Platon bis Noam Chomsky* (S.7-13). München: C.H. Beck.

Habermas, Jürgen (1999a). Hermeneutische und analytische Philosophie. Zwei komplementäre Spielarten der linguistischen Wende. In J. Habermas, *Wahrheit und Rechtfertigung. Philosophische Aufsätze* (S.65-101). Frankfurt a.M.: Suhrkamp.

Habermas, Jürgen (1999b). Wege der Detranszendentalisierung. Von Kant zu Hegel und zurück. In J. Habermas, *Wahrheit und Rechtfertigung. Philosophische Aufsätze* (S.186-229). Frankfurt a.M.: Suhrkamp.

Humboldt, Wilhelm v. (1981a). Über die Verschiedenheit des menschlichen Sprachbaues. In W. v. Humboldt (edited by A. Flitner und K. Giel), *Werke in fünf Bänden, Band III* (S.144-367). Darmstadt: Wissenschaftliche Buchgemeinschaft.

Humboldt, Wilhelm v. (1981b). Brief an Schiller: Über Sprache und Dichtung. In W. v. Humboldt (edited by A. Flitner und K. Giel), *Werke in fünf Bänden, Band V* (S.195-200). Darmstadt: Wissenschaftliche Buchgesellschaft.

Humboldt, Wilhelm v. (1981c). Über Denken und Sprechen. In W. v. Humboldt (edited by A. Flitner und K. Giel), *Werke in fünf Bänden, Band V* (S.97-99). Darmstadt: Wissenschaftliche Buchgesellschaft.

Kant, Immanuel (1988). *Kritik der reinen Vernunft* [edited by Wilhelm Weischedel] (10. Auflage). Frankfurt a.M.: Suhrkamp.

Krämer, Sybille (2001). *Sprache, Sprechakt, Kommunikation. Sprachtheoretische Positionen des 20. Jahrhundert*. Frankfurt a.M.: Suhrkamp.

Majetschak, Stefan (1996). Ludwig Wittgenstein. In T. Borsche (Hrsg.), *Klassiker der Sprachphilosophie. Von Platon bis Noam Chomsky* (S.365-384). München: C.H. Beck.

Wittgenstein (1960). *Tractatus logico-philosophicus*. Frankfurt a.M.: Suhrkamp.

Wittgenstein, Ludwig (1989a). *Werkausgabe in acht Bänden, Band 1*. (6. Aufl.). Frankfurt a.M.: Suhrkamp.

Wittgenstein, Ludwig (1989b). *Werkausgabe in acht Bänden, Band 5 (Das Blaue Buch)* (6. Aufl.). Frankfurt a.M.: Suhrkamp.

B. Chinese Medicine & Historiography, Western Medicine

Zhu Ming

The Framework of Holism in TCM and Western Medicine

Influence of Natural Philosophy on Medicine

Cosmology

Great philosophers like Thales, Empedocles, Pitargores, Sacrates, Aristotle, etc. in Greek built up the fundament of western philosophy. Some concepts developed from them, for instances, »apeiron« from Anaxiamander of Miletus, »air« from Anaximenes of Miletus and »pneuma«, which share similar connotations with Chinese concepts of »Primary Qi« (Yuan Qi) or »Vital Energy«.

Actually there are many Chinese philosophers emerged almost at the same epoch like Laozi, Confucius, Mengzi, Zhuangzi, Mozi, Xunzi, Hanfeizi, etc. who have found their own philosophic schools.

Philosophical schools

There are many Greek philosophic schools such as Platonic School, Epicurean School, Stoic School, Cynic Schools at that time, until the later time with the influence of peripatetic school. In another aspect, almost all medieval Muslim philosophers up to the end of the twelfth century, and perheps even later, were practising physicians… Exactly as Galen said: A good physician should also be a philosopher.

Medical schools

Around 5th century before Christ, there were three large medical schools distributed in three main islands of ancient Greek, forming a prosperity of medicine at that time. These three medical schools are recorded as Knidas, Sicily and Kos schools. Hippocrate, who is in regard to nowadays the father of western medicine, is the chief representative for Kos medical school. From this group of physicians, their medical achievements have been written into the medical classics as »*Corpus Hippocraticum*«.

There are also three main medical schools in China almost in the same era, which has been recorded in one of Chinese classics (*Li Ji • Qu Li*) as »Fu Xi« by whom Acupuncture was invented and manufactured, »SU NÜ« who developed pulse-diagnostics and »Shen Nong«, who made discovery on herbs and applied them to clinical treatments. There is old saying like »Never take the medicines prescribed by whom does not belong to any of the three medical schools.«

The Five-Element Theory in TCM and the Four-Humor Theory in Western Medicine

Let's compare the Five-Element Theory in TCM and the Four-Humor Theory in Western Medicine by giving the following tables:

The Five-Element Theory in TCM

Element	Organ	Colour	Season	Emotion
wood	liver	green	spring	Anger
fire	heart	red	summer	Happy
earth	spleen	yellow	later summer	over-thinking
metal	lung	white	autumn	Sorrow
water	kidney	black	winter	Terror

The Four-Humor Theory in Western Medicine

Element	Organ	Colour	Season	Emotion
air	heart	red	spring	Sanguineous
fire	liver	yellow	summer	Bilious
earth	spleen	black	autumn	Melancholic
water	brain	white	winter	Phlegmatic

From this point of view, the two systems share remarkable similarities in the framework of holism in both medicines.

Alimentary therapy

Avicenna thinks that there are four orders of medicaments, i.e. the four degrees:

1. imperceptible to the senses
2. without perceptible interfering with the body functions
3. evident interference with the body function
4. causing destruction or death of tissues

From above, Avicenna displays that the food are ranged from the moderate quality till something toxic in nature. There is no strict boundary between the medicinal food and the alimentary medicament, so is TCM.

As TCM states, the medicament usually bears an extreme quality (like very hot or sharp pungent, etc.) which can influence the viscera; while the alimentary food tends mostly to be even and moderate in nature. Nourishing the body is based upon the food; healing of illness relies on the herbal medicament (quoted from *»Herbal Prescriptions Precious Worth a Thousand Gold • Preface on Alimentary Therapy« written by Sun Simiao in the Tang Dynasty).* In the history of western medicine, medicinal foods and drinks such as wine, garlic, egg-yolk, gours, meat-juice, etc.

- Drugs with warm or hot nature such as garlic, wine, aconite, sulphur
- Drugs bearing cool or cold nature like: lettuce, peony, etc.
- Drugs with toxic effects such as leeches, viper, scorpion Venor, hyposcyamus, aconite, sulphur, etc.
- Herbs for balneology such as pine nut, cherry bay, etc.

There are many common species both as food and medicaments in TCM such as hawthorn, lotus' seed, lily, Chinese date, ginger, garlic, pepper, peony, Chinese cinnamon, lettuce, caraway, almond, variety of nuts, medlar, rhubarb, goat-liver, black chicken, duck, etc. Stated by the China Public Health Ministry in 2002, 87 sorts of herbs recorded as general food including honey, corn mint, chrysanthemum flower, black sesame, chicken's stomach, yam, etc. In another aspect, a cold must be treated by warm medicine, this is known by both medical systems as a common application of healing principle.

On apoplexy

Galen thought that apoplexy can be clinically categoried into Blood Plethora and Cac'ochymia two types, and this illness was only blamed for the temperament of cold and moisture. So did Avicenna. In addition, he added one type of apoplexy due to the deficiency of »natural heat« (or called »lodging warmth«) in spite of the clinical excessive types.

TCM regards that apoplexy is resulted from internal-wind which can be aroused by strong emotional stimulations, overactivity of liver-Yang and deficiency of the kidney-Yin, etc. By the influence of the emotions, blood-stasis and phlegm accumulation may appear; of course, it comes with Qi stagnation simultaneously. In another case, liver-wood is too dry to catch fire in upper flaming with the brain damage due to kidney-water insufficient.

On sub-health state of both medicines

In western medicine from historical background: There are three states of the human body, according to Galen:

1. Health – a state in virtue of which the human body presents that particular temperament and configuration whereby all its functions shall proceed unembarrassed.
2. Disease – a state which is exactly contrary to Item 1.
3. A third state that is neither health nor diseases. There are three variants: (a) the health is not perfect and yet there is no actual illness. For instances, the state in old persons, and in juveniles, and in those convalescent from illness. (b) Both states occur simultaneously in the same member (i.e. the organ): either in two quite different respects (as when the temperament of a person is normal, but there is compositional abnormality; he may be healthy in regard to two passive qualities, but not in regard to two active ones). (c) Both states occur in one person, but at different times of the year (as when a person is well in winter but ill in spring) (see *The Canon of Medicine of Avicenna, Book I, Item 196*).

TCM emphases precaution for diseases, as it is saying: a high level doctor treats patients in early stage, even when the disease has not yet formed. Therefore the preventive measures in calming down the disturbances or proper regimen for restoring the health should be applied at the right moment. Otherwise, treating the disease after it has already taken place is just like digging a well until one is thirsty, or casting the weapon after the war has begun. (*Plain Questions • Chapter Si Qi Tiao Shen Da Lun, Yellow Emperor's Inner Classic*)

The third state is contemporarily so-called »Sub-Health« in China. In such a state, preventive medicine is strongly addressed to regain Yin-Yang equilibrium, to dredge energy-meridians, to replenish the viscera and to ease emotional stimulants and tensions of the mind.

Unity of body and soul

Life is a co-ordinated form of the physical, mental and spirital faculties. HEALTH means a sustainable state in balance of above three aspects.

According to Aristotle the heart is the source of allmental and emotional functions. In Canon of Medicine of Avicenna, he elaborated that there were three kinds of faculty, and therefore of functions proceeding therefrom, i.e.the vital faculty (haywaniat); the natural faculty (taby yat) and the animal faculty (nafsaniat). In addition, he followed Galen's opinion, and thought that each faculty has its own principal member (internal organ or viscera), which forms its storehouse, and from which its functions emerges. These three faculties have been since then developed as only three powers or parts of the soul are commonly assigned – namely, the vegetable soul, the sensitive soul and the rational soul... There are five genera of powers of the soul – the vegetative, the sensitive, the appetitve, the locomotive and the intellecture. Again, Avicenna pointed out that the soul (nafs) is the source of the senation and movement.The proof of the existence of above three faculties, and of its being single or multiple, is a question for natural science, which is as well part of philosophy (quoted from »*The Canon of Medicine of Avicenna*« *Book I, Item 137-167*).

Enlightened by above medical holistic points of view between the body and soul, latterly many psychologists like Sigmund Freud (1856-1936 A.D.) and his student Carl Gustav Jung were the pioneers in the field of abnormal psychology and clinical psychology.

The interactions between King-Fire (Jun Huo) and Potential-Fire (Xiang Huo) elaborated by Zhu Zhenheng (1281-1358 A.D.) in the Jin-Yuan dynasties, who is both a well-known physician and erudite philosopher in TCM history. The Zhu's theory is showing that there is another center co-existing with the heart-fire (the brain) as the motivation of life power. It lodges in the lower part of the body where the liver-blood and kidney-essence offer its nourishment and the matter supply. The two forces interact with each other in order to remain the normal life as well as mental activities of the human. This indicates that people underworld for sexual pleasure and forget health-preservation principle, just as that lamp will go out at the exhaustion of lamp-oil and fish will die when water is dried up. According to TCM, the life of vitality is governed by the kidney-essence and liver-blood, alike that lamp depending on oil for light and fish replying on water for life.

Avicenna's theory and TCM on the primary and the secondary of the diseases

As far Avicenna's text at the end of the first book of his *Canon of Medicine (O.Cameron Gruner, p.529)*, it reminds us of the well-known rule formulated by the Chinese physicians concerning the treatment of two simultaneously occurring diseases one of which is primary (Ben), the other is secondary (Biao), i.e. so-called in Chinese »biao ben qing zhong huan ji«.

As *Huang Di Nei Jing (Yellow Emperor's Inner Classic)* has mentioned in consequence the following different conditions:

1. When the disharmony of Qi and blood is caused by a certain disease, the disease is primary, and the disease should be treated first; when the disease is re-

sulted from the disharmony of Qi and blood, the disharmony of Qi and blood is primary, and it should be treated first.

2. When the patients contracts other disease first and then the diarrhea occurs, treat the disease first; when the patient has diarrhea first and then another disease occurs, adjust the indigestion and treat diarrhea as the primary reason, and then treat the disease later.
3. When another disease is affected firstly and then the abdominal flatulence occurs, the secondary symptom of abdominal flatulence should be treated first. In addition, when the abdominal flatulence appears first, and then the heart irritation happens, under this circumstance the abdominal flatulence should be also treated firstly as it is the primary reason.
4. When another disease happens first and then the retention of feces and urine appear, the secondary symptoms of the retention of feces and urine should be taken into consideration as the emergent case and be treated at first. If there is no retention of feces and dysuria, the primary disease which occurs first should be treated at the beginning.
5. Before healing of the disease, inspect discreetly whether the disease is a slight one or a severe case, and then adjust it accordingly. When the disease is a light case, both therapeutic methods of reinforcing and reducing can be applied at the same time; when the disease is a severe case, treat the primary first or treat the secondary first according to its specific condition. For an instance, when the disease happens first and then fever occurs, the secondary fever should be treated first.

The above healing-principles are mentioned in *Huang Di Nei Jing (Plain Questions • Chapter 65, On the Primary and Secondary in Transfering the Sequence of the Disease*)

Avicenna put forward that, when several maladies occur together, we should deal first with that which fulfils one of three conditions.

1. When the one must be cured before the other can be relieved. For instance, if inflammation and ulceration occur simultaneously, the former must be attended to first until the intemperament on which it depends is remedied. The ulcer will never be healed until that is put right. The ulcer is then treated.
2. When the maladies are related as cause and effect. Example: obstruction and fever. The former must be treated first. If the obstruction will only yield to a »hot« remedy, we should not be able to cure the fever. We may treat phthisis with desiccants, but we shall not cure the fever, because its cause is beyond our reach. The cause would be amenable to desiccant treatment, but this would keep up the fever.

3. When it is absolutely essential to deal with one of the maladies. Thus suppose relapsing fever and palsy should occur concurrently. There is no question about treating the former, and venesection is the proper treatment. But this will not cure the palsy.

The disorder and the symptom to which the malady owes its name may occur together. In such a case one would begin by dealing with the malady itself. But if the symptom became urgent, we should turn our attention to it. And leave the disease itself alone for the time. Thus, in a case of colic (ji fu tong), we should turn our attention first to relieve the violent pain, even though the condition causing it is thereby adversely affected. Again, we should postpone a venesection (otherwise indicated) if the stomach were in a feeble state or if there were diarrhea, or if were nausea.

Sometimes we should do a venesection (for instance) without hesitation even though that would not remove the whole trouble. For instance, in a case of spasmodic disease, we should not empty out all the morbid humor, but we should leave some behind rather than risk losing some of the healthy humor, in the hope that this itself would cure the spasmodic movements.

Western medicine and TCM on heat

According to the Atomistic Structure of Matter, it was taught that the four elements are fire, air, water and earth. Each element follows the subsequent one. Water, however, does not enclose the whole earth. For by divine wisdom to the general advantage water uncovers some parts of the earth so that animals and plants can exist. Heat is actually a factor during the process of rarefication. Vaporization is the first effect caused by heat. Gold cannot be divided by heat into particles because they are extremely adhesive. Water is more readily affected by heat than earth. Homogeneous particles become joined by heat, but heterogeneous particles become separated.

The origin of heat is life, and life is maintained also by fluids. This has been told by Rashid ad-Din (1247-1318, A.D.), one of the greatest medieval Muslim physicians and historians. During the Mongol invasion of Persia he became Prime Minister (vizier) of three rules of the Ilkhand dynasty. His interest in Chinese medicine is attested by his book *Tansuqnamah,* which is so far regarded as the earliest translation of Chinese medical literature in middle-east. He also gave the book the subtitle »*Ilkhans's Treasure Book of Chinese Sciences*«, and organized scholars to compile it. Rashid ad-Din wrote another book »*Treatise on Heat*«. In this book he summarized his discourse by emphasizing that there are various kinds of heat: natural heat, elementary heat, and the heat of the sun. Each sort of heat has its own peculiar effect. The natural heat exists together with the primary fluid, and both of them constitute life.

According to Chinese medicine, heat and dryness belong to Yang; while cold and moisture belong to Yin. Yang has the function of forming up and increasing the Qi, while Yin bears the function of shaping up the body. As things which have reached their extremes turn into their opposites, e.g. extreme cold will lead to heat and extreme heat will bring on cold. Cold energy condenses water and results in turbidity; while heat energy makes water vaporizating and produces lucidity.

In TCM, there are as well many sorts of heat (fire). For instances, fire (heat) is one of the six pathogenic factors by the climatic influences. (*Fundamentals of Traditional Chinese Medicine, Beijing: Foreign Language Press, 1992.pp.126. Chief Editor: Yin Hui-he*). As a Yang pathogenic factor characterized by flaring up and ascending, it usually causes high fever, polydipsia, perspiration, full and frequent or rapid pulse. In addition, pathogenic heat is likely to consume the body fluids, which may result in thirsty, dry throat, dark-red urine and indulgence in drinking, etc.

Besides the climatic influences, there is also the heat (or fire) generated internally in the body. According to the Five Element theory, heat pertains to the heart and the heart charges the mental activities, therefore, as *Plain Questions (The Yellow Emperor's Inner Classic*) states: »Anxiety and mania are due to pernicious heat«, and »febrile unconsciousness and convulsions are due to fire«. Laterly a conclusion has been drawn by the famous physician Liu Wan-su (1100-1200, A.D.) in the Yuan dynasty, who was living a little earlier time than Rashid ad-Din. Liu stated: »Six climatic influences (i.e. wind, cold, summer heat, dampness, dryness and fire) turn into fire (heat)«, and »Five emotional changes (i.e. happiness, angry, worrying, sorrow and terror) turn into fire«. (*cf. Ren Ying-qiu, et al.. Various Academic Schools of Traditional Chinese Medicine, Shanghai Press of Sciences and Technology, 1984: pp 45*)

In *Huang Di Nei Jing* (*Yellow Emperor's Inner Classic, Chapter »Yin Yang Ying Xiang Da Lun", in meaning to the Corresponding Relation between the Yin and Yang of Man and all Things and That of the Four Seasons*), there is a famous item: »Violent-fire consumes Qi (vital energy); gentle-fire cultivates Qi«, which means that some food or drug like pepper bears a strong property of hot and pungent, which may take the body energy away; while some other like ginger has a medium-warm property which can build up vital energy and make the body strong. The significance of this item has been later explored by Li Dong-yuan (1180-1251 A.D.), who was a great physician in the Jin-Yuan dynasties. Li added one new meaning in pathology to this item: the violent-fire can be also the hot weather or strong hectic influences including excessive emotions which exhaust vital energy; while the gentle-fire like a gorges sunshine or easy-going surroundings may warm up the body and cultivate vital energy as well as nourish the soul.

The oil of the lamp reflects the body – a trope by both medicines

Avicenna has said that an old man's temperament is contrary of a young man, for in the course of aging it changes. For an example, when wood is burnt it turns to coal. But the essence of wood is not like the essence of coal. Likewise the essence of grapes, wine, raisins and sirup is not the same, although they are of the same origin. But because they underwent a change they ended up at the extreme opposite. This holds true with view to the young man whose temperament changes very much to the opposite when he grows old.

When a child is born, his natural heat is strong and his body-fluid is abundant. During all stages of life, from childhood to the old age, man's natural heat declines and his body-fluids decrease. We know by experience, Rashīd ad-Dīn says, that old and sick people have less natural heat and that their bodies are colder compared with those of young men. As mentioned in the context above, Rashīd ad-Dīn elucidated that natural heat constitutes the life while cold is opposed and contrary to life. No one can have a temperament that is both warm and cold. Hot drugs must be taken moderately. Otherwise they act like oil in a lamp: the more oil is added to a lamp the more its light will decrease until it extinguishes entirely. A drug that is hotter than it should be makes the body dryer than it should be, and a drug that is colder that it should be makes the body moister that it should be.

Based upon TCM, the oil of lamp is showing totally another picture, just as mentioned in the text of Zhu Zhenheng's theory (see the Part II: Unity of the Body and the Soul). Zhu said: »At the sight of pretty women the sexual desire is aroused«, »the rising of sexual desire leads to the flame of Potential-Fire (Xiang Huo) and the consumption of the essence and blood«, which means exactly the over-burning of the lamp-fire and exhaustion of the lamp-oil. Therefore he does suggests: »Man should keep away from women for a period of time and take good care of themselves so as to save the essence of the life from abuse.« (*cf. On Inquiring the Properties of Matter by Zhu Zhenheng*). The follower in his medical school, Long Zunxu, a physician in the 16th century (the Ming dynasty), addressed »abstinence from indulgence in sexual activities to conserve the essence«, and »Man has his body from the endowment of essence and blood from his parents. When he comes of age, however, he with the increasing of sexual urge drains the endowed essence in the river of love and the ocean of lust. He who has exhausted his essence young will die young; he who has exhausted his essence later will accordingly die later; and he who has exhausted his essence later still will not be able to enjoy the full life span.« (cf. His book *Admonitions for Men and Women Nan Nu Kun Yan).* This means that the body essence both for men and women should be saved and remained like the full lamp-oil to achieve longevity and life-long bright-light (the healthy-state).

At the end let's remind us of the old saying from the *Yellow Emperor's Inner Classic (Plain Question)* of TCM:

»The changing-principle of the cosmos can adapt to the human beings; insight-comprehension of history helps us to understand the present better; all things are no exception of reflection of the vital-energy (Qi).«

Plain Questions·Chapter Qi Jiao Bian Da Lun, Huang Di Nei Jing

References

(1) Needham, J. (1975). *Science and Civilization in China.* Cambridge: University Press.

(2) Yongyan, W., Ming, Z., et.al. (1999). *Internal Medicine Textbook of TCM.* Beijing: Public Hygiene Press.

(3) Klein-Franke, F., Ming, Z., et al. (2001) The Passage of Chinese Medicine to the West. *American Journal of Chinese Medicine, Vol.29, Nos3-4*, pp.559-565

(4) Hongjun, Zhao (translator) (1982). *Hippocrate's Collections.* Hebei Press of Science & Technology.

(5) Gruner, O. C. (translator) (1929). *The Canon of Medicine of Avicenna (Book I).* UK: Burleich Press.

(6) Klein-Franke, F., & Ming, Z. (1999). *Avicenna's Links with Chinese Medicine – A Chapter of the History of Sino-Arabic Relations during the Middle Ages.* Asian Medicine (London: Wellcome Trust).

(7) Wu, Nelson Liansheng, & Wu, Andrew Qi (1997). *English-Text of Yellow Emperor's Canon Internal Medicine* (黄帝内经), China Science & Technology Press; Beijing.

(8) Klein-Franke, F. & Ming, Z. (2003). The Book of Heat from Rashid ad-Din's Chinese Medicine from a Source in 14th Century Persia. *The American Journal of Chinese Medicine, Vol.31, No.6*, 1-6.

(9) Enqin, Zhang, et al. (1990). *Health Preservation and Rehabilitation.* Publishing House of Shanghai College of Traditional Chinese Medicine (pp.130-135).

Timon Cheng-Yi LIU, Jian-Ling JIAO, Xiao-Yang XU, Jian LU, Xiao-Yuan DENG & Song-Hao LIU

Process Theory – The Bridge of the Eastern and Western Culture

Abstract

Eastern culture is based on process theory. In this paper, a process was studied from viewpoint of quantum mechanics and process-specific time was put forward to redefine the *yin* and *yang* of traditional Chinese medicine (TCM) and extend TCM *yin-yang* rules to systems of modern sciences such as cells, autonomic nervous system and sports processes. As TCM is an important part of Eastern culture and modern sciences are important parts of Western culture, our discussion showed that process theory should be an important candidate theory to bridge the gap between the Eastern and Western culture.

Eastern culture draws its inspiration and insight directly from the perennial pattern of nature, which is why the Tao (Way) transcends all cultural boundaries and consistently withstands the tests of time. The principles of balance and harmony run throughout the Eastern culture. Traditional Chinese science was based on the »theory of birth-to-death« and characterized by the »cycle-production« model (Wang et al 2001). The Traditional Chinese medicine (TCM) is a typical example of the Eastern culture. Influenced by the thinking model of traditional culture, the TCM takes *Qi* as its core conception to describe and summarize the live activities of human body, and uses *yin-yang* and the *Five Elements* as its basic model to establish a system of physiology, pathology, diagnosis and therapy of diseases (Xu 1996, Fan 2002). While Western medicine is, to a great extent, based on anatomy and quantitative analysis, TCM describes the life regulation with different perspectives including society, culture, physiology and psychology. The human body is understood as an »energetic composition«, through which energy flows. The unobstructed flow of energy through the meridians (pathways of energy) is considered a prerequisite for both a healthy body and mind. If these energy streams are interrupted, it will result in either physical or emotional disturbances, or possibly both. In this regard, ancient TCM views a disease in a holistic and dynamic way, which is rather foresighted even in the light of today's medical science. The Eastern culture has been very extensively documented traditions that are, unfortunately, out of reach of most Western researchers. This is not due to a separation by physical distance or even the language barrier in our viewpoint. It is due to their philosophical gap.

Process thought (Whitehead 1978) in general seeks to elucidate the *developmental* nature of reality, emphasizing *becoming* rather than static existence or being. It seeks the-many-becoming-one in a sequence of integrations at every level and moment of existence. Reality is the process of creative advance in which many past events are integrated in the events of the present, and in turn are taken up by future events. Events particularize ultimate creative power. The world is the realization of a selection of creative potentials. Though an outgrowth of Western philosophy, process philosophy has many affinities with the Chinese tradition (Neville 1977). Process theory was used to bridge the gap between Eastern and Western culture in this paper.

1. Process-specific time

In this section, the process-specific time will be introduced to represent the degree of difficulty (DD) of a process so that the higher the DD of a process, the more difficult the process occurs.

A process consists of many sub-processes. The simplest process is the elementary process. From the viewpoint of quantum mechanics, an elementary process is just a collision process. There are many kinds of collision processes. Firstly, we discuss the collision process of a particle and a photon which process-specific time is called radiation time. The radiation time can be calculated in terms of its cross section σ which is positively related to its transition rate (Liu et al 1996 & 2003):

$$t = 2(\sigma / \pi)^{1/2} / v_e \tag{1}$$

where v_e is the root-mean-square speed of the electron in the initial states. For the absorption process, σ is the absorption cross section. For the non-resonant absorption, we have (Liu et al 1996 &2003): $\omega\uparrow$, $t\uparrow$, so that:

$$t(\text{hot color}) < t(\text{cold color}) \tag{2}$$

where red, orange and yellow are called hot color, and green, blue and violet are called cold color. For the resonant absorption, we have (Liu et al 1995) $\omega\uparrow$, $t\downarrow$, so that:

$$t(\text{cold color}) < t(\text{hot color}) \tag{3}$$

We then discuss the collision process of particles which process-specific time is called collision time. Let the root-mean-square relative speed of the ith nucleus of the collision system in the initial state be v_i, and the minimum root-mean-square relative speed v be defined as $v = \min\{v_i\}$. Collision time can be calculated in terms of the collision cross section σ_c (Liu et al 1996 & 2003):

$$t_c = 2(\sigma_c / \pi)^{1/2} / v \tag{4}$$

As σ_c represents the possibility of the occurrence of the collision, and v represents the energy needed by the collision, we have (Liu et al 1996 & 2003):

$$t_c \downarrow, \mathrm{DD} \uparrow \tag{5}$$

A process consists of many elementary processes, but not all the elementary processes occur very easily. There is a key elementary process that occurs the most difficult. The DD of the key elementary process represents the DD of the whole process, which is called the key process principle and can be generally demonstrated (Liu et al 1996 & 2003). For example, the elementary process that the key enzyme catalyzes is the key elementary process of a metabolism process. Let the collision time of the ith elementary process be t_{ci}. According to the key process principle, the specific time of a process, t_p, can be defined as $t_p = \min\{t_{ci}\}$. From Eq. 5, we have:

$$t_p \downarrow, \mathrm{DD} \uparrow \tag{6}$$

As a typical example, we discuss the cellular signal transduction pathways. They can be classified into two classes, the one mediated by the G proteins, and the other one mediated by receptor-linked enzyme which is one of gualylate cyclase, tyrosine kinase and serine/threonine kinase and so on. The receptor of the former pathway strides membrane seven times. However, the receptor of the latter pathway strides membrane only one time. In terms of Eq. 6, we have:

$$t_p(\text{receptor - linked enzyme}) > t_p(\text{G protein}) \tag{7}$$

In the pathway mediated by G_s , G_i or G_q, the migration of the α subunit is the key elementary process that is of the shortest collision time t_c. Let $t_m(\alpha)$ be the migration time of the α subunit. From Eq. 6, we have $t_p = t_m(\alpha)$. As molecular mass (α_s) > molecular mass (α_q) > molecular mass (α_i), we have from Eq. 6:

$$t_p(G_i) > t_p(G_q) > t_p(G_s) \tag{8}$$

2. Time parallel principle

According to time parallel principle, the change of the process-specific times of two weakly nonlinearly coupled processes is parallel (Liu et al 1996 & 2003):

$$T_1\uparrow,\ T_2\uparrow \tag{9}$$

The time parallel principle can be shown by a simple model, two pendulums coupled by one nonlinear oscillator (Liu et al 1996 & 2003). It holds for the biological co-evolution in the level of species or molecules.

As a typical example, we discuss photobiomodulation on cells (Liu et al 1996 & 2003). In this case, the interaction of laser irradiation with a membrane receptor in the cell which is represented by radiation time t and the corresponding signal transduction pathways which are represented by the process-specific time t_p are weakly nonlinearly coupled so that we have according to our time parallel principle Eq. 9:

$$t\uparrow,\ t_p\uparrow \tag{10}$$

The cellular signal transduction pathways can be classified into two kinds: pathway 1 mediated by Gs protein: cAMP↑, and pathway 2 is mediated by G_i protein, G_q protein, or one of receptor-linked enzyme: cAMP↓. From Eqs. 2, 7, 8 and 10, we may have hot color laser ~ pathway 1, cold color laser ~ pathway 2. In other words, we have the biological information model of photobiomodulation (BIMP) (Liu et al 1996 & 2003):

Cold color activates pathway 2, Hot color activates pathway 1 (11)

This has been supported by its successful application in the cellular level, animal model level and clinic level (Liu et al 1996 & 2003).

3. Traditional Chinese medicine

The role of processes or function in TCM is the same as the one of states or structure in modern sciences so that TCM might be called process medicine. As process philosophy become more popular, TCM become more important. In this section, TCM will be discussed from viewpoint of process-specific time.

Yin-yang is one of the basic models of TCM to establish a system of physiology, pathology, diagnosis and therapy of diseases (Shuai 1992). It should be pointed out that the *yin-yang* model is only used to discuss TCM objects such as whole body, five *zangs* or six *fus*. However, the *yin-yang* concept is widely used in the cellular level for modern sciences (Tan 1993, Hunter 1995, Akam 1998, La Thangue 2003, Ou et al 2003). For example, Ou et al (2003) propose that *yin-yang* balance is antioxidation-oxidation balance with *yin* representing anti-oxidation and *yang* as oxidation. At this point, the *yin-yang* model of TCM should be extended to discuss cellular processes (Liu et al 2000 & 2002).After comparative research with TCM *yin-yang* model (Shuai 1992), we define *yin* and *yang* in terms of DD represented by process-specific time (Liu et al 2000 & 2002): the process of low DD is defined to be *yang* and the process of high DD is defined to be *yin* for the two nonlinearly coupled processes of a system, which is called DD *yin-yang* model. This definition is not only in agreement with TCM *yin-yang* model for TCM objects (Liu et al 2000 & 2002), but also in agreement with the *yin-yang* model for cellular processes (Tan 1993, Hunter 1995, Akam 1998, La Thangue 2003, Ou et al 2003). At this point, the *yin-yang* balance of TCM can be stated as following, a system is healthy if its *yin* and *yang* are balanced, and a system is in sub-health or disorder if its *yin* and *yang* are not balanced.

According to DD *yin-yang* model, time parallel principle, Eq. 8, is in agreement with TCM *yin-yang* parallel principle for TCM objects (Shuai 1992) so that it is called DD *yin-yang* parallel principle: the *yin* process of one system is related with the *yin* process of the other system and the *yang* process of one system is related with the *yang* process of the other system between the processes of two weakly nonlinearly coupled systems. As Ou et al (2003) have stated, the *yin*-tonic traditional Chinese herbs have, on average, about six times more antioxidant activity (*yin*) and polyphenolic contents than the *yang*-tonic herbs. As Ko et al (2004) have pointed out, although *yang*-tonic herbs tend to boost body function possibly through enhancing the mitochondrial oxidative processes (*yang*), the *yin* property (i.e. antioxidant potential) of these herbs can also play a role in safeguarding mitochondrial ATP generation, and the pharmacological basis of ›*yang*-invigoration‹ by Chinese tonic herbs might be due primarily to the enhancement of mitochondrial ATP generation.

4. Photobiomodulation

Photobiomodulation is an effect of low intensity monochromatic light or laser irradiation on biological systems, which stimulates or inhibits biological functions but does not result in irreducible damage. At the cellular level, monochromatic light or laser irradiation at low intensity can generate significant biological effects, including cellular proliferation, collagen synthesis, and the release of growth factors from cells (Karu 1998). There are two recent studies investigating cellular mechanisms of photobiomodulation using most advanced contemporary experimental techniques, a fluorescence resonance energy transfer technique (Wang et al 2005), cDNA microarray technology (Zhang et al 2003) and single cell confocal microscopy (Alexandratou et al 2002), which might open a new page in investigation of cellular mechanisms of photobiomodulation and the improvement of understanding of clinical usefulness of this therapeutic modality as Karu (2004) has pointed.

Whether there is photobiomodulation depends on the initial state of a cell or tissue. According to Karu's theory (Karu1998), there is no photobiomodulation on a cell which redox potential is so that the cell normally functions; the lower the redox potential of a cell comparing with the normal redox potential, the stronger the photobiomodulation. As Tunér et al (1999) have summarized, the light energy is thought to reap the greatest benefit where it is most needed. In other words, a healthy cell is in DD *yin-yang* balance so that there is no photobiomodulation, and there is photobiomodulation on a non-healthy cell until the cell is healthy so that photobiomodulation can be called cellular rehabilitation which has been discussed by King et al (2001).

Yin and *yang* are antagonistic, but they will transform into each other under some condition (Shuai 1992), which can be extended to other systems such as cells according to DD *yin-yang* model so that it is called DD *Yin-Yang* inter-transformation. This holds for BIMP (Liu et al 1996, 2002 and 2003). According to DD *yin-yang* model, we have cellular *yin* and *yang* from Eqs. 7 and 8:

Pathway 1 belongs to *yin*, and pathway 2 belongs to *yang* (12)

The *yin* and *yang* of laser irradiation or monochromatic light depend on its dose. At dose 1, the lowest dose for photobiomodulation, Eq. 2 holds so that we have:

Hot color belongs to *yin*, and cold color belongs to *yang* (13)

According to DD *yin-yang* parallel principle, we have Eq. 11 from Eqs. 12 & 13. At this point, Eq. 11 is called BIMP1. If the dose is at dose 2 which is larger than the threshold of dose 1, the *yin-yang* properties of laser irradiation or monochromatic light will transform into each other according to DD *Yin-Yang* inter-transformation so that we have:

Hot color belongs to *yang*, and cold color belongs to *yin* (14)

According to DD *yin-yang* parallel principle, we have from Eqs. 12 & 14:

Cold color activates pathway 1, Hot color activates pathway 2 (15)

This equation is called BIMP2. Generally, we have Eq. 14 according to DD *yin-yang* inter-transformation if the dose is at dose 2n (n = 1, 2, 3, ...) which is larger than the threshold of dose 2n-1 if it does not damage membrane or cell compartments such as mitochondria, lysosomes, endoplasmic reticulum so that Eq. 14 is called BIMP 2n, and we have Eq. 15 according to DD *Yin-Yang* inter-transformation if the dose is at dose 2n+1 (n = 1, 2, 3, ...) which is larger than the threshold of dose 2n if it does not damage membrane or cell compartments such as mitochondria, lysosomes, endoplasmic reticulum so that Eq. 15 is called BIMP 2n+1. BIMP n (n = 1, 2, 3, ...) has been supported by its successful application in the cellular level, animal model level and clinic level (Liu et al 1996 & 2003).

Yin and *yang* are antagonistic. Yova et al (1994) have shown that the effects of low intensity He-Ne laser irradiation at dose 2 and adrenalin on red blood cell deformability are antagonistic. Adrenalin can elevate the intracellular cAMP level, and belongs to *yin*. However, low intensity He-Ne laser irradiation can lower the intracellular cAMP level according to BIMP2, and belongs to *yang*. The observed result is due to the *yin-yang* antagonism. One has the same results when the HeLa cells were simultaneously irradiated with narrow-band red light at dose 2 and a wide-band cold light at dose 2 (Karu 1998). In these cases, the red light belongs to *yang*, and the cold light belongs to *yin* according to BIMP 2, and the DNA synthesis rate was near control level due to the *yin-yang* antagonism.

Karu (1998) has studied the stimulation of DNA synthesis in HeLa cells after consecutive irradiation with blue and red light at dose 2, and she found, the sequence 633 nm followed by 404 nm had no effect on DNA synthesis, but the sequence 404 nm followed by 633 nm stimulated it. DNA synthesis mediated by pathway 2 in HeLa cells belongs to *yang* according to Eq. 12, and the stimulation of DNA synthesis in HeLa cells is to reinforce *yang*. Karu's results (Karu 1998) shows that the sequence reinforcing *yang* followed by replenishing *yin* can not reinforce *yang* due to the *yin-yang* antagonism, only the sequence replenishing *yin* followed by reinforcing *yang* can reinforce *yang* due to *yin-yang* interdependence.

The objects of TCM are whole body, five *zang*s or six *fu*s. It can be extended to cells in view of our successful discussion. Cells are extensively and deeply studied in modern life science. Cellular TCM might be a discipline to bridge a gap between TCM and modern life sciences. As cellular model is a popular approach to study life science, cellular TCM suggests that TCM rules might hold for life science, which might become a new discipline of modern sciences. Of course, the further research should be done.

5. Photon TCM

In recent year, photonics has made marvelous progress, and the biological information function of photons was used in the diagnosis and treatment of TCM. At this point, Liu et al (2000) have put forward an interdiscipline of photonics and TCM, photon TCM (PTCM), which studies TCM, such as the diagnostics, therapeutics, indistinct disease theory, rehabilitation, health care and so forth, by using photonics. Photobiomodulation is one field of PTCM as it is discussed from cellular TCM in the previous section. Some treatments mediated by autonomic nervous system will be discussed in this section.

As parasympathetic subsystem (PSS) is activated more difficult than sympathetic subsystem (SS) is, and SS is developed more early than PSS according to develop biology, we have according to Eq. 6 and DD development discussed in the next section:

$$\text{SS belongs to } \textit{yang}\text{, and PSS belongs to } \textit{yin} \tag{16}$$

Eq. 3 holds since the interaction of monochromatic light with vision pigments is resonant. We then have according to DD *yin-yang* model:

$$\text{Hot color belongs to } \textit{yang}\text{, and cold color belongs to } \textit{yin} \tag{17}$$

For TCM chromophototherapy (Liu et al 1995), color vision and autonomic nervous system are weakly nonlinearly coupled in hypothalamus so that we have the color-autonomic-nervous-subsystem model (CAM) (Liu et al 1995) according to Eqs. 16 and 17 and DD *yin-yang* parallel principle cold color excites PSS, and hot color excites SS. For low intensity laser acupuncture, photobiomodulation on acupoint cells and autonomic nervous system are weakly nonlinearly coupled in hypothalamus through the corresponding meridian so that we have according to Eqs. 13, 14 and 16 and DD *yin-yang* parallel principle (n= 1, 2, 3, …) (Jiao et al 2003).

- At dose 2n-1, cold color excites SS, and hot color excites PSS
- At dose 2n, cold color excites PSS, and hot color excites SS

CAM and above models were supported by their successful applications (Liu et al 1995& 2000, Jiao et al 2003).

6. Sports Science

Modernized sports emphasize the product, the measurable results of competition. Some Eastern exercises such as Taiji Quan (Lan et al 2002) have not been Olympic sports yet. It might be because their exercise processes are so complex that their representation and modulation has been little studied. For example, the coaching process is vulnerable to differing social pressures and constraints, the humanistic nature of the coaching process remains a little understood and under researched area (Potrac et al 2000, Jones et al 2002). Hochstetler (2003) has examined the processes in sports. Further research will be done in this section in the viewpoint of DD *yin-yang* model.

Athlete performance can be studied from the viewpoint of DD *yin-yang* model so that the performance score of an athlete is suggested in this paper to consists of a set of the degree of difficulty (DD) of his performing processes: $\{DD_i\}$, and a set of the degree of *yin-yang* balance (DY) of these processes: $\{DY_i\}$. $\{DD_i\}$ have been used and can be modified from the viewpoint of DD *yin-yang* model. $\{DY_i\}$ are suggested for the first time, which might be the key point that some Eastern exercises such as Taiji Quan become Olympic sports.

System development is from *yang* to *yin* because the DD of its new process is higher than the ones of its old processes so that the process occurring more early is *yang* and the process occurring more lately is *yin*, which is in agreement with TCM development for TCM objects (Liu et al 2000 & 2002) so that it is called DD development. Motor process development is from *yang* to *yin* according to DD *yin-yang* model. One of Japanese motor learning programs (Li et al 1998) is according to DD development so that it is from *yang* to *yin*. However, the ordinary motor learning is from basic subprocesses to whole process since a motor process consists of basic subprocesses. The statistical test has shown that the effect of the Japanese way is significantly better than the ordinary way (Li et al 1998).there are many ways for TCM practitioner to learn from TCM, but the best way should be process training according to DD *yin-yang* parallel principle, i.e. apprenticeship education (Chen et al 2000). Athlete training is similar to TCM practitioner training so that its best way should be apprenticeship education, that is, general athletes learn from elite athletes through their coaches. Chinese training of some female sports such as table tennis is according to apprenticeship education: female athletes learn from elite male athletes, which is the secret that Chinese table tennis team is always at the top level in the world (Yang et al 2000).

7. Discussion

As TCM is understandable from modern science by means of process-specific time, it can be used to understand Western culture. Paralogy of postmodernism is easily understood by DD *yin-yang* balance since different developing theories have different *yin-yang* property. Popular vegetarianism is easily understood by *yin-yang* parallel principle since vegetable belongs to *yin*, and can be used to enforce *yin* processes such as PSS to help human being to develop. Since social development is from country to city so that country belongs to *yang* and city belongs to *yin* according to DD develop, citizen likes going to country and countrymen likes going to city in order to be in *yin-yang* balance, which enriches tourism. Of course, these explanations are very primary, and further research should be done.

Acknowledgements

The first two authors have been very pleased to receive Wallner's visiting Guangzhou in 2002 and thank him for his inviting to write this paper. This work has been supported by National Science Foundation of China (60178003, 60278012, 60478048&30470495), Team Project (20003061), Key Project (2001 1480) and General Project (20031526) of Guangdong Science Foundation, the 2000, 2001 and 2002 summer student research grants of the American Society of Lasers in Surgery and Medicine, a Chinese Scholar Visitorship of the Croucher Foundation, Visiting Foundation of State Key Laboratory of laser Technology in Huazhong University of Science and Technology, and Guangdong Qianbaishi Fellow Foundation (Q02087).

References

Akam, M. (1998). The *Yin* and *Yang* of Evo/Devo. In *Cell 92* (2): 153-155.

Alexandratou, E., Yova, D., Handris, P., Kletsas, D., & Loukas, S. (2002). Human fibroblast alterations induced by low power laser irradiation at the single cell level using confocal microscopy. In *Photoch Photobio Sci 1* (8): 547-552.

Allison, J. P., & Krummel, M. F. (1995). The *Yin* and *Yang* of T-cell costimulation. In *Science 270* (5238): 932-933.

Chen, P. J., & Wu, H. Z. (2000). Modal discussion of medical education in ancient China. In *Education of Chinese Medicine 19* (2): 47-48 (in Chinese).

Fan, Q. L. (2002). *Science of Prescription*. Shanghai: Shanghai TCM University Press.

Hunter, T. (1995). Protein-kinases and phosphatases – the yin and yang of protein-phosphorylation and signaling. In *Cell 80* (2): 225-236.

Jiao, J. L., Liu, T. C. Y, Li, C. Z., & Liu, S. H. (2003). Information biology of laser acupuncture. In *PROC SPIE 5254*: 131-138.

Jones, R. L., Armour, K. M., & Potrac, P. (2002). Understanding the coaching process: A framework for social analysis. In *QUEST 54* (1): 34-48.

Li, J., & Mao, Z. G. (1998). Motor learning and teaching of physical education. In *Chinese School Physical Education* (4): 73.

Karu, T. (1998). *The Science of Low-Power Laser Therapy*. Amsterdam: Gordon and Breach Science Publishers.

Karu, T. (2004). High-tech helps to estimate cellular mechanisms of low power laser therapy. In *Lasers Surg Med 34* (4): 298-299.

King, L. B., & Monroe, J. G. (2001). Immunology – B cell receptor rehabilitation – Pausing to reflect. In *Science 291* (5508): 1503-1505.

Ko, K. M., Mak, D. H. F., Chiu, P. Y., & Poon, M. K. T. (2004). Pharmacological basis of ›*Yang*-invigoration‹ in Chinese medicine. In *Trends Pharmacol Sci 25* (1): 3-6.La Thangue, N. B. (2003). The *yin* and *yang* of E2F-1: balancing life and death. In *Nat Cell Biol 5* (7): 587-589.

Liu, C. Y., Liao, C. J., & Liu, S. H. (1995). Theoretical research on color indirect effects. In *Proc SPIE 2393*: 346-356.

Liu, S. H., Liu, T. C. Y., Li, Y., & Meng, Y. Y. (2000). Introduction to photon traditional Chinese medicine. In *Proc SPIE 4224*: 179-185
Liu, T. C. Y., Gao, Y. Q., & Liu, S. H. (1996). Light-cell interaction: quasi-hormone model and time theory. In *Proc SPIE 2887*: 140-151.
Liu, T. C. Y., Duan, R., Li, Y. & Cai, X. W. (2002). Traditional Chinese medicine on the effects of low intensity laser irradiation on cells. In *Proc SPIE 4536*: 137-140.
Liu, T. C. Y., Jiao J. L., Duan, R., Li Yan, Yeung, Y. Y., & Liu, S. H. (2003). Membrane mechanism of low intensity laser biostimulation on a cell. In Simunovic Z (ed.), *Lasers in Medicine, Surgery and Dentistry. Croatia: European Medical Laser Association.* 83-105.
Lan, C., Lai, J. S., & Chen, S. Y. (2002). Tai Chi Chuan: an ancient wisdom on exercise and health promotion. In *Sports Med 32*(4): 217-24.
Neville, R. (1977). Wang Yang-Ming's ›Inquiry on the Great Learning‹. In *Process Studies 7*(4): 217-237.
Ou, B. X., Huang, D. J., Hampschl-Woodill, M., & Flanagan, J. A. (2003). When east meets west: the relationship between *yin-yang* and antioxidation-oxidation. In *FASEB J 17* (2): 127-129.
Potrac, P., Brewer, C., Jones, R., Armour, K., & Hoff, J. (2000). Toward a holistic understanding of the coaching process. In *QUEST 52* (2): 186-199.
Shuai, X. (1992). *Fundamentals of Traditional Chinese Medicine*. Beijing: Foreign Languages Press.
Tan, Y. H. (1993). *Yin* and *yang* of phosphorylation in cytokine signaling. In *Science 262* (5132): 376-377.Tunér, J., & Hode, L. (1999). *Low Level Laser Therapy*. Graengesberg: Prima Books in Sweden AB.
Wang, F., Chen, T. S., Xing, D., Wang, J. J., & Wu, Y. X. (2005). Measuring dynamics of caspase-3 activity in living cells using FRET technique during apoptosis induced by high fluence low-power laser irradiation. In *Lasers Surg Med 36*(1): 2-7.
Wang, J., Zhang, L. G, & Meng, S. H. (2001). Chemical, pharmacological and organizational considerations of combination Chinese medicines. In *J Chin Materia Medica 26*: 799–804.
Whitehead, A. N. (1978). *Process and Reality*. New York: Free Press.
Xu, G. (1996). *Chinese Herbal Medicine*. Vermilion: London.
Yang, S., & Zhang, X. (2000). Scientific chanrateristics of Chinese table tennis trainning. In *Sports Science 20* (2): 30-33 (in Chinese).
Yova, D., Haritou, M., & Koutsouris, D. (1994). Antagonistic effects of epinephrine and helium-neon (He-Ne) laser irradiation on red blood cells deformability. In *Clinical Hemorheology 14* (3): 369-378.
Zhang, Y. O., Song, S. P., Fong, C. C., Tsang, C. H., Yang, Z., & Yang, M. S. (2003). CDNA microarray analysis of gene expression profiles in human fibroblast cells irradiated with red light. In *J Invest Dermato 120* (5): 849-857.

Susanne Weigelin-Schwiedrzik

Recent PRC Scholarship on Liang Qichao and the Globalization of the Research on Modern Chinese History

Historiography and globalization

The writing of Chinese history has so far been split into an inner and an outer perspective. Chinese historians have written their histories without referring to what historians write about Chinese history from outside China, and historians from outside China tend to write their histories by referring directly to primary sources, regarding the Chinese discourse on Chinese history more as a field of political debate than of sound scholarship. This is not to say that there are not hidden influences that indirectly guide the respective views on Chinese history, and, of course, I am not trying to deny that western concepts of history writing have been discussed by Chinese historians and integrated into their concepts of Chinese history. Vice versa, Western historians have always been dependent on the scholarly production of Chinese historians, especially on new compilations of primary sources, but also, though to a lesser degree, on the master narrative of Chinese history as written by Chinese historians. But the inner and the outer perspectives on Chinese history have not yet developed to form a common field of discourse in which both sides of the spectrum respect each other as equally equipped to pursue the common task of writing Chinese history. That is why we seldom encounter references to Chinese secondary sources in Western publications on Chinese history, and even more seldom do we find Chinese historians referring to Western scholarship in their writings on Chinese history. There are rare exceptions from this rule, and these exceptions seem to be more obvious in recent publications on Chinese history than in former years. But not only in China does the writing of history lag behind the process of globalization. History writing and identity building is closely linked to each other, and the process of identity building is based on defining in group and out group which with necessity implies the difference of inner and outer perspectives. At the same time, the writing of history is part and parcel of the process of nation building, a process which some among us see as having reached its limits with the world going through a phase of globalization.

If globalization is more than overcoming national boundaries with regard to the exchange of goods and services, it will lead to a restructuring of the intellectual discourse and the hierarchy of the field accompanying it. Taking the PRC as an example, we observe that it was the field of literary production that internationalized itself at a pretty early stage after the 1978 decision on reform and opening in China. Writers soon realized that international acclaim was instrumental in enhancing their position in the Chinese field in terms of the artistic freedom they enjoyed, but also with regard to their social status and economic situation. With awarding the Nobel Prize to Gao Xingjian the international field of literary production has accepted Chinese literature as a ›global player‹, and the sometimes over critical reaction against this decision shows that Chinese literature even though it still occupies a minor position in the international literary field has at least grown to become a disturbing factor on the world market of literary production.

If compared to literature, the field of historiography is still pretty much confined to the boundaries of the nation state. I would take the risk to say that in most countries of the world (and the US obviously is one of the exceptions) the number of academic historians writing the history of their own nation by far outgrows the number of those working on the history of foreign countries. Except for extreme rare cases the position in the scholarly field of those historians working on the histories of their respective countries is much higher than those doing research on other parts of the world. This is especially true for the PRC for quite obvious reasons: Even though the role of Sino-Marxism is not as prominent as it used to be, the highest positions in the field of Chinese historians are still occupied by a generation of historiographers deeply influenced by Marxism and unable or unwilling to leave historical and dialectical materialism behind as the foundation of their *weltanschauung;* the ability to converse and write in foreign languages is still and even among the younger generation of Chinese historians not developed to a point where they can easily voice their opinions internationally; and last but not least, the central position of historiography within the debate on politics and morale which history writing has occupied traditionally has lead historians in the PRC to believe that giving up their role as consultants and censors of the political elite would inevitably lead to an extreme downgrading of their social status as well as to a marginalization of their discipline (For further explorations into this field see: Bourdieu 1992, Cohen 1984, Weigelin-Schwiedrzik 1999, Hockx 1999). Joining the international field of historiography carries the risk of loosing the ear of those leading politicians in China still waiting for history writing to play a role in the process of nation building.

In this paper, I would like to discuss the example of recent PRC scholarship on one of China's most prominent 20th century scholars Liang Qichao in the context of globalizing the historical discipline. The historiography on Liang Qichao seems especially apt at going about this undertaking because of three reasons: First of all, we can observe an upsurge of scholarly writings about Liang Qichao in the PRC. Some of these publications refer more openly than others to non-Chinese sources. Mainstream historians have shown in their recent discussions of Liang Qichao that they are aware of the international scholarly debate on Liang. This gives us the chance to understand the way PRC scholars discuss and use non-Chinese historiography. On the top of that, Liang Qichao's own writings on historiography can be understood not only as an early attempt to link historiography to nation building, but also as a maybe too early attempt at overcoming the boundaries of nation state historiography. It is interesting to see that neither Liang's notions on historiography as propelled in his early writings nor the arguments as proposed in his later writings even though highly influential at the time of their first publication seem to have had a long lasting effect on the concept of history writing in China. In the last part of my paper I would therefore like to discuss Liang Qichao in the context of PRC historiography asking for the reasons why even today he cannot serve as a model with the help of which to define the rules of the game in the globalizing historiographical field.

Cui Zhihai on Levenson, Zhang Hao and Huang Kewu

To my knowledge, Cui Zhihai[1] is the first PRC scholar having dedicated an article to the discussion on the outer perspective on Liang Qichao (Cui Zhihai 2000). He starts out with Joseph R. Levenson's book *Liang Ch'i-ch'ao and the Mind of Modern China* (Levenson 1959) which has been available in a Chinese edition by Sichuan Renmin Chubanshe since 1986, a translation that he characterizes as »not ideal« (Cui Zhihai 2000,fn.1, p.483). Based on his reading of the English edition, he comes up with several criticisms of Levenson's approach to Liang Qichao.[2]

1 Cui Zhihai is professor at the Institute for Modern History (Jindaishi Yanjiusuo) of the Academy for Social Sciences in Beijing. In 1998 he spent a sabbatical at the Center for Chinese Studies at the University of California, Berkeley.

2 Liang Qichao has attracted the attention of Chinese intellectuals and scholars from the West at least since the nineteen fifties. Liang was a scholar trained in the traditional educational system of China, a disciple of Kang Youwei and together with him one of the proponents of the 1898 reform movement. As this movement met with the resistance of those factions inside the Qing court who obeyed to Ci Xi, Liang was forced to leave China and lived in Japan for the next years to come. From there he wrote an enormous amount of articles transferring Western knowledge from Japan to China. As part of this process, he introduced most of today's vocabulary in the fields of social sciences and politics into the modern Chinese vernacular and greatly influenced the Chinese conception of the modern state and the modern nation. After a long trip to Europe in the aftermath of WW I, Liang seems to have lost his hope. He no longer believed that China could overcome her difficulties by learning from the West. Instead he started dong research on the respective strengths and weaknesses of the Eastern and the Western traditions trying to convince his readers of the necessity to develop a world culture based on the strengths of different civilizations. Joseph R. Levenson wrote his book on Liang in the nineteen fifties and has since then been a major challenge to anyone writing on Liang from an outside perspective. Zhang Hao followed into his steps, but at the same time tried to overcome the strictly »Western« perspective Levenson had shown in his book, drawing on a methodology which is called

First of all, he reproaches Levenson of a »Eurocentrism« underlying his argument on the tension between history and value[3] as the main explanation for Liang's intellectual development. To Cui Zhihai, Levenson's argument is rooted in an understanding of Western civilization and Chinese tradition as fundamentally opposed to each other. As a consequence of this, he is unable to discover internal possibilities of change and revival. He regards any attempt to cling to Chinese tradition as irrational and emotional while looking for help and stimulus from the outside is unquestionably rational and adequate. This notion, according to Cui, underestimates the plurality and vitality of Chinese tradition as well as the internal differences within the Western civilization, reflecting a mechanistic view on the dichotomy of »tradition versus modernity« (Cui Zhihai 2000, p.487). Due to Levenson's overstressing the incompatibility of Western civilization with Chinese tradition, he cannot understand Liang's attempt to reconcile the two in his later writings, interpreting them rather unilaterally as a sign of Liang Qichao overcoming his alienation from Chinese tradition in his last phase of intellectual development (Cui Zhihai 2000, p.488).

Another consequence of Levenson's mechanistic juxtaposition of ›tradition‹ and ›modernity‹ is his inability to make out an inner logic to Liang Qichao's sometimes self contradicting arguments on democracy, war, the role of the individual or the hero in history etc. To see all this as a reflection of Liang Qichao's inner tension between history and value does not convince Cui. He would rather like to view Liang mainly as a propagandist willing to reformulate his argument if needed to reach the aim he was out to reach (Cui Zhihai 2000, p.489). »All in all, the articles Liang Qichao wrote in his capacity as a propagandist are not works he published as the result of profound reflection, this is something we have to keep in mind when analyzing Liang Qichao's thought.« (Cui Zhihai 2000, p.490). Nevertheless, Cui recommends Levenson's book as a main contribution of Western historiography on Liang Qichao giving applause especially to Levenson's introducing the categories of ›culturalism‹ versus ›nationalism‹[4]. Cui believes that these two categories cannot only help to understand the ever changing nature of Liang Qichao's thought, but are also instrumental in analyzing a whole range of ques-

---

»sino-centric«. Huang Kewu is a scholar from Taiwan who as his critic Cui Zhihai belongs to a younger generation shouldering the task of rewriting 20th century Chinese history.

3 For Levenson, the changes in Liang Qichao's thought are due to a tension between history and value »Every man has an emotional commitment to history and an intellectual commitment to value, and he tries to make these commitments coincide« (Levenson, Confucian China and its Modern Fate, p.1).

4 According to Levenson, the kind of nationalism proposed by Liang Qichao is based on a notion of cultural unity strongly influenced by the *tianxia* conception of the Chinese empire. Whoever agrees to the Chinese cultural values is part of the nation.

tions related to the discussion of Western ideas in the context of the intellectual debate in early 20th century China (Cui Zhihai 2000, p.490).

Cui regards Zhang Hao's book *Liang Ch'i-ch'ao and Intellectual Transition in China, 1896-1907* (Chang Hao 1971) which he himself translated into Chinese together with Ge Fuping in 1993 (Cui Zhihai 2000, fn.1, p.491) as an indirect critique of Levenson's work. This is shown, according to Cui, mainly by Zhang Hao (i.e. Chang Hao) repudiating the dichotomy of tradition versus modernity and by putting the ›challenge and response‹ paradigm[5] aside (Cui Zhihai 2000, p.491). But, what seems to be even more important to Cui, is the fact that Zhang Hao's book overcomes Levenson's Eurocentrism and instead prefers a ›China centered approach‹ which stresses internal factors of development instead of external challenges (Cui Zhihai 2000, p.491). Besides these fundamental differences, Cui also sees Zhang Hao overcoming Levenson by showing more respect and understanding for Liang's rapid change of ideas interpreting this tendency not so much as a lack of ability to rationally cope with the intrusion of Western ideas but as due to an inherent logic of Liang's thought (Cui Zhihai 2000, p.496). Comparing the two publications, Cui comes to the conclusion that Zhang Hao's book is not as refreshing and inspiring as Levenson's, but »Zhang Hao's point of view is no doubt more objective, all embracing and closer to the facts than Levenson's« (Cui Zhihai 2000, p.498).

Nevertheless, Cui also comes up with a number of criticisms regarding Zhang Hao's interpretation of Liang Qichao's development. First of all he deplores a lack of historical and political context in Zhang's approach to Liang characterizing Zhang's interpretations as »moving from thought to thought« (Cui Zhihai 2000, p.499). But while applauding Zhang's sense of understanding for Liang Cui also criticizes Zhang's putting too much stress on the continuity in Liang's thought. Even though Zhang takes great pain in analyzing the influence of Western thought on Liang he does not pay due attention to the Japanese influence which, according to Cui, should not be overlooked. Liang spent so many years in Japan and not only read a wide variety of Japanese books on Western learning but – according to Cui – got in contact with Western thought through the interpretations inherent in the Japanese translations (Cui Zhihai 2000, p.500-501). Finally, Cui Zhihai deplores Zhang's concentration on the period between 1896 and 1907. Cui is neither convinced by the argument saying that Liang Qichao was the central thinker of the years 1896 to 1907 (Cui Zhihai 2000, p.502), nor does he follow Zhang in arguing that the period between 1896 and 1907 could be more important

5 The so called ›challenge and response paradigm‹ has been the basis of interpreting China's urge for modernity. According to this paradigm, there was no indigenous tendency toward modernization in China before the intrusion of the West. China's modernization can therefore only be conceived as a response to the challenges set by the West.

than the May Fourth Movement (Cui Zhihai 2000, p.503). These two criticisms lead him to repudiate Zhang of not having understood the importance of Liang's later development and for not having been able to give a full account of the complexity of Liang's thought (Cui Zhihai 2000, p.503).

In the last part of his article, Cui Zhihai turns to Huang Kewu's book *A rejected choice: A study of Liang Qichao's accomodative thinking* published in Taiwan in 1994 (Huang Kewu 1994). This book poses the biggest challenge to Cui Zhihai as it focuses on the question of reform and revolution in Liang's thought and thus takes up a topic, which touches a fundamental paradigm of PRC historiography[6]. Huang Kewu criticizes the tendency of mainstream research on Chinese modern history to support the so called ›classical faction‹ with its demand for fundamental and rapid change based on a broad and idealistic vision of the future and downgrade the step by step pragmatic approach to social change as propagated by the so called ›historical faction‹. According to Cui, Huang Kewu uses Liang Qichao's thought as a model for an alternative strategy of change in China. According to Cui, Huang argues in favor of rewriting modern Chinese history demanding a change of paradigm. He no longer believes that the decision for revolutionary change was unquestionably correct, but tries to argue in favor of reform as the right solution for China's problems. Cui strongly opposes this strategy of Huang Kewu's on two grounds: First of all, he comes up with historical evidence showing that the opposition between reform and revolution was not as fierce in the early decades of the 20th century as Huang would like his readers to believe. According to Cui both factions were basically pragmatic in their strategic choices. The difference between reform and revolution was not due to a difference of *weltanschauung,* but rather a consequence of the two factions assessing the situation in China differently and therefore coming up with different strategies of change. In both cases, the choices the respective factions took were based on ›reality‹ and not on a visionary belief (Cui Zhihai 2000, p.510-512).

Secondly, Cui strongly opposes Huang's criticism of the Xinhai Revolution based on Liang Qichao's writings. Cui not only doubts that Liang's writings were as influential as Huang thinks them to be, he also criticizes Huang for interpreting Liang unilaterally. Even though Liang strongly opposed revolution before 1911 Cui rejects the possibility to use Liang's writings as a total repudiation of the Xinhai Revolution. Liang himself was more adaptable to the results of the revolution than his earlier articles would one expect him to be (Cui Zhihai 2000, p.512-514). To sum up his arguments against Huang's interpretation Cui reproaches Huang of trying to replace the ›revolution paradigm‹ by the ›modernization paradigm‹

6 Conventional PRC historiography argues that reform of the dynastic system could not help China to meet the challenges of Western intrusion. The Revolution of 1911, although deficient, serves as an example and starting point for a long time period of revolution leading eventually to the founding of the PRC in 1949.

which according to Cui is a step back towards a renewed form of Eurocentrism (Cui Zhihai 2000, p.515).

Cui Zhihai rounds up his discussion of non-PRC research on Liang Qichao by voicing his fundamental criticism of the outer perspective on Chinese history. His first step is to ask the question of how to combine philosophy and history. He demands that historians should refrain from forcing their philosophy on history and should instead see history as a testing ground for the validity of philosophical ideas. By this Cui implies that some of the research on Liang Qichao is too strongly shaped by theoretical prejudices, and he cites Paul Cohen with his criticism of Western research on Chinese history as a strong support for his argument (Cohen 1999). Quite clearly this argument is mainly directed against Levenson and his long lasting effect on the outer perspective research on Liang Qichao. In order to get rid of the Levenson shadow (Cui Zhihai 2000, p.521), Cui supposes to step into new fields of research on Liang. Instead of reinterpreting the same articles time and again, he suggests that researchers should pay more attention to Liang's ideas on China's economic development (Cui Zhihai 2000, p.521) and on his scholarly works rather than his political essays. On the top of that, he reiterates his disappointment about researchers focusing on Liang's early thought rather than trying to understand his later development. »All in all, the research on Liang Qichao's thought as pursued outside China should leave Levenson behind, because time has come to write a book covering the whole life and thought of Liang Qichao with all his works.« (Cui Zhihai 2000, p.522)

Cui Zhihai's in depth review of the Liang Qichao research from an outer perspective tells us a lot about his intentions regarding both the relationship between inner and outer perspectives in the research of modern Chinese history and the argument he wants to make about Liang Qichao. Cui defines the inner perspective as the PRC perspective and selects with Levenson a non-Chinese historian, with Zhang Hao a Sino-American and with Huang Kewu a historian from Taiwan to make clear what he thinks the different components of the outer perspective could be. Although he openly addresses the outer perspective as »*haiwai*« or non-Chinese he does not explicitly refer to the difference between inner and outer perspectives. This together with the fact that he takes the pain to write this lengthy review which in the context of PRC historiography is quite an unnecessary undertaking in terms of career planning shows that he is aimed at internationalizing the PRC discourse on Liang Qichao. He can do this without greater risks because even though he clearly transgresses the boundaries as set by conventional PRC historiography his detailed criticisms show that his notion of internationalization is based on concepts which do not contradict conventional historiography in the PRC. In Levenson's and Huang Kewu's cases, the outer perspective is according to Cui characterized by a pre-existent theoretical concept in which Liang only serves as an example for proving the validity of the theory. While this is the argument that Western historians usually come up with when criticizing

PRC historiography it is now used against themselves implying that the outer perspective is not based on the thorough study of primary sources and ›historical facts‹. Instead it selects from the variety of Liang's writings only those that fit into the theoretical concept. Both Levenson and Huang Kewu are being criticized for Eurocentrism as the basis of their theoretical concepts with Eurocentrism being responsible for their inability to understand the specifics of the Chinese historical development. For Cui, Eurocentrism is the theoretical conception that undermines any attempt to look at Liang Qichao from an ›objective‹ and ›all embracing‹ point of view which – if put the other way round – means that only those who look at China from a Chinese perspective can avoid forcing theories on the facts and thereby giving a truthful picture of history. Alas, this turn around of arguments falls short of its brave intentions when it falls into the traps of paradigms seemingly of anti-colonial origin and therefore beyond scrutiny.

This is especially true for the revolution paradigm that Huang Kewu is trying to overcome in his book on Liang Qichao. For Cui, the revolution paradigm is unquestionable and cannot be counted among those theories that are forced on Chinese history as it is not a pre existent theoretical concept but a historical fact. But, as a matter of fact, for Cui it is more than a fact, it is his basic belief that China could not be rescued from colonial exploitation and destruction without restructuring its society by means of revolution. Cui does, of course, not admit, that writing the chronology of Chinese revolutions in the 20th century and thus acknowledging revolution as a fact of modern Chinese history is not entirely the same as his belief in the necessity of revolution. Consequently, he finds his own argument against Huang seeing revolution as the focus of China's tragedy in the 20th century totally convincing. While the outer perspective on modern Chinese history would regard the revolution paradigm just as theoretical as the modernization paradigm, Cui argues that the necessity of revolution is inherent in 20th century Chinese history and therefore a theory that is extracted from the facts while the Eurocentrism of the outer perspective is a theory pre-existent to the facts.

The revolution paradigm is part of the specifics of the historical development in 20th century China, which again can only be understood by those able to see this development as different if compared to the rest of the world. Whoever wants to participate in the Chinese discourse on Chinese history has to submit to the idea of the particularity of historical development in China, this is what Cui's criticism of Levenson and Huang Kewu is all about. And by quoting Paul Cohen Cui shows that he is aware of the fact that there are historians outside China willing to submit to this precondition.

Quite clearly Zhang Hao is the book that Cui likes the best, and the reason for this is that Zhang Hao takes a ›China centered approach‹ based on »imaginative participation« (Cui Zhihai 2000, p.491). Thus Zhang Hao, in spite of the criticism Cui voices with regard to his book can serve as a positive example of how the outer perspective on Chinese history can conform to the rules of the game as preferred by Cui Zhihai. These rules imply that Chinese history can only be understood ›from a Chinese perspective‹ at the center of which stands the notion of the particularity of historical development in China. This methodology is based on the necessity to develop theories about this development from ›within‹ China derived from the facts of Chinese history. It is opposed to the methodology of applying theories of Western origin to Chinese history.

Cui Zhihai's selection of Western scholarship on Liang Qichao might be incidental and should therefore not lead to speculations why he left out some and preferred others. Nevertheless, it seems quite implausible to assume that he does not know Tang Xiaobing's book on Liang Qichao (Tang Xiaobing 1996). The reason why Tang Xiaobing's *Global Space and the Nationalist Discourse of Modernity – The Historical Thinking of Liang Qichao* does not show up in Cui's review is more than coincidence, as it seems to me. If Cui is out to define the rules of the game for internationalizing the discourse on Liang Qichao he inevitably comes across the problem of defining the position of the younger generation of PRC historians having left the country to pursue their research from outside the PRC. These historians are ›in‹ and ›out‹ at the same time and could play a major role in internationalizing the discourse on Chinese history. As a matter of fact, they are in an even better position to attract international attention for Chinese scholarship than those historians publishing in the PRC. Maybe this is the reason why it seems wise for Cui Zhihai to meet them with disregard instead of debating openly with them.

Their strategy of internationalization is opposite to what Cui is aiming at: They submit to the rules of the game as set outside China, they accept Western theories as the starting point of their research and do not necessarily submit to the notion of China's particularity. Looking at it from this perspective, the field of internationalization is already under fierce contention with two different strategies on the side of the younger generation of Chinese historians trying to set the standards: Chinese historians from outside the PRC want to dominate the field by internationalizing the writing of Chinese history moving from West to East, while PRC historians as Cui Zhihai try to define the rules of the game going form East to West.

At this point the problem of hierarchy in the international field meets with the problem of a future hierarchization of the historical field in the PRC. That is why at the same time Cui is trying to define the rules of the game for the international discourse on Chinese historiography he is out to define a profile for PRC historiography on Liang Qichao. He clearly diverts from mainstream PRC historiography on Liang Qichao by stressing Liang's qualities as a scholar, a politician and a propagandist, by downgrading the importance of Liang's opposition against the revolution of 1911 and by stressing the value of Liang Qichao's writings after 1919 as opposed to the critique of most PRC historians with regard to Liang's reactionary tendencies in his later development.

Recent PRC scholarship on Liang Qichao's historical theory and methodology

The history of Chinese historiography has recently become a major field of research among the younger generation of PRC historians (see also Zhang Yanqian and Yu Zhiguo 1996, He Yongchuan 1984, Wu Jun 2001, p.2-5). The focus of their interest is the historiography of early Chinese modernity, and Liang Qichao has attracted quite some attention as he is seen as standing right at the turning point from traditional to modern historiographical thinking. However, the interest in Liang is pretty much confined to academic circles in the PRC, the generally interested reader of Chinese history seems to have forgotten him. Nevertheless, statistics testify to some 360 articles and 20 books (this information was given to me by Li Hongyan, Chinese Academy of Social Sciences; for the most important book length publications see: Li Xisuo and Yuan Qing 1993; Geng Yunzhi and Cui Zhihai 1994; Chen Qitai 1997; Chen Pengming 1999; Huang Minlan 1999) that have been published in the PRC between 1986 and 2001.

Liang Qichao is so complicated and multi-facetted a personality that the research on him has developed to form a field of discourse in which cultural conservatism is voiced just as frequently as progressive liberalism (for the PRC discussion on the question of cultural conservatism see among others: Li Shenzhi 1998, Hu Sheng 1995). Liang can be fitted into different frames of thought: he can be interpreted as having understood in the course of his intellectual development that Western thought is of no help for China; but at the same time, he can also be seen as the model for a 20th century Chinese intellectual open to introducing Western thought as the basis of modernization in China (Huang Minlan 1999, p.359).

Up until the 1990s, PRC historians pretty much agreed on their basic assumptions about Liang Qichao. Their research was guided by Sino-Marxism leading them to a slightly positive evaluation of Liang's earlier repudiation of Chinese tradition, especially during the years before the 1911 Revolution. Research was concentrated on Liang's writings about traditional Chinese historiography, while his later writings reflecting Liang's doubts about the possibility to objectively assess historical development were rejected for their idealistic, unscientific and reactionary tendencies. Representative of this strain of arguments is Bai Shouyi's assessment published in 1999:

»Liang Qichao's academic interests are broad, but generally speaking suffer from superficiality. From time to time he came up with interesting insights about historiography, yet seldom went into depth, but kept changing his ideas. To be superficial and ever changing is the particularity of his scholarship. And very often these changes moved him backwards, which tells us that he had not really understood some of his earlier insights. [...] Liang Qichao did not necessarily take a very serious attitude towards his own arguments concerning historiography, even towards important ones, which is why he later on did not mind changing them. [...] Liang Qichao's historiographical thinking is located at the borderline between feudal and bourgeois historiography, it reflects the class character of the landlord and bourgeois classes [...]. In his earlier phase, his historiographical thinking had some progressiveness to it, but could not exert any influence. Later on, as times progressed, he moved on in the opposite direction and threw all the progressive things away, going step by step backwards. After May 4th he became in what he said and what he did an enemy of Marxism. Nevertheless, his historiographical thinking was quite representative and influenced some people.« (Bai Shouyi 1999, p.298-300)

To carefully praise Liang's early activities (Jiang Ling, Zou Guanxiu and Guo Jianpo 1992, Gong Guoqing 1995) and to criticize Liang for his backward tendency of intellectual development is still quite frequently seen in recent publications (Li Yuhua 1986, Bing Zhangchu 1995). Historians deplore Liang rapidly changing his ideas and the fact that he came out with a lot of brilliant insights without ever developing them into a coherent body of scholarly research (Wu Huaiqi 1996, p.340). Nevertheless, there are some articles which try to understand Liang's later development without labeling him as reactionary. Even though the introduction of Marxism-Lennism is still regarded as the major achievement of the May 4th period, authors like Ma Shaohua acknowledge much to the contrary of earlier research on Liang that his later contributions to historiographical methodology were instrumental in overcoming the mechanistic world view of the evolution theory and to modernizing historical research by introducing positivism. In his writings on historical theory and methodology, so the argument goes, Liang did not only express his doubts about evolution theory as the basis of historical interpretation, he also questioned the validity of causality as the basis of historical explanation and denied the possibility to derive laws and regularities from the research of history. While Ma as other authors regret that Liang lost his confidence in establishing the truth about history, he interprets this not so much as a sign of growing reactionary tendencies but as an attempt to get rid of historical determinism and to correctly assess the role of the individual in history (Ma Shaohua 2001, about the same opinion is expressed by Wu Jun 2001, p.91, for an even more positive assessment of Liang's contributions to the theory of historiography see Wang Yeyang 1994).

Geng Yunzhi and Cui Zhihai do not go so far in rehabilitating the late Liang Qichao. They trace back his doubts about causality and historical laws to the influence of Bergson and Rieckert which made Liang overlook that people's minds were shaped by the conditions under which they develop. While rejecting this tendency of Liang Qichao (calling it »totally wrong«, Geng Yunzhi and Cui Zhihai 1994, p.423, Wu Jun speaks of »total nonsense«, Wu Jun 2001, p.91) they appraise Liang for having seen the necessity to differentiate between humanities and natural sciences at a very early stage (Geng Yunzhi and Cui Zhihai 1994, p.423). Geng Yunzhi and Cui Zhihai even go so far as to criticize the mechanistic worldview of materialism dominant at the time and see Liang much more positively in comparison to mainstream thought of his times.

Another interesting topic of discussion, which has come up lately is focused on Liang's attitude towards positivism. While some authors tend to interpret his later ideas as a sign of historical relativism opposed to positivism, others stress the fact that Liang had from his first explorations into historiography on, especially during his exile in Japan, already come in touch with positivism. This implies that his later publications on historiography have in fact to be seen in the continuity of his earlier writings admitting that his article on *The Research Method of Chinese History* (Liang Qichao 1923) is much more outspoken in its support for the school of positivism (Wang Dong 2001). Zhang Shuxue, on the contrary, argues that Liang's articles of the twenties reflect his opposition to the school of positivists. According to this author, Liang Qichao was the head of a scholarly network favoring historical relativism (Zhang Shuxue 2000).

The Japanese influence on Liang's thought, which had long been neglected by PRC historians has lately gained some importance. In March of 2001, a Chinese translation of a Japanese conference volume on Liang Qichao was published (Hazama 2001), and several articles discuss the Japanese factor in Liang's intellectual development. Zhang Mingfu argues pretty much on the same line as Matsuo that most of what Liang wrote during his time in exile was not more than a summary of what he had read in Japanese books and he explicitly tries to show this for Liang's famous article on the *New Historiography* (Liang Qichao 1902). Zhang comes to the conclusion that most of what has up to now been attributed to Liang's genius should be seen as a mere copy or translation of what he had read in Japan (Zhang Mingfu 2001, Jiang Jun 1993, Matsuo 2001; for a less radical view see: Jiao Runming 1996). Liang was good in destroying the past, but not creative enough to invent the future.

Another topic relevant for the research on Liang's historical thinking is the influence of Buddhism on his intellectual development. Authors taking up this topic generally agree that Buddhism had a deep and long lasting influence on Liang, but became more important in his later years when Liang started voicing his doubts about the concept of causality and gradually replaced it by the concept of interrelatedness and mutual dependence. Liang's knowledge of Buddhism is regarded as elaborate and sophisticated exerting its influence also on his alienation from evolution theory (Tian Xiang 1993, Gao Zhennong 1982).

To sum up, PRC scholarship on Liang Qichao has become much more diverse and less conventionalized than it used to be in earlier years. Nevertheless, the topics that had been discussed in earlier high-tides of Liang Qichao research, especially in the 1960s and the 1980s, still dominate the discussion, and even though the publications are generally based on a closer reading of Liang's works than in earlier years, only very few authors tend to question the basic assumptions as reiterated by Bai Shouyi in his 1999 statement (Bai Shouyi 1999). They have problems in regarding Liang as a positive factor in 20th century Chinese history of ideas, as they cannot come to grips with his habit of rapidly changing ideas as well as with his doubts regarding the objectivity of historical research. Liang Qichao does not fit into the canon of the historical development as defined by official historiography in the PRC, he is no supporter of the Xinhai Revolution, nor does he easily fit into the spectrum of May 4th intellectuals, he is outspoken in his critique of traditional Chinese historiography and the founder of the so called ›new historiography‹, but he does not fit into the model of bourgeois intellectuals radicalizing themselves to eventually become fellow travelers of the Communists. Thus he cannot be used to serve any of the models PRC historiography has established so far for the overall historical as well as individual development. This it what makes it difficult for PRC historians to come to a positive assessment of his contributions to early 20th century Chinese discourse and inhibits them from developing the kind of ›imaginative participation‹ that Cui likes about Zhang Hao's book (Cui Zhihai 2000).

Concerning the above raised question of globalizing historical scholarship on 20th century Chinese history, the fact that up to now most of the research on Liang Qichao still tackles with questions asked by official historiography in the PRC shows that the historiographical field these historians have in mind is still mostly confined to the PRC. Even though in some cases we do find references to Levenson's ›history and value‹ paradigm non-Chinese scholarship is usually not discussed and the questions PRC historians deal with are those questions that have for long dominated the PRC discourse on Liang Qichao.

Two exceptions from the rule

There are very few publications that do not follow the mainstream of Liang Qichao scholarship as introduced above. The two cases I would like to discuss here are both publications aimed at rereading ›classical‹ Liang Qichao texts on historiography. Huang Minlan published an article prior to her well known book length publication on Liang Qichao (Huang Minlan 1999) under the title of *The True Significance of Liang Qichao's ›New Historiography‹ and Historiographical Misinterpretations* (Huang Minlan 1994). For Huang Minlan the much discussed text *New Historiography* is a political pamphlet and not a scholarly publication on theories and methodologies of historiography. The main topics Liang is dealing with in this text are, according to Huang Minlan, questions concerning the legitimacy of political power structures, the relationship between state and government, between nation and individual as well as between culture and scholarship on the one hand and the interests of the nation on the other. The main issue Liang is interested in is the issue of how to understand the ascent and descent of a nation and the kind of responsibility intellectuals as well as normal citizens have to burden in the development of a nation. For Huang, Liang Qichao only uses the critique of traditional Chinese historiography to propel his ideas, but as historiography plays a key role in building the nation, it is quite plausible for him to develop his ideas on a future political order in China in the context of criticizing traditional Chinese historiography. Vice versa, discussing Western ideas on historiography means using it in order to reject the kind of autocratic regime still prevailing in China at the time, which is why, according to Huang, he mostly praises Western historiography for its support to the process of nation building and democratization. Thus in writing his *New Historiography* he in fact is discussing the failure of the 1898 reform movement and the future possibilities for China to enhance its internal coherence and international status by overcoming the autocratic dynastic order.

To Huang Minlan, Liang's critique of traditional Chinese historiography serving the needs of the dynastic order is in effect a critique of the traditional Chinese political system lacking the support of the people. With traditional historiography not differentiating between state and government and by treating the state as the property of the ruler it disguises the true essence of the autocratic regime. Thus Liang Qichao's praise of Western historiography is focused on praising democracy as the only means to legitimize political power on the grounds of its support by the people. Only a nation state with a democratic order is a strong nation state. But China, in effect, is not only ruled by an autocratic regime lacking the kind of legitimacy it needs in order to be strong, the people itself lacks the kind of refinement (suzhi) needed to form the basis of a strong nation state. This is shown by the Chinese nation running short of solidarity among the people, a problem that can only be solved by educating the people with the help of a new kind of culture and scholarship. This kind of new culture and scholarship has to serve the aim of defining China's national identity and historiography is the most important discipline in this context.

If read in this manner, Liang's *New Historiography* develops, according to Huang Minlan, a quite coherent system of political thought which is easily overlooked as he develops his argument by discussing traditional historiography and defining the tasks of the ›new historiography‹. Liang's main criticism of traditional historiography is aimed at historiography not playing an adequate role in fulfilling its political task. He is not really interested in questions related to the methodology of historiography and in looking at historiography as a field of pure and politically uninterested research. If he mentions evolution theory, he is not out to discuss the philosophical meaning of the evolution theory for historiography, but he is in fact discussing the possibility of future development for China in political terms. However, for over 90 years, Liang's text has been interpreted to display his ›new historiography‹ as a critique of traditional historiography. Historians have tended to overlook the fact that Liang was mainly a political activist at the time he wrote his *New Historiography* and that only from the year 1918 on did he become more and more interested in academic questions. That is why, according to Huang, the difference between his early and later works on historiography are much more due to a difference of perspective than to a fundamental change of mind.

Huang deplores that misunderstanding Liang's *New Historiography* as a scholarly text criticizing traditional Chinese historiography has had the effect of developing a highly simplified view on traditional Chinese historiography in which the sometimes polemical arguments Liang propels to serve his political aims are taken for an in depth understanding of what traditional historiography in China was all about. This again has inhibited China's younger generation of historians to adequately assess the strengths and weaknesses of traditional Chinese historical scholarship.

The second article I would like to discuss here was written by Wang Yeyang under the title of *Liang Qichao's Explorations into Historical Epistemology* in 1994. Wang focuses on the later Liang Qichao and praises him to be the first Chinese scholar to have seriously discussed the question of historical epistemology. Especially in his articles on *The Research Method of Chinese History* (Liang Qichao 1922) as well as in his supplements to this text (Liang Qichao 1926), Liang, according to Wang, focuses on the relationship between subject and object in the process of history writing and discusses the nature of historical events as compared to the kind of data on which natural scientists base their findings on the laws and regularities of nature. He defines the relationship between subject and object as being relative meaning that the object of historiography, i.e. events in the past, only exists in relationship to the subjective which is defined as either the historiographer or the reader of historiographical texts. As the subjective approach to the object of research has such a dominating influence on the outcome of the research process historians have to discipline themselves and concentrate on refining their methodology of how to establish a chronology of events, how to endow facts with meaning and how to explain them. The aim of historical research has to be finding out whether »the truth is right or false« which implies, according to Wang, that historical research has to be independent of politics. Research has to occupy an autonomous zone of itself and must not be instrumentalized for propagandistic purposes. Wang summarizes Liang's achievements in this field of historical epistemology, as he calls it, by saying: »Liang Qichao is in our country the first to have stressed and researched the importance of subjectivity in the context of historical epistemology. He was the first to have elaborated on the subjective consciousness on a high level of abstraction assessing its positive role in the context of historical epistemology« (Wang Yeyang 1994, p.90-91). But as Liang was clearly conscious of the strong relationship between history and politics he knew that he had to make a difference between research in the field of natural sciences as compared to historical research saying: »The aim of [writing] history is to bestow the reality of the past with new meaning and new value so as to supply man with a mirror of his actions« (Liang Qichao 1922). For Wang Yeyang this means that Liang Qichao had realized at a very early point that the way people look at history is always shaped by the surroundings in which they live and which compel them to confront the past with a myriad of questions that change as times change. Liang not only realized this kind of relationship between object and subject, but he also went so far as to acknowledge that this is what history writing was all about and that the subjectivity is not a deficiency of the historical discipline. To the contrary, Liang held the opinion that historiography could only fulfill its task if written with the aim of application (zhiyong), while at the same time historiography's aim of application could only be reached if based on a scientific methodology controlling and limiting the subjectivity of the historian: »Only historiography (shixue) which is really scientific can have the kind of enormous social effect which it should have« (Liang Qichao 1922).

Historical events were for Liang Qichao the reflection of human will. That is why historical events are unique. While natural sciences deal with repeatable objects of research and are aimed at extracting the laws of nature from their data, the writing of history must not be aimed at finding out the general principles of a historical development. General principles of development are, as Wang interprets Liang, of no interest for a historian. If historians were aimed at the general, they would have to leave out everything, »the soul« as Liang Qichao put it (Liang Qichao 1923), that makes history interesting to them and their readers. Thus in the context of historiography, the methodology of induction is only of use if applied to the establishment of an order of sources and facts.

At this point, Wang draws a clear line between his own theories and those found in Liang's text. He thinks that Liang's understanding of the difference between humanities and natural sciences and his argument on the unique and the general should be critically assessed. On the one hand, he agrees to Liang seeing induction as a methodology to bring order into the chaos of facts transmitted through history, on the other hand, he strongly opposes Liang in his fundamental repudiation of the general in the context of historical studies. This shows that Wang is not prepared to get rid of the basic understanding of historiography as held by the mainstream of PRC historians claiming that the aim of history writing should not only be to reconstruct the truth concerning the events of the past, but also to extract the rules and regularities of historical development on the basis of knowing history »as it really was«.

All in all, Wang wants to make the point that Liang's writings in the last phase of his life should be regarded as of scholarly value and should be assessed in the context of the discourse at the time. If seen against the background of what Liang's contemporaries voiced on questions of historical epistemology, Liang's insights were farsighted and profound.

Both articles seem to be of quite some importance when assessing the possibilities of globalizing the research on Chinese history. Huang Minlan's contribution is outspoken and thought provoking as she openly discusses a question the discourse on which seems to be taboo although everybody knows about it. Huang Minlan discusses Liang's text as a political pamphlet and criticizes her colleagues for overlooking this important fact implying that the close relationship between history and politics which most Chinese historians tend to count among the positive aspects of Liang's historical methodology has nothing to do with historiography *per se*, but should be understood as the direct outcome of Liang discussing politics. If we turn this argument against the mainstream of academic historians in the PRC, this means that the historical discipline as profiled by these people is a field of political discourse and has still not developed to define itself as a field of academic research. As a matter of fact, Huang Minlan applies the methodology of ›allegorical reading‹ which most Western scholars dealing with the relationship between historiography and politics in the PRC deploy when analyzing the historiographical discourse as a political debate. It is exactly this kind of reading the subtext to the text which most PRC scholars hesitate to share with their readers. They might have reasons that do not only relate to the tradition of text analysis in China but also to bad experiences during earlier political campaigns. Quite obviously, »allegorical reading« was too often misused as part of political campaigns in the past. Nevertheless, Huang Minlan does not shy away from this method. Her ›allegorical reading‹ of Liang Qichao produces new insights in the texts as well as impulses for the development of the historical discipline in China.

Huang Minlan's 1994 reading of Liang Qichao is very near to Tang Xiaobing's as published in his 1996 book *Global Space and the Nationalist Discourse of Modernity*. In Tang's discussion of Liang's *New Historiography* he stresses that this text is mainly an »an essay that deals not so much with the possibility of historical knowledge as with the necessity and usefulness of the past in a nationalist project of rejuvenation« (Tang Xiaobing 1996, p.50). Even though Tang would not go as far as Huang in interpreting the *New Historiography* as a political pamphlet, he does come to the conclusion: »Indeed, history writing for the New Historian (i.e. Liang Qichao, SWS) was first and foremost a political statement and intervention« (Tang Xiaobing 1996, p.64). Both Tang and Huang stress the political ambitions and strategies Liang propagates in his *New Historiography* and acknowledge that Liang is focused on the social function of historiography rather than dwelling on specific problems of historical methodology. However, Tang's question is put differently from Huang. Huang wants to hit mainstream PRC historiography and therefore discusses the relationship between history and politics; Tang wants to come to a thoroughly positive assessment of Liang Qichao by discussing the relationship between national and global space as the territory of historiography.

By characterizing Liang as a postmodernist thinker at the beginning of the 20th century, Tang Xiaobing wants to attract our attention to Liang's contemporaneity. This also seems to be Wang Yeyang's point when he stresses that Liang was the first in China to discuss questions of historical epistemology and methodology and made contributions to this field at a very early stage that still deserve consideration. Wang wants to attract PRC historians to Liang because he sees in him an orientation for historiography searching for theory and methodology beyond Marxism and Mao Zedong Thought. And he is quite similar to Tang in his interest concerning the late Liang's attitude towards China and the world. Defending Liang against PRC mainstream historiography's attack on his late ›conservatism‹ Wang writes in another 1994 article on Liang's assessment of traditional Chinese historiography: »After reaching maturity Liang understood and evaluated traditional historiography from a global (shijie) and contemporary (dangdai) point of view. Acknowledging the successes of traditional historiography was [therefore] not [a sign of] conservatism, but open minded.« (Wang Yeyang 1994a, p.50) Wang goes on to explain how Liang was out to prove that East and West could complement each other and that as a precondition for this mutuality both sides had to come to an adequate assessments of their respective strengths and weaknesses (Wang Yeyang 1994a, p.49): »The fact that Liang Qichao changed his attitude from believing in the revolution of traditional historiography to criticizing, continuing and reforming as well as renewing it is, as we have to admit, a relatively correct attitude. [The same is true for] him regarding Chinese and Western cultures as complementary to each other and producing strength by combining their strengths in order to create something new for mankind« (Wang Yeyang 1994a, p.51). This again is what Tang Xiaobing calls »a global imaginary of difference« (Tang Xaobing 1996, p.216) which according to Tang was the new insight Liang pronounced in his later writings on historiography.

The »global image of difference« is based on the assumption that globality is composed of the sum total of particularities. While the term ›particularity‹ implies – strictly speaking – that there is some kind of universality somewhere, Tang Xiaobing does not seem to be interested in the possibility of universality on a meta-level of understanding. His answer to colonial historiography is the historiography of difference and particularity. While Tang Xiaobing praises Liang Qichao exactly at this point, Cui Zhihai and Wang Yeyang voice their doubts as both of them want to regard the particularity of Chinese history as integrated into world history. They insist on history being a scientific undertaking aimed at finding out the objective truth about the past including the rules governing historical development. This is where they have to branch off from Liang Qichao's chain of thought. Liang did not believe in the rules of history. He reconciled, according to Wang, the particularity of Chinese history with world history on the meta-level of epistemology. Chinese history is different and particular if seen in the light of the dominating Western model, but the methodology and epistemology this research is based on is universal.

As a matter of fact, without Tang Xiaobing mentioning Huang and Wang and vice versa, the two articles discussed above show quite some interesting similarities. Most of the points Tang raises when discussing *New Historiography* and *The Research Method of Chinese History* also come up in Huang's and Wang's discussions of the two texts. This shows that while using different methodologies and theoretical approaches, scholars in and outside the PRC seem to pursue similar questions. The reason why they do not relate to each other is difficult to assess, but it seems quite possible that PRC scholars working in the US are not encouraged to discuss findings and arguments propelled by their colleagues inside the PRC. It does not help them to establish their position in the field while PRC scholars inside China neglect publications from outside the PRC because of similar reasons. Nevertheless, the similarity of questions asked shows that instead of tabooing the existence of PRC historians pursuing their research outside China, PRC historians should understand them as a bridge between two otherwise quite separate spaces of research on Chinese history. Simultaneously, PRC scholars outside China should discuss the findings of their colleagues from China so as to fulfill a bridge function between the above mentioned inner and outer perspectives on Chinese history. In both cases this would mean running against the tide and taking the risk to be isolated from the mainstream. However if seen against the background of globalization in the field of historiography, this would be a worthwhile undertaking for both sides!

Liang Qichao and the question of post-nationalist historiography

As a matter of fact, Liang Qichao like quite a number of Chinese intellectuals who were his contemporaries did have a post-nationalist flavor to his thought. This flavor might go back to his relationship with Kang Youwei who designed in his book *On Great Harmony* a world empire instead of a nation state for China's future. But it might also go back to his experience in post WW I Europe where he became witness of the destructive forces of nationalism. Both experiences made him different from the May 4th generation of intellectuals and their strong inclination towards nationalism. In times of anti-imperialism and national salvation it seems even from today's perspective quite unusual for Liang Qichao to come up with an eclectic approach towards the dichotomy of East and West saying: »From now on, we should with all our strength import European and American thought, we should try to understand it, we should digest it, and if we think that our former scholarship is not good enough to solve our problems or if we think that their scholarship is not good enough to solve their problems, this should bring about change, because only then do we have the chance to create something new.« (Liang Qichao as cited in Wang Yeyang 1994a)

As Tang Xiaobing points out, this vision of Liang's never had the chance to become reality. Liang's vision of a future historiography transcended the possibilities of his contemporaries as their minds were strongly shaped by the experience of colonialism and nationalism. But in contrast to Tang Xiaobing who interprets Liang's vision as postmodernist, I would suggest that the tension between national and global space as to be observed in Liang's writings on historiography are not a tension between present and future but much more between past and present. In early 20th century China's development from empire (tianxia) to nation (guo), Liang Qichao's so called post-nationalist thinking was indeed more pre-national than post-national as it reflected a persistence of his understanding of China as empire instead of nation state. Although Liang was a supporter of the idea of nation state in the early 20th century, he expressed his doubts about a narrow understanding of nationalism in his later writings. It is in this context that he voiced his hopes that after going through a phase of nationalism China could eventually regain its unique position in the world by contributing to a worldwide civilization: »If we do not build our nation to become rich and strong, so that our nation can contribute to all of mankind, then our nation will be built in vain. Understanding this truth means to understand that our nation carries a very big responsibility in front of itself. What kind of responsibility? It is the responsibility to enlarge our civilization by taking from the Western civilization and to enlarge Western civilization by taking from our own civilization so that they merge and become a new civilization.« (Liang Qichao 1918)

This way of looking at China's position in the world seems to have long been forgotten. Even though China has been integrated into world economy and world politics, there is no sign of a common civilization emerging from this. Even in a field as universal as scientific research, there is – as we saw from the first part of this article – no common discourse when it comes to writing history. Understanding each other's history means in the first place understanding and respecting each other's way to write history. As long as historians believe that they can write history without taking the dichotomy of inner and outer perspectives into account there is no chance for a common discourse to emerge. If the field of history writing wants to actively join the process of globalization instead of passively waiting to be victimized it is time to imagine what historiography beyond the nation state could be like. It is in this context that rereading Liang Qichao's contributions to the methodology and theory of historiography is certainly inspiring and highly necessary.

Bibliographical Notes

Most of the articles cited below can also be drawn from a CD called: Liang Qichao zhushu ji yanjiu wenxian quanwen guangpan. This CD is part of a series called Ershi shiji zhongguo wenhuashi zhuming xuezhe ziliaoku, Peking, Beijing Daxue Chubanshe, Beijing Weiming Keji Wenhua Fazhan Gongsi 1998.1.

Bai Shouyi (1999). *Tantan jindai zhongguo shixue* (Talking about modern Chinese historiography). In: Bai Shouyi 1999a, p.294-327.

Bai Shouyi (1999a). *Zhongguo shixueshi lunji* (Volume on Chinese historiography). Peking: Zhonghua Shuju.

Bing Zhangchu (1995). *Liyi yu huigui: Wuxu bianfahou Liang Qichao liang ci sixiang zhuanbian* (Alienation and return: The two changes in Liang Qichao's thought after the 1898 reform). In: Qiushi xuekan 1995.5, p 86-95.

Bourdieu, Pierre (1992). *Homo academicus*. Frankfurt/Main: Suhrkamp.

Chang, Hao (1971). *Liang Ch'i-ch'ao and Intellectual Transition in China, 1890-1907.* Cambridge, Masachusetts: Harvard University Press.

Chen Pengming (1999). *Liang Qichao xueshu sixiang pingzhuan* (An evaluative biography of Liang Qichao and his scholarship). Peking: Beijing Tushuguan Chubanshe.

Chen Qitai (1997). *Liang Qichao pingzhuan* (An evaluative biography of Liang Qichao). Nanning: Guangxi Jiaoyu Chubanshe.

Cohen, Paul (1984). *Discovering History in China.* New York: Columbia University Press.

Cui Zhihai (2000). *Ping Haiwai sanbu Liang Qichao sixiang yanjiu zhuanzhu* (Review of three monographies on Liang Qichao's thought). In: Zhongguo Shehui Kexueyuan Jindaishi yanjiusuo 2000, p.482-522.

Gao Zhennong 1982: Liang Qichao de foxue sixiang (Liang Qichao's Buddhist thought). In Zhongguo zhexueshi yanjiu 1982.4, p.98.

Geng Yunzhi and Cui Zhihai (1994). *Liang Qichao.* Canton: Guangdong Renmin Chubanshe.

Hazama, Naoki (ed.) (2001). *Liang Qichao, Mingzhi riben, xifang: Riben Jingdu daxue renwen kexue yanjiusuo yanjiu baogao* (Liang Qichao, Meiji restauration, the West: A Research Report of the Institute for the Humanities at Kyoto University). Peking: Shehui Kexue Wenxian Chubanshe.

He Yongchuan (1984). *Jianguo yilai Liang Qichao yanjiuzhong jige wenti de gaishu* (Summary of some questions concerning the research on Liang Qichao since the founding of the PRC). In: Zhongshan Daxue Xuebao 1984.1, p.84-95.

Hockx, Michael (1999). *The Literary Field of Twentieth Century China.* Honululu: Hawaii University Press.

Gong Guoqing (1995). *Liang Qichao xin shixue yu »jiu dang shi zhi wu«* (Liang Qichao's new Historiography and the [principle] of doing research on history for contemporary use). In: Lishi jiaoxue 1995.2, p.35-38.

Hu Sheng (1995). *Jinian »Lishi Yanjiu« zazhi chuangkan 40 zhou nian zuotanhui shang de fayan* (Intervention on the occasion of the symposium commemorating the founding of the »Lishi Yanjiu« magazine 40 years ago). In: Lishi Yanjiu 1995.1, p.3-4.

Huang Kewu (1994). *Yige bei fangqi de xuanze: Liang Qichao tiaoshi sixiang zhi yanjiu* (A rejected choice: A study of Liang Qichao's accomodative thinking) Taipeh: Zhongyang Yanjiuyuan Jindaishi Yanjiusuo.

Huang Minlan (1994). *Liang Qichao »xin shixue« de zhenshi yiyi ji lishixue de wujie* (The true significance of Liang Qichao's ›New Historiography‹ and historiographical misintepretations). In: Jindaishi yanjiu 1994.2, p.219-235.

Huang Minlan (1999). *Zhongguo zhishi fenzi di yi ren Liang Qichao* (The first Chinese intellectual: Liang Qichao). Wuhan: Hubei jiaoyu chubanshe.

Jiang Ling, Zou Guanxiu and Guo Jianpo (1992). *Liang Qichao dui fengjian shixue de pipan (Liang Qichao's critique of feudal historiography).* In: Shanghai Shifan Daxue Xuebao 1992.1, p.57-59.

Jiang Jun 1993: *Liang Qichao zaoqi shixue sixiang yu Futian Hemin de »Shixue Tonglun«, (Liang Qichao's early thinking and Fukuzawa Yukichi's »General Introduction to Historiography«).* In: Wen shi zhe 1993.5., p 28-34.

Jiao Runming (1996). *Liang Qichao de ribenguan (Liang Qichao's perception of Japan).* In: Jindaishi yanjiu 1996.1, p.202-215.

Levenson, Joseph R. (1959). *Liang Ch'i-ch'ao and the Mind of Modern China.* Berkeley: University of California.

Levenson, Joseph R. (1958-1965). *Confucian China and its Modern Fate.* London: Routledge.

Li Shenzhi (1998). *Shenme shi zhongguo xiandai xueshu jingdian (What is classic in the context of modern Chinese scholarship?).* In: Shanghai Wenhuibao 1998/8/28, p.8.

Li Xisuo and Yuan Qing (1993). *Liang Qichao zhuan* (Biography of Liang Qichao). Peking: Renmin chubanshe.

Liang Qichao (1985). *Yinbingshi wenji* (Collected essays from the ice-drinker's studio). Taipeh (Chung Hwa Book Company).

Liang Qichao (1902). *Xin Shixue (New Historiography).* In: Liang Qichao 1985, 4:9, p.1-32.

Liang Qichao (1918). *Zhongguoren duiyu shijie wenming zhi da zeren* (The great responsibility of the Chinese people towards global civilization). In: Liang Qichao Quanji, p.2985-2987.

Liang Qichao (1922). *Zhongguo lishi yanjiufa (The Research Method of Chinese History*). In: Liang Qichao Quanji, p.4087-4153.

Liang Qichao (1923). *Yanjiu wenhuashi de jige zhongyao wenti.* In: Liang Qichao 1985, 14:40, p.1-6.

Liang Qichao (1926). *Zhongguo lishi yanjiufa bupian* (Supplements to The Research Method of Chinese History). In: Liang Qichao Quanji, p.4797-4880.

Liang Qichao Quanji (1998). *Liang Qichao Quanji.* Peking: Beijing Chubanshe.

Ma Shaohua (2001). *You cheng wu bai: Liang Qichao de yinguo siwei yu zeren de lishiguan* (No success without defeat: Liang Qichao's thought on causality and his historical theory on the responsibility of man). In: Hainan Tianya dianzi zazhi 2001.6 (http://www.ehawkcn.com/my%20webs/a01/009/046. htm).

Matsuo, Youji (2001). *Liang Qichao yu shizhuan - Dongya jindai jingshenshi de benliu* (Liang Qichao and historical biography – the moving around of the history of the modern Asian spirit). In: Hazama 2001, p.244-288.

Sen Jizi (2001). *Liang Qichao de foxue yu riben* (Liang Qichao's Buddhism and Japan). In: Hazama 2001, p.184-217.

Tang Xiaobing (1996). *Global Space and the Nationalist Discourse of Modernity. The Historical Thinking of Liang Qichao.* Stanford: Stanford University Press.

Tian Xiang (1993). *Liang Qichao de fojiaoshi yanjiu* (Liang Qichao's research on the history of Buddhism). In: Xueshu yanjiu 1993.2, p.83-88.

Wang Dong (2001). *Shizheng zhuyi yu zhongguo jindai shixue* (Positivism and modern Chinese historiography). In: Shanghai Hebei Xuekan 2001.2, p.19-23.

Wang Yeyang (1994). *Liang Qichao dui shixue renshilun de tantao* (Liang Qichao's research on historical epistemology). In: Changchun Changbai xuekan 1994.2, p.88-93.

Wang Yeyang (1994a). *Liang Qichao dui zhongguo chuantong shixue de renshi* (Liang Qichao's understanding of Chinese traditional historiography). In: Tianjin Lishi jiaoxue 1994.9, p.49-51.

Weigelin-Schwiedrzik, Susanne (1999). Die chinesische Historiographie in den 90ger Jahren: Zwischen Erkenntnistheorie und Marktwirtschaft. In H. Kaelble & D. Rothermund (eds.), *Comparativ. Leipziger Beiträge zur Universalgeschichte und vergleichenden Geschichtsforschung. 11.Jahrgang, Heft 4, 2001: Nichtwestliche Geschichtswissenschaften seit 1945*, pp.53-79.

Wu Huaiqi (1996). *Zhongguo shixue sixiangshi* (A history of Chinese historiographical thought). Hefei: Anhui Renmin Chubanshe.

Wu Jun (2001). *Xixue yu Liang Qichao shixue* (Western learning and Liang Qichao's historiography). Unpublished Doctoral thesis of Beijing Shifan Daxue, May 2001.

Zhang Mingfu (2001). *Di san jie quanguo qingnian shixue gongzuozhe xueshu huiyi zongshu* (Summary of the third symposium of young academic historians from the whole country). In: Xinan Shifan Daxue Xuebao 2001.2, p.108-113.

Zhang Shuxue (2000). *Zhongguo xiandai shixue zhuchao lungang* (An outline of mainstream modern historiograpghy in China). In: Shandong Daxue Xuebao 2000.6, p.37-43.

Zhang Yanqian and Yu Zhiguo (1996). *Dongtai yu zongshu: Jinian lai Liang Qichao yanjiu zongshu* (Trends and Summaries: Summary of recent research on Liang Qichao). In: Wen shi zhe 1996.2, p.94-99.

Li Yuhua (1986). *Duanlun Liang Qichao shixue sixiang de bianhua* (Short comments on the changes in Liang Qichao's historiographical thought). In: Henan Shixue yuekan 1986.1, p.59-63.

Zhongguo shehui kexueyuan jindaishi yanjiusuo (ed.) (2000) *Qingnian xueshu luntan* (Discussionforum for young scholarship). Peking: Shehui kexue wenxian chubanshe.

Gustavo Bueno

Medicina y Biología

La idea de Medicina anda confundida una y otra vez con la idea de Biología. Gregorio Marañón fue uno de los responsables de esta confusión en varias de sus obras: no sólo en su libro *Las ideas biológicas del Padre Feijoo* (en donde, a fin de cuentas, suscita cuestiones que efectivamente pueden llamarse biológicas) sino también en otros, como en su *Ensayo biológico sobre Enrique IV de Castilla y su tiempo.* Marañón utilizaba el adjetivo «biológico» fascinado sin duda por el prestigio que había alcanzado este término en unos años en los cuales, por cierto, los estudios universitarios no incluían explícitamente a la Biología entre sus Facultades; es decir, en una época en la que Marañón, médico de profesión, podía, sin peligro de ser acusado de intrusismo, considerarse como biólogo, a la manera como un Ortega, en unos años en los que no estaban institucionalizadas las Facultades de Sociología, podía ser considerado como «sociólogo» al margen de cualquier reproche de los Colegios correspondientes. Pero los estudios biológicos de Marañón y, en particular, el ensayo «biológico» sobre Enrique IV, no son propiamente estudios biológicos. Su ensayo sobre Enrique IV es sencillamente una suerte de «historia clínica», llevada a cabo con los conceptos propios de la profesión médica, que le conduce a un «diagnóstico morfológico» del rey castellano («displásico eunucoide con reacción acromegálica») y aun psiquiátrico («esquizoide con timidez sexual»). No hay ni un solo atisbo de aplicación de metodologías propias de la investigación biológica (la época no permitía tampoco análisis genéticos, por ejemplo). Las observaciones «raciológicas» de Marañón en este ensayo (el «prognatismo racial» de los Austrias, con génesis castellana, tendría el alcance de un antecedente clínico) así como el concepto de «curso degenerativo» de ciertos rasgos propios de los Trastámaras tienen más bien el alcance de antecedentes médico-psiquiátricos del diagnóstico.

A muchos les sonará a cuestión secundaria la diferenciación entre la perspectiva médica que atribuimos a Marañón y la perspectiva biológica en la que él quería situarse. A fin de cuentas, dirán, ambas perspectivas se ocupan de los organismos vivientes, tanto vegetales como animales (parece que fueron Lamarck y Treviranus quienes, hacia 1806, acuñaron el término «Biología», precisamente con la intención de reunir en una misma disciplina los estudios de Botánica y los de Zoología). Sin embargo, las diferencias entre Medicina y Biología son importantes, y no son diferencias de detalle sino de esencia. Desde luego una selección de los textos de Feijoo sobre cuestiones biológicas no podría superponerse a una selección de textos sobre cuestiones médicas. Y no se trata meramente de las diferencias que puedan mediar entre el género y la especie, como podría pensar quien trazase la línea fronteriza de este modo: la Biología se ocupa de la vida orgánica en general, mientras que la medicina se circunscribe a la vida orgánica humana. Hablando en el lenguaje cotidiano: la Biología es una ciencia, mientras que la Medicina es un arte que aplica los conocimientos generales de la Biología a los intereses humanos.

Ahora bien, esta diferencia popular nos orienta ya sobre el verdadero alcance de la distinción. Porque las actitudes de la Biología y de la Medicina ante la vida en general y ante la vida humana en particular son muy distintas y en muchos puntos contradictorias. La Biología, en tanto se rige por la teoría de la evolución, contempla a los organismos vivientes (y por tanto a los hombres entre ellos) como momentos de un proceso evolutivo que tiene lugar a lo largo de los siglos de un modo diferenciado y que las diferentes taxonomías se encargan de establecer. El biólogo, por tanto, saludará con interés, como un acontecimiento interesante, cualquier mutación que se produzca en un organismo. Cuando un embrión humano aparece con seis dedos o con un corazón trascolocado, el biólogo podrá ver en estos casos ejemplos de «mutaciones [8] prometedoras» en busca de su adaptación. Dixon ha escrito un libro en el que expone diferentes morfologías posibles hacia las cuales pudieran derivar las morfologías actuales y les da nombres más o menos pintorescos, como volufante, &c. Más aún, el biólogo está llamado a ensayar, mediante la ingeniería genética u otros arbitrios posibles transformaciones de las especies orgánicas actuales (del homo sapiens entre ellas), ya sea con fines pragmáticos (producción de alimentos transgénicos, por ejemplo) ya sea como ejercicio puro de experimentación científica. El biólogo experimental puede también quitar la vida a los organismos vivientes cuando ello sea necesario para poder profundizar en su estructura.

Pero la Medicina, en cuanto disciplina práctica, no puede mantener la perspectiva propia que atribuimos a la Biología. Tiene cerrado el paso a cualquier «experimento» en ese sentido. ¿Por qué? Sin duda porque considera a los organismos normales de la especie humana como organismos «perfectos», puntos finales o terminales de la evolución de las especies, que no requieren modificación estructural alguna, sino, por el contrario, el cuidado más exquisito para su conservación. La Medicina, como disciplina práctica, así podría ser definida, se acerca a la vida de los organismos humanos, entendidos como sujetos corpóreos operatorios (y por ello la psiquiatría es una disciplina genuinamente médica) con el objetivo de imprimirles transformaciones precisas, no cualesquiera (ni siquiera la transformación que condujera al superhombre), sino únicamente de estos dos tipos, orientados ambos a hacer prevalecer ciertos valores morfológicos y fisiológicos sobre otros acaso biológicamente posibles:
(1) El primero engloba a toda clase de transformaciones orientadas a «convertir», si le es posible, al individuo enfermo en individuo sano (medicina curativa) o a convertir al individuo malformado (respecto del canon elegido, pongamos por caso, el canon de Policleto en la tradición helénica) en individuo bien formado

respecto de ese canon (eugenesia, cirugía estética). Tiene prohibida en cambio la Medicina las transformaciones inversas a las de este primer tipo: la Medicina no puede transformar al individuo sano en enfermo, ni siquiera experimentalmente, y menos aún puede transformar al individuo sano o enfermo en cadáver. Ni siquiera la eutanasia clínica es admisible por la profesión médica.

(2) El segundo tipo de transformaciones engloba a las que pudiéramos considerar como «transformaciones idénticas», es decir, a las transformaciones del individuo sano en individuo sano; una fórmula que podría parecer a alguien tautológica o vacía, pero que sin embargo constituye una buena definición de lo que se conoce como medicina preventiva.

La naturaleza constitutivamente práctico-operatoria de la Medicina, respecto de su campo propio (los vivientes humanos), no excluye la posibilidad de la proyección de las categorías médicas a los organismos humanos que ya no viven, a los cadáveres, ya sea como un medio auxiliar de ampliación de sus conocimientos prácticos, como en las autopsias reales, ya sea «a fondo perdido», como en las autopsias históricas; de la misma manera a como la arquitectura, que se ordena constitutivamente a la construcción de cuerpos tridimensionales, puede proyectar sus categorías sobre una superficie, sea como medio auxiliar y a veces imprescindible para conseguir la ampliación de sus posibilidades técnicas (trazas, rasguños, planos) sea «a fondo perdido», como la arquitectura imposible de las escaleras virtuales de Escher.

Se comprende que la Medicina, así definida, sea una disciplina esencialmente «humanística». Suele llamar la atención la frecuencia de los médicos de profesión que, al mismo tiempo, experimentan una gran preocupación por las «humanidades». Pero, según lo dicho, más aún debiera llamar la atención el que un médico careciera de este interés humanístico, puesto que el interés por las humanidades se inscribe en su mismo terreno profesional. Más aún, por su condición de humanismo práctico, la Medicina se constituye como una disciplina esencialmente ética, si entendemos la ética por su ordenación a la asistencia de la vida del cuerpo humano individual, en lo que se opone a la moral, que se ocupa más bien, y a veces en conflicto con la ética, por la asistencia a la supervivencia del grupo. De cualquier modo, la Medicina, así [9] definida, habrá de comportarse siempre dentro de las normas éticas: no porque el médico, además de serlo, «debe» mantener una conducta ética, sino porque de no mantenerla dejaría de ser automáticamente médico, para convertirse, por ejemplo, en biólogo.

Ahora bien, de la concepción según la cual el médico está inclinado, por naturaleza, a preservar la vida humana y a ejercitar por tanto las virtudes éticas fundamentales, no se infiere la recíproca, a saber, que un humanista, en cuanto tal, haya de interesarse por cuestiones de medicina. No lo tiene vedado, sin duda, y una larga tradición demuestra la probabilidad de que un filósofo o un humanista se interese por la medicina, y sobre todo, si es epicúreo o con la salud delicada, propenda a llegar a ser médico de sí mismo. Pero también es verdad que la tradición del humanismo espiritualista considerará excesivamente grosero el cuidado excesivo por la «parte animal» del hombre, aunque considere este cuidado como una pesada carga derivada de la situación de unión coyuntural de n espíritu inmortal con un cuerpo mortal capaz de enfermar. Por ello es tan digno de admiración que un fraile benedictino como lo era Feijoo, aun siendo delicado de salud, se interesase sistemáticamente, y sin abandonar ni un instante la perspectiva de su humanismo filosófico, por la materia médica. Esta colección de escritos del padre Feijoo sobre cuestiones de Medicina puede constituir por tanto, para los médicos que se acerquen a ella, un motivo abundante para sus reflexiones, y no sólo en la dirección histórico arqueológica «a fondo perdido», sino también en la dirección de la ampliación de los planteamientos y soluciones de los problemas de nuestro presente. Todo el mundo podrá comprobar que las reflexiones médico filosóficas que el padre Feijoo escribió desde su convento benedictino de Oviedo hace doscientos cincuenta años conservan, cambiando lo que haya que cambiar, su plena actualidad.

Hermann Schuster & Johann Muhr

A Rural Transylvanian German-Rooted Elementary School Becomes a Hospital for All and a Home for Aged People

First of all we would like to emphasise that we wrote this contribution to honour the 60th birthday of the founder of Constructive Realism, Fritz G. Wallner.[1] Wallner is a philosopher of science teaching at the University of Vienna who has excellent contacts with a lot of scientists all over the world with international reputation. F.G. Wallner's Constructive Realism is able to answer to the new challenges for philosophical thinking. It must be stated that by application of Constructive Realism on the one hand philosophers initiate reflection in science and on the other hand scientists reflect their disciplines. Strangification is Wallner's most powerful constructive realistic method. Therefore we will relate our scientific investigations to the ideas of Constructive Realism and we will show possible benefits of reflection by strangification for our discipline.

1. Constructive Realism – an introduction

1.1. Preliminary note: Constructive Realism concedes any scientific community to generate and position its own norms and standards[2]. This means in detail:

1.2. Before exploring the world on a scientific basis, humans already have – to some degree – »insight« into the world. Thus, the existence of a pre-scientific »knowledge« can be safely assumed[3]. Scientific and every-day knowledge are intertwined with each other and according to Wallner there is the possibility that by applying the method of Constructive Realism these two forms of human actions can be brought together, can be closely described and also differentiated from each other[4]. In other words: First humans are caught up in every-day thinking and by carrying out every-day acts humans will create their picture of the (given) »world«. Then, according to Wallner, humans transport these acts onto their methods of gaining scientific »knowledge«, »regional scientific knowledge« etc[5].

As far as our issues of the hospital sector and the care e.g. for the elderly and for old people (partly also elementary school) in Transylvania/Romania are

1 H.S. would like to dedicate this contibution to Corina, Leopoldine, Martha.
2 see Wallner (2002, p.27)
3 see Wallner (1992, p.39)
4 see Wallner (1992, p.13, p.39, p.47)
5 see Wallner (1992, p.39)

concerned, Wallner states that in every day life humans are informed about these topics to a certain degree via newspapers, magazines[6] etc. The same goes for people with German roots living there, for ethnic Romanians, so-called Romas (gypsies) and also Hungarians (and Székler) in Transylvania.

1.3. Next Wallner differentiates between *knowing* (*Können*) and *knowledge* (*Wissen*)[7]. An example for *knowing* is baking a cake or skiing. Some people bake extremely well-tasting cakes or ski very well by applying the rules of baking[8] or skiing, but without having any scientific knowledge of why these rules work. Concerning the term *knowledge* we can say that when reconstructing the »world« (environment) we become constructivists. This concept is based on the idea of producing reality: [...] Knowledge is somehow the deconstruction of a given entity [...]«. In our case we primarily use rules of qualitative methods[9] of social research but also some other methods of social research that help to construct reality.

1.4. The concept of construction therefore goes from *knowing* to *knowledge*[10]. In Wallner's words »[...] any activity to obtain *knowledge* changes the world [...]«.[11] Moreover, Wallner stresses that »[...] Constructive Realism has a strict interdisciplinary structure [...]«.[12]

1.5. Wallner coins a new term for scientific constructions replacing the term theory: »microworlds«[13]: »Scientific reality is the total complex of microworlds«[14]. According to Wallner, reality can be transformed to (the) world (environment) by applying strangification, the method of Constructive Realism[15].

1.6. What does strangification (»Verfremdung«) mean? Strangification is a special kind of translating anything involved by understanding[16]. The procedure of strangification reads: one (logical) system of propositions is transferred from its original context Â into another context Â*:[17] This is our »tool«. By means of

6 see Wallner (1992, p.39)
7 see Wallner (1997b, pp.16-17)
8 see Wallner (1997b, p.17)
9 see Girtler (1992a, pp.49ff, pp.149ff) and Girtler (1996 (1996, pp.218-221) – further e.g. Diekmann (1995, pp.449-450, pp.450-459)
10 by means of argumentum e contrario: e.g. see Wallner (1997b, p.21)
11 see Wallner (1997b, p.22)
12 see Wallner (1997b, p.46)
13 e.g. see Wallner (1997b, p.46)
14 see Wallner (1997b, p.47)
15 e.g. see Wallner (1997b, p.47)
16 see Wallner (1997b, p.36)
17 see Wallner (1992b, pp.87-89), Wallner (1997a, pp.25-27) and Wallner (1997b, pp.44-46)

strangification we are able to introduce notions in a different way to find a more differentiated way to understand the background of our own insight[18].

According to Construcitve Realism, the given world never will be understood, but by constructing reality respectively microworlds we are at least able to handle the world[19]. Thus Constructive Realism regards (scientific) knowledge as a product of functional microworlds (and vice versa).[20] In this sense scientific practise is much more often »more intelligent« than scientific theory: Contructive Realism is an activity![21]

2. What is »regional science«?

The following anticipation should be made: Wallner stresses that it is not precise to use undifferentiatedly the term »science« – it is more concrete to speak about e.g. »European science«.[22] We, the authors of this article, define in this sense »regional science« as a kind of science related to a specific ethnic region that influences scientific insight and experience. In course held in January 2004 Wallner mentioned that Siebenbürgen can be seen as an example for a separate culture (»Sonderkultur«). According to a relativist viewpoint we emphasise that every culture develops its »special science«.[23]

3. Siebenbürgen as an example of »regional science« and separated culture

In Siebenbürgen we are obviously dealing not with only one, but with a number of special cultures and therefore with a plurality of »sciences«, founded on impressions and experiences the two authors made at the local social field. Following Wallner's ideas, we bare in mind that the introduction of (scientific) ideas and entities depends on the cultural background, and it is the use of these ideas and entities that generates scientific experience and insight.[24]

»Regional science« – in our case the one of Siebenbürgen – states something completely different than the current scientific mainstream like Western science practised e.g. in Germany or Austria. In the case of other, regional cultures (like in Siebenbürgen) we must assume a very different knowledge and meaning

18 see Wallner (1997a, p.26)
19 see Wallner (1992, p.43; pp.46ff; p.78; p.94)
20 see Wallner (1992, p.50)
21 see Wallner (1992, p.62)
22 see Wallner (1997a, p.13 – in note 1) and Wallner (1992, p.39)
23 see Wallner (2002, p.25)
24 see Wallner (2002, p.254)

of the »world«.[25] In this article both science and regional science – with respect to the perspective of human acting – shall be taken into consideration from the viewpoint of Constructive Realism.[26]

The »impression« that the Siebenbürgen Saxons create in respect of the culture of Siebenbürgen can be read as follows: The Siebenbürgen Saxons imported culture into the country starting in the 12th century.[27] A short overview over the history of culture and science in Siebenbürgen shows[28] that cultures in Siebenbürgen are primarily formed by the following essential cultural influences:

- the region around Mosel and Main, West and East of the lower Rhine, Flandern, Luxembourg, Saxony (through the Siebenbürgen Saxons) and other regions of the German Nation's Roman Empire
- Hungary
- the Habsburg Monarchy: (among others) settlement of about 4.000 »transmigrants« (for the most part of evangelic religion, later on so-called »Landler«[29] of Siebenbürgen) between 1734 and 1776
- the settlement of migrants from the »Wallachic« and »Moldawic« regions
- from Turkey (and Greece)
- Bulgaria, Russia and some other countries
- not to forget the influence of Jewish people.

Until 1918 the dominant voices in Siebenbürgen were: (1) the Hungarians, (2) the Széklers (the »eighth hungarian tribe«, H.S.), and (3) the Siebenbürgen Saxons. On the contrary the »East Romans« (the ethnic Romanians – in the terms of the Saxons and Landler: the »Wallachs«) were broadly excluded from political activities. The Roma (»Tigani«) were completely expelled from any political process.

Starting in 1989/90 a steadily increasing emigration (resp. re-migration) of the German-rooted Romanians to Germany and to a smaller dimension to Austria

25 see Wallner (1992, p.39)

26 see Wallner (1992, p.39)

27 This image was always experienced by the authors during their (empirical) field research starting in 1997 (Schuster) respectively 1994 (Muhr).

28 Cultural influences also by the Teutonic order (dating from 1211 to 1225) – see Kraljic (2001).

29 According to our impressions there are only three remaining of about 20 Transsylvanian »Landler«-villages: Großpold (in Romanian: Apoldu de Sus; in Hungarian: Nagy Apold), Grossau (in Romanian: Cristian, in Hungarian: Kereszteny-Sziget), Neppendorf (in Romanian: Turnisor, in Hungarian: Kis Torony) (Neppendorf is now a district of Hermannstadt, in Romanian: Sibiu, in Hungarian: Nagy Szeben), see e.g. Girtler (1992b, p.9), Girtler (1997, pp.10-13) and further Muhr & Schuster e.g. in Girtler (2002, p.249).

took place that seems to be (with respect to the technique of migration) a repetition of the biblical exodus of the Israelites out of Egypt.

The historic inter-/multiculturality in Siebenbürgen[30] can be demonstrated by the fact that nearly every small village was triple named and – as the authors could find on the spot – still are at least double-named,[31] in the following languages:

- Romanian (for example »Laslea«)
- German (»Gross-Lasseln«)
- Hungarian (»SzászSzent-Lászlo«)

4. Ad »school«: free interview and free participating observation with the Schotsch family (a family of bee-keepers)

On the occasion of a free interview (»free« is defined by the fact that the interviewer and the interviewed person speak as egalitarian and equivalent partners) between the Schotsch family, now resident at Reichsdorf/Ro that is located about 28 km distant to Gross-Lasseln, and one of the authors (i.e. H.S.), Mr. Schotsch sen. presented his view of reality: His father was a full-keeper (this means »full farmer«) in Gross-Lasseln in the fifth (of seven) neighbourhood(s). Within the family they talked the idiom of »Siebenbürgen Saxon«, a dialect very similar to the idiom around Mainz/Germany.[32] But at school, in the evangelical church and in the kindergarten the language of speaking and learning was High German.

The number of inhabitants of Gross-Lasseln counted then a maximum of about 2.000 Saxons, 200-300 Romanians, and about 1914 only one family of gypsies (Roma) lived there. Actually, the inhabitants are for the most part gypsies (more than 1.000) living together with 500-800 Romanians and about 20 Saxons.

It is worth mentioning here that in 1948 one of the first collective agriculture in the »People's Republic Romania« was instituted in Gross-Lasseln. On this occasion, as the Schotsch Family remembers, very high decorated communist functionaries came to visit Laslea and the event ended in a big party with music playing and everybody having fun.

---

30 see Wallner (1997b, pp.60-62)

31 This means that very often two, three or even four cultures lived more or less closely together in one region. In normal times, i.e. in peace, there hardly arose any problems in this respect (according to the impressions made by the authors on the spot). See further e.g. the »map of transsylvania« (1999), Szent Petery/Karney (1990) and Verseck (1998, p.197).

32 This hints at a cultural transfer from the mother country West and East of the lower Rhine to Siebenbürgen/Romania by immigration of Saxons of German origin after the 12th century (see Schullerus 1926, p.IX; foreword H.S.).

Asked concretely about school, Mr. Schotsch presented his knowledge like this:

- the just mentioned school in Gross-Lasseln was assumed to be about 500-600 years old;
- before Ceausescu's reign seven classes were installed, during Ceauscescu's reign (dating to 1989) ten classes for compulsory school. After the revolution there were eight classes and nowadays again ten. At the times of the seven-class education, the school building was divided into seven classrooms (four for lower, three for upper graded scholars); furthermore, there was a laboratory, a gymnasium for physical exercises and a door-keeper.

According to the narration of the Schotsch family the school in Gross-Lasseln was – as usual in Siebenbürgen –a confessional school of the local evangelical community until 1947. And there was a hostel for scholars from the neighboured villages.[33] In 1948 this primary school was nationalised and since then no more German class was installed. Thus, the new »National School« turned to be a mere Romanian institution despite of the fact that about one hundred children of (obligatory) school age were still German native speakers. Later on a second building for primary school was built.

Until 1989/91 the »old« school building was used for educational purposes. Caused by the »emigration« of the most Siebenbürgen Saxons back to Germany beginning at the »turn« in 1989, a big part of the building was left and abandoned. In the view of Mr. and Mrs. Schotsch the (r)emigration, especially of the Saxon teachers and priests, was »the beginning of the end of the old culture«, and this decline is still going on.

Here the question rises: Why wanted German-rooted people leave Siebenbürgen resp. Romania by all means? Dating from 1948 to about 1952 »people without land«, among them extremely poor families of Roma, were quartered on families in Gross-Lasseln like in the place of the Schotsch Family: the German-Rooted hosts (sometimes up to eleven persons in one family) had to be content with one single room for living, but, however, in some cases they even were forced to leave the place. Until about 1952 the German-rooted inhabitants were

33 One of these villages is Valchid (in German: Waldhütten; in Hungary: Váldhíd) where the Transsylvanian Saxon Rudolf Salanscki lives. For some time he spent as patient in the complex of the »Lukas Hospital Lalea«, and according to him who is a friendly man he was well treated by the excellent medical head Dr. Opreran and the entire staff. Mr. Salanscki got psychotherapeutic treatment and care that he appreciated very much. We would like to mention that in the farm of the Salanscki family one of the authors (i.e. H.S.) established a museum of culture, sanity and aviation (in the house Valchid Nr.76). A further dependence of this museum is located in the farm of the Fodor family (in the house Valchid Nr.165).

seen as having »no rights and no possession«.[34] That's surely the main reason why they left the country.

As the research results of one of the authors (i.e. H.S.) suggest, some »Landler« children went to the former school in Laslea about two centuries ago.

5. Constructs: medicine and national health

Preliminary note: What can or should be understood by (human) medicine? According to the perspective of the authors medicine deals with human (well)being. W. Schell points it out like that: »Medicine is the science of the healthy and the sick people«.[35] According to Aristotle the aim (τελοσ) of medicine is the »good« of human health.[36] Is the only reason for a »good" like health the fact that we can make an experience of it? Or is health eventually a construction – for example in form of a »picture«?[37]According to the statutes of the WHO (World Health Organisation) the definition reads: »Health is the state of complete physical, psychic and social well-being and not only the absence of illnesses and defect…« (health as an »ideal aim«).If medicine and health turn out to be human constructs, they will be seen dependant on the culture and the region in which they are »practised«. Wallner explains that every science is basically a »regional science«.[38] If we pass from a pre-scientific knowledge on to a scientific one, science will usually show up as regional science.[39]

6. Facts about the »Lukas Hospital Laslea«

In the following, some mostly »qualitative« empirical studies on the spot in Siebenbürgen with the main focus on the Lukas Hospital in Laslea[40] shall be examined from the viewpoint of Constructive Realism:

In 1994 (J.M) respectively in 1997 (H.S.) the authors were »in the field« in Siebenbürgen for the first time. The aim of these stays was to make examinations – especially in rural/agricultural regions – of the local inhabitants, including the

---

34 see Girtler (1992b, p.42) and Längin (1997, pp.26-27)

35 see Schell (1995, p.91)

36 e.g. see Lüth (1972, p.73)

37 see Wittgenstein (1989, p.39)

38 e.g. see Wallner (1992, p.39)

39 see Wallner (1997a, p.13/note 1 – H.S.)

40 By means of free speeches applying the qualitative methods of Girtler (1992a, pp.149ff); or by means of free participating observation applying the methods of Girtler (1992a, pp.43ff) and by means of other qualitative research methods and other empirical methods (see Diekmann 1995, pp.371-544).

old Austrian population, in particular from a perspective of social and cultural studies. The sectors of rural school education system, health care and the care for older people were the main focus of the examination, which started from the German rooted inhabitants. In the course of the studies of the Siebenbürgen Saxons and Landlers and after extended investigations, the authors found near the beautiful town of Schässburg (in Romania: Sighisoara, in Hungarian: Segesvár) the Lukas Spital in Laslea as an ideal place for their studies. The institution »Lukas Spital« consists of a hospital, a medical consulting room, a home for older people (inhabited usually by Siebenbürgen Saxons) located in the former school building and – locally separated – a place for a special project called »Wohnen am Hof' for a care-taken and supervised living for older patients. Gross-Lasseln was a Siebenbürgen-Saxon community where in 1758 41 Siebenbürgen Landler lived;[41] but nowadays we found not a trace of them. It can be mentioned here that from the 2.000 German-rooted persons (Siebenbürgen Saxons) living here until 1989, only 20 remained on the spot in 2002/2003.[42]

Now we will apply Wallner's method of strangification to the former rural school.

6.1. A note to the old Austrian Landlers who were also German-rooted inhabitants of Siebenbürgen: The Siebenbürgen Saxons have been wearing the shirt on the outside, a strong span (about 20 cm) below the body-belt (in summer time). This way of dressing was a special traditional fashion in Siebenbürgen to show unity and solidarity amongst the German-rooted persons (especially the youngsters) on official occasions, but initiated by the Saxons so that the Landlers refused to wear their shirt on the outside with the statement: »We don't give up our belief.«[43]

The special health social-gerontologic project »Wohnen am Hof« (living on the farm) by the Lukas Spital Laslea: On a locally separated »farm« with a court and a garden in Laslea, about seven older persons should live in accordance to their everyday life, based on their own initiative and cooperation, but under permanent medical and caretaking surveillance.[44] In the context to elder people research L. Rosenmayr (2002) (working at the Boltzmann Institute in Vienna) points out that:

41 see Buchinger (1980, p.433)

42 That is the result of the field research done by H.S. (interview with the evangelical priestess of Großlasseln/Laslea, Ms Ilse Totea who is a Siebenbürgen Saxon).

43 see Schullerus (1926, pp.50f). This is a case of strangification: Belief for dressing manner. Both authors got the idea that the old Austrian evangelical (A.B.) Landler were transmigrated (i.e. deported) by force in 1734-1776 according to their convincing religious faith.

44 The newest plan schedules to accommodate Alzheimer patients here in near future.

- »Nature doesn't like the age (the seniority).« (P.B. Baltes, a German gerontologist)
- In that sense a creature is »relevant« in a biological sense only if it is still able to reproduce itself (respectively to reproduce its species).
- The principle of seniority was only valid and of force in some special historic segments and under certain conditions and circumstances. The principle is founded on the exchange of women (»fresh blood« for the own and the other tribal community), which was under supervision of the seniors and is, concerning the topic »The Culture of Ageing in LONGEVETY«, very important.[45]

Let's have a look to percentage of »seniors of various countries« (related to the years 2000 and 2050);[46] people of »more-than-65-years-old« counts:

- in Germany: 18% in 2000; estimated 28% in 2050
- in Italy: 18% in 2000; estimated 35% in 2050
- in Austria: 18% in 2000); estimated 35% in 2050
- dates of Romania are not available (H.S.)

6.2. Empirical research on the spot (Lukas Spital Laslea) – Facts, Resultates, and Strangification: The hospital made an extraordinary well-groomed impression, nearly like a laboratory for electronic computer components, as one of the researchers (H.S) could convince himself exploring the building in 2002/2003. The park and resort can be described as very well cared of. Hygiene is a very important aim of the hospital: the consultation room, rooms for the patients, floors, sanitary installations, the day-room and the kitchen are extremely hygienic. From reports and information (»narrations«) made by the caring staff, the authors draw the conclusion on an extended complex of sanitary measures (especially in intensive-caring, medical treatment and visit, ecological-lasting removal of medical and other refuse).

According to our view the medical and sanitary standard of the hospital and of the home for patients is adequately correspondent to that one in Germany or Austria. It can be said with Wallner that interculturality[47] and »scientific exchange« is realising itself in that point: »...scientists change the world in their laboratories, but this has no consequences for the world outside the laboratories. However, if science is applied to technology, you can see the results.«[48]

---

45 see Rosenmayr (2001pp.1-8)

46 e.g. see Kytir (2001) (some calculations done by H.S.); and see United Nations statistics in »Land ohne Leute«, in *Die Zeit* (May, 10th 2001, dossier p.15).

47 see Wallner (1997b, p.53)

48 see Wallner (1997b, p.54)

6.3. Dialogue[49]: The relation between people (1) doctor – patient, (2) caring staff – patient[50], and (3) other staff – patient can be qualified as exemplary professional concerning the relationship doctor-patient. The doctor as the »health expert« is in a dominant position. This corresponds to a »moderate« position of a »via media« (a »medium way« like in Germany and Austria). The local emergency medicine would be on actual state of science, as reported in free interviews by the competent persons of the place.

6.4. Socio-medical problems in Siebenbürgen: According to the authors special problems of social medicine and in the field of prevention[51] in Siebenbürgen are

- alcohol (partially a very high consumation rate of vodka)
- smoking (very widely spread)
- negative distress caused by monotony, severe poverty (very big charges caused by expenses while having a very poor income)
- lethargy and depression caused by the disappearance of old (rural) values (e.g. elder single German-rooted persons witness the Siebenbürgen Saxon and Landler culture vanish)

As a further result of the field research we saw that prophylactic medicine is practised very successfully in the Lukas Hospital Laslea, in respect of both the life of patients and protection of environment. Important to mention here in 1988 the highest mortality rate (standardised on age) in Europe in respect of cardiovascular diseases was to be found in Romania; Germany was ranked on range 13th and Austria on range 12th.[52]

Remarks on the management of the Lukas Spital Laslea: Four of five people of the personnel body are responsible for administration; the staff consists of both German-rooted and Romanian-rooted persons. The direction of the Hospital is leaded by a very competent and efficient ethnic Romanian, Dr. Oprean, so that inter-/multiculturality is guaranteed in that respect.

After his exploration tour through the hospital (2002/2003) one of the authors (i.e. H.S.) came to construct following »images« about the patients: One female Romanian patient turned to be a permanent case for nursing because of a plunge out of the window. One young Roma woman showing serious psychic and

---

49 As Lüth (1972, p.275, p.336, p.338) stresses dialogue (or conversation) is a decisive factor of human therapy.

50 The problems of social contacts between nursing staff and patients in Austria is described by Hofer (1997, pp.76-83; pp.107-111).

51 in general see Berufsverband Deutscher Präventologen, e.V. Hannover 2001 (Leaflet given to H.S.)

52 see WHO statistics dating back to 1991; but in 2002 an Italian cardiologue informed H.S. about the fact that the statistics didn't change so much.

physical infirmities, a permanent nursing case, too, who needs consistently physical and psychological treatment. All the patients in the hospital are cared for in a first-class manner by a competent caring staff applying excellent social relation as H.S. convinced himself extensively on the spot. As reported by the interview partners, the staffs consist of 50 – 60 persons. The kitchen and the store rooms for keeping food was in an excellent order and, as mentioned before, the standard can be compared with Western Europe standard. The complex house-keeping (about 13 persons) is managed by a very friendly and competent Romanian woman (before her a Franconian woman called »Sister Margit« was in charge).

7. Some examples of strangification (as found in literature)

In the following we would like to specify examples for strangification/alientaion in respect to medicine and public health in Siebenbürgen:

7.1 According to A. Schullerus (1926, pp.40-42) the (rural) Siebenbürgen Saxon consider health as very important. In cases of bad health or accident the typical Siebengürgen Saxon consults the doctor who has his full confidence: The dotor is the one who perceives and knows first the disease and who makes the ordination of a remedy. Further the Siebenbürgen Saxon trusts in the »medicine« (the medical remedy itself) qualified either in relation to its prize (Sbg. Saxon: »e hued en deier Medizin verschirwen«) or to its visible effects (»dat wor en stark Medezin, se hued en gepackt, gescheddelt...«). The recovering is giving thanks to the doctor: »Wo der Härr Dokter ned erous kam, bäs na lag schi lang angder'm Dresch [=Driesch]« (»angder'm Driesch« = in the grave).

For lighter or special illness (e.g. constipation or rheumatism) the »Amtfrä« (the midwife) is the responsible and proper person acting with the »Sprätz« (the syringe) or with ointment (»zemzän«). The authors confirm that the patients showed an extremely high trust in the medical system, in the doctors and in the first-aid-nurses. In former times at least one of them lived near to every village in Siebenbürgen what can be found to smaller extension until nowadays.

As frequently reconfirmed by local inhabitants of Siebenbürgen (in free interviews and free participation observations) there is still a kind of »popular medicine« widely spread. In the same way Schullerus states that especially the German-rooted are said to have tried to extract or to eradicate the »spirit of the disease« by medium of mystic popular-medical rituals. He quotes an old poem as an example:

The mother of the mountain and the gnome
go together across a mountain.
What should you do?
You shall go to N.N.
And break his legs
And stinge his back.

I shall make a dead out of him?
No, not that shall you do.
Come with me into a green forest
There are two cold springs
Of one of them you shall drink
And you shall drown to the ground.

7.2 As conclusion we would like to quote some remarks about the relation of the Roma/Zigani to the complex of »doctor and hospital« in general.

In der Maur (1978, p.266) states: »The gypsy is always avoiding doctors«. And the more: »The Roma/Zigan is lacking any relation to medical science. This is grounded on the fact that he is complete belonging to a natural population who comprehends sickness very different to the high civilised: out of his relationship to the demons…« He continues: »...if nevertheless they (the Roma) were consulting a hospital or eventually – for example in case of contagious diseases by official initiative – are brought there, they are looking in a sly manner for their early release in order to practise their own-generated remedies…«

8. Acknowledgements

We would like to thank all the kind persons, especially the ones living in Transsylvania, but also everyone elsewhere who gave us any assistance and help.

Bibliography

Balas, H. (1997). Betagte Landler. In R. Girtler (ed.), *Die letzten der Verbannten. Der Untergang der alt Österreichischen Landler in Siebenbürgen* (pp.111-118). Wien.
Buchinger, F. (1980). *Die »Landler« in Siebenbürgen. Vorgeschichte, Durchführung und Ergebnis einer Zwangsumsiedlung im 18. Jh.* München.
Cassirer, E. (1954). *Philosophie der symbolischen Formen.* Darmstadt.
Diekmann, A. (1995). *Empirische Sozialforschung.* Hamburg.
Girtler, R. (1992a). *Methoden der empirischen Sozialforschung.* Köln/Weimar.
Girtler, R. (1992b). *Verbannt und Vergessen. Eine untergehende deutsch-sprachige Kultur in Rumänien.* Linz.

Girtler, R. (ed.).(1997). *Die Letzten der Verbannten. Der Untergang der alt Österreichischen Landler in Siebenbürgen/Rumänien.* Wien.
Girtler, R. (2002). *Echte Bauern. Der Zauber einer alten Kultur.* Wien.
Groth-Schmachtenberger, & Mayer-Krausz (o.J.). *Damals im Südosten. Siebenbürger Sachsen, Donauschwaben in alten Fotos.* O.O.
Haring, Karsch & Schuster (1975). *Urban Economics* (manuscript for a book concerning aspects of regional science). Los Angeles/Wien.
Hofer, K. (1997). *Pflegebedürftig. Von der Betreuung zu Hause und im Pflegeheim.* Wien.
In der Maur, W. (1978). *Die Zigeuner – Wanderer zwischen den Welten.* Wien/München.
Kaelke, A.-K., & Steffen, M. (1999). *The »Global Village Grossopold«? Information und Kommunikation in einem Siebenbürgisch-Deutschen Dorf: Forschungsbericht.* Unpublished.
Kralljic, F. (2001). *Der Einsatz des Deutschen Ordens in Ungarn.* Unpublished paper.
Kytir, J. (2001). Der demographische Hintergrund. In *Zukunfts-enquete: die gewonnene Generation* (11.06.2001). Akademie der Wissenschaft – Österreichischer Seniorenbund (paper given to H.S.).
Längin, B.G. (1997). *Unvergessene Heimat Siebenbürgen.* Augsburg.
Lüth, R. (1972). *Kritische Medizin.* Reinbek bei Hamburg.
Lukas Hospital Laslea (ed.).(o.J.). *Lukas Spital Laslea* (leaflet biven to H.S. in 2003).
Map of Transsylvania (Erdely Helysegnevtare, 2.Kiadas) (1991) copyright: Fodor, A./Kovats, Zs. Budapest.
Muhr, J., & Schuster, H. (2002). Auf den Spuren weiterer Landlerdörfer. E.g. in R. Girtler (ed.), *Echte Bauern. Der Zauber einer alten Kultur* (p.249). Wien.
Panoff, M., & Perrin, M. (1982). *Taschenwörterbuch der Ethnologie.* Berlin.
Redelberger, G., Quintus, H., Muhr, H., Schuster, H., & Grieb, D. (2002). *Vorwort zu Wissenschaft jenseits von Soziologesisch (für R. Girtler* (ed. Lex Liszt). Oberwart.
Rosenmayr, L. (2001). The Culture of Aging. In *Zeitschrift für Geriatrie 34*, 2-8.
Rosenmayr, L. (2002). *Generationen in der Natur und in der frühen Menschheitsgeschichte* (talk in the Austrian radio in 2002; paper handed to H.S.)
Schell, W. (1995). *Grundzüge der Hygiene und Gesundheitsforschung.* Hagen.
Schullerus, A. (1926). *Siebenbürgisch-sächsische Volkskunde.* Leipzig.
Schuster, H. (1968/1998 rev.). *Old Austrians of the former Austro Hungarian monarchy.* Unpublished paper.
Schuster , H. (1991). *Ost-West joint ventures österreichischer Betriebe in Osteuropa* (masters thesis at the Technische Universität Wien). Unpublished paper.
Schuster, H. (1996-97). *Essays* for the international Garry Becker price on the unintended consequences of welfare state and related issues (Contributions to a competition).
Schuster, H. (1999). *Holzarbeit und Weintrinken.* Unpublished.
Schuster, H. (2002a). *Arzt und Hygiene* [revised]. Unpublished paper.
Schuster, H. (2002b). *Qualität im alltäglichen Gesundheitswesen* [revised]. Unpublished paper.
Schuster, H. (2003a). *Die innere Sicherheit am Beispiel Siebenbürgen (Reichesdorf). Contribution to a FM4-competition [revised].* Wien.

Schuster, H. (2003b). *Eine kulturwissenschaftliche Wanderung in Siebenbürgen (Neudorf, Waldhütten). Contribution to a literature competition organised by ›Verein Exil‹ [revised]*. Wien.

Schuster, H. (2003c). *My Museum of Culture, Sanity and Aeronotics in Waldhütten/Valchid in Transsylvania* (leaflet).

Schuster, H. (2003/2004). *Gesundheitswissenschaften – Pflegewissenschaften/Soziologie der Pflegewissenschaften und C.R.* (Papers e.g. for the cooperation in the course »Soziologie des Pflegedienstes« in the summer term 2004 at the University of Vienna) Unpublished.

Schuster, H. (2004). Konstruktiver Realismus und die Regionale Wissenschaft mit Beispiel: Historisches Tibet bis 1950. In M. J. Jandl & F. G. Wallner (eds.), *Umwelt in Reflexion. Beiträge aus Philosophie, Wissenschaft und Politik* (pp.117-126). Hamburg.

Szentpetery, T., & Kerny, T. (1990). *Gottes feste Burgen – Sächsische Wehrkirchen des Mittelalters in Siebenbürgen*. Ungarn.

Trupp, A., Schuster, H., & Fabsits, M. (2000). *»Wie funktioniert Wissenschaft?« Ein Ethnologiemediziner legt sein diesbezügliches Bild dar*. See andreas.trupp@aon.at.

Verseck, K. (1998). *Rumänien*. München.

Wallner, F. (1992a). *Acht Vorlesungen über den konstruktiven Realismus*. Wien.

Wallner, F. (1992b). *Wissenschaft in Reflexion*. Wien.

Wallner, F. G. (1997a). Aspekte eines Kulturwandels. In F. G. Wallner & B. Agnese (eds.), *Von der Einheit des Wissens zur Vielfalt der Wissensformen* (pp.25-28). Wien.

Wallner, F. G. (1997b). *How to Deal with Science if You Care for other Cultures. Constructive Realism in the Intercultural World*. Wien.

Wallner, F. G. (2002). *Die Verwandlung der Wissenschaft. Vorlesungen zur Jahrtausendwende* (ed. by M. Jandl). Hamburg.

Wittgenstein, L. (1989). Philosophische Untersuchungen. In *Werkausgabe Band I* (6. ed.). Frankfurt a.M.

Martin Voracek, Oliver Bernecker & Gernot Sonneck

Suicide Myths and Misconceptions in Medical Students. Preliminary Report

Background

Basic suicidological knowledge is crucial for all health care practitioners, constituting an important facet of mental health literacy (cf. Goldney, Fisher, & Wilson, 2001). For instance, psychological autopsy studies repeatedly have demonstrated that a significant portion of suicide victims consult medical doctors prior to their committing suicide. However, little is known about medical students' knowledge about suicide facts.

Methodes

We investigated upper-division (fourth-year) medical students' suicidological knowledge, relative to a control group (first-year psychology students), with an extended (42-item) RFOS version (»Revised Facts on Suicide Quiz«; Hubbard & McIntosh, 1992; McIntosh, Hubbard, & Santos, 1985) in Austria (N = 546; 383 females and 163 males; 289 of them medical undergraduates, 257 psychology undergraduates). Subjects' age was M (Md) ± SD = 26.3 (24) ± 7.2 yrs.

Results and discussion

Age-adjusted analysis of covariance (with factors: participants' major × gender) results evidenced rather modest knowledge levels (for medical vs. psychology students, in order, M = 19.3 vs. 16.6 out of 42 items correct).
Major accounted only for a modest portion ($p < .001$; partial $\eta^2 = .056$) of total variability in RFOS scores.
Age was positively associated with knowledge ($p = .001$; partial $\eta^2 = .019$).
Gender differences were trivial ($p = .47$; partial $\eta^2 = .001$); interestingly so, even on gender-specific items.
(Partial η^2, an effect size metric, is the proportion of the total variability attributable to an analysis of (co)variance factor; conventional benchmarks are: values around/lower than .01 small effects, around .06 medium effects, and around/higher than .14 large effects; cf. Cohen, 1988.)

Participants scored best:

- on items targetting clinical/interpersonal knowledge (e.g., »Suicide rarely happens without warning«: 74.2% correct answers, 22.3% false, 3.5% »don't know«);
- less so on demographic/epidemiological facts (e.g., »There is a strong correlation between alcoholism and suicide«: 49.6% correct answers, 22.1% false, 28.2% »don't know«);
- and worst on facts about time-dependent (chronobiological) suicide risks (e.g., »The season of least suicides is...«: only 4.3% correct answers; i.e., winter).

The figures show the results for two RFOS items concerned with time-dependent suicide risks, i.e., guessed peaks and troughs of monthly and weekly suicide occurrence. Percentages for peak/trough categories (»guessed peak/trough«), as chosen by the subjects, are plotted against respective population figures (»actual distribution«) for Austria (based on 55,009 officially registered suicides during the period 1970-99). Dotted reference lines indicate uniform distribution.

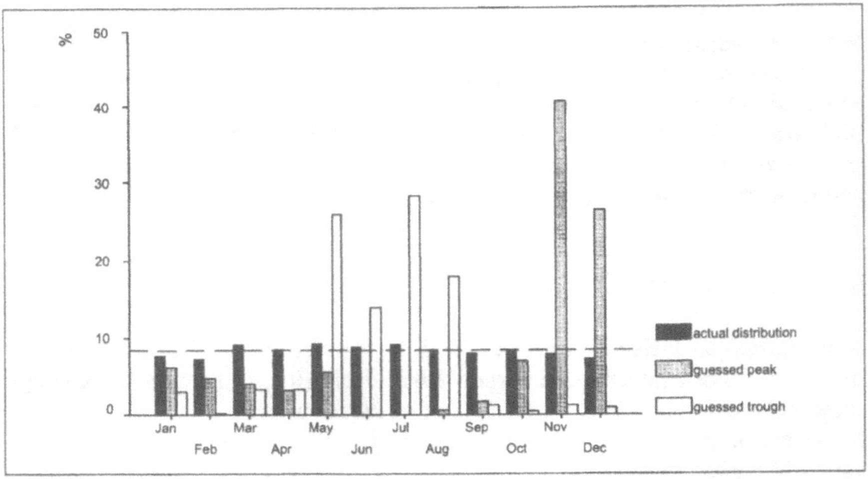

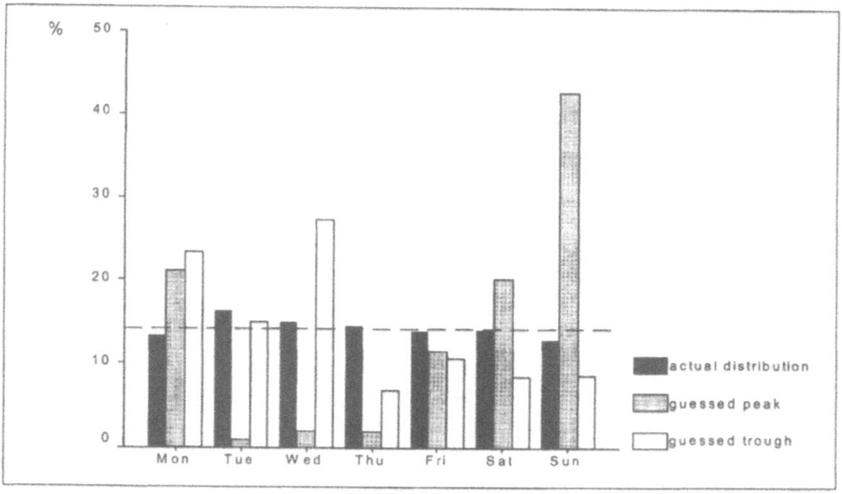

Conclusion: The relatively modest overall knowledge level, coupled with the specific finding that fourth-year medical students, relative to first-year psychology students, achieved only marginally better scores, calls for further implementation of suicidological knowledge contents in medical curricula.

The most pervasive suicide myths concern time-dependent suicide risks. Thus, facts on suicide seasonality, clearly counter-intuitive to everyday reasoning (Northern Hemisphere suicides peak in May/June, not in November or around Christmas), should be addressed in medical and health professional training.

References

Cohen, J. (1988). *Statistical power analysis for the behavioral sciences* (2nd ed.). Hillsdale, NJ: Erlbaum.

Goldney, R. D., Fisher, L. J., & Wilson, D. H. (2001). Mental health literacy: An impediment to the optimum treatment of major depression in the community. *Journal of Affective Disorders, 64,* 277-284.

Hubbard, R. W., & McIntosh, J. L. (1992). Integrating suicidology into abnormal psychology classes: The revised facts on suicide quiz. *Teaching of Psychology, 19,* 163-166.

McIntosh, J. L., Hubbard, R. W., & Santos, J. F. (1985). Suicide facts and myths: A study of prevalence. *Death Studies, 9,* 267-281.

C. Humanities

Karl Klement

Educational Situations, Educational Research and the Reflective Practitioner

About Wallner

A man who lives his own ideas seldom can be found… Fritz Wallner is the living example of an academic showing and performing his own theory – the Constructive Realism (CR). Wherever he appears – in every single area – he is the one who uses familiar forms in an unfamiliar ways: he became the master of ›estrangement effects‹. Unfortunately his surroundings does not always realise the educational attitude of these effects and often answers with a lack of understanding. So Fritz Wallner as an educator polarises and provokes but he always forces to reflect by creating educational situations. On the other hand he is a meticulous observer in which way »practice answers« to his estrangement effects and he exercises »reflection on action« in a very strict way. So he explains how professionals make sense of the world they inhabit by showing that educators and teachers as well learn from the act of reflection itself. He argues that ways of thinking about his own work results in improvements to practice…

About educational situations

Whatever may be the task of philosophers of education, the typical task of the teacher is a practical one: that is, he is constantly preoccupied with what to do in a situation requiring him to do something. This does not at all mean that thinking and reflecting is a less important part of his business, for, as the old controversy aroused by pragmatism showed, theory is not opposed to practice but essential to it. The teacher, however, needs a type of thinking particularly suited to practical problems – it might be called practical thinking, in contrast to that which arose without a practical end in view. Without it, the way a teacher acts can be inconsistent, indecisive, or mechanical and rigid. Nor is it likely that he can free himself from these hindrances to effective work unless he forms, in the course of his practical thinking, what may be called a »concept« of education – that is to say, a set of ideas, characterised by their common capacity to contribute to his practical work.

These may be combined in various ways according to the practical problem concerned, and they consist of a number of procedures appropriate to the carrying out of the teacher's work, plus a number of aims in pursuit of which those procedures are operated. This »set of ideas« – in the sense of Fritz Wallner is a set of »Verfremdung« (»strangification«) looking at familiar forms in an unfamiliar way in order to perturb and to show their structures in a new, unknown kind of thinking. As to be seen an »educational situation« in the sense of Fritz Wallner is first of all a situation of uncertainty and confrontation with something unexpected...

About the research paradigm

The interpretative researcher – like Fritz Wallner – cannot accept the idea of there being a reality »out there« which exists irrespective of people, for reality is a construct of the human mind. People perceive and so construe the world in ways which are often similar but not necessarily the same. So there can be different interpretations of what is real. Concepts of reality can vary from one person to another. Instead of reality being »out there«, it is the observers who are »out there«. They are part of the world which they are observing and so, by observing, may change what they are trying to observe. The interpretative researcher sees language as a more or less agreed symbolic system, in which different people may have some differences in their meanings; in consequence the sharing of accounts of what has been observed is always to some extent problematic. Because of differences in perception, in interpretation and in language it is not surprising that people have different views on what is real.

Interpretative researchers reject the positivist's view that the social world can be understood in terms of casual relationships expressed in universal generalisations. To them human actions are based on social meanings, such as beliefs and intentions. People living together interpret the meanings of each other, and these meanings change through social intercourse. Interpretative researchers recognise that by asking questions or by observing they may change the situation which they study. They recognise themselves as potential variables in the enquiry and so, in writing reports, may use personal pronouns.

To the interpretative researcher the purpose of research is to describe and interpret the phenomena of the world in attempts to get shared meaning with others. Wallner's Constructive Realism in this way is a very communicative method! Interpretation is a search for deep perspectives on particular events and for theoretical insights. It may offer possibilities, but no certainties, as to what may be the outcome of future events. The word »hermeneutics« is sometimes used to describe work in this paradigm. It means the art of interpretation.

Interpretative researchers inevitably study singularities, but they differ in their views on the extent to which the collated evidence from many singularities can be expressed in the form of generalisations. The data collected by interpretative researchers is usually verbal- fieldwork notes and transcripts of conversation. Sometimes this can be analysed numerically but more usually it is not open to the qualitative statistical analysis used by positivists. Hence it is described as qualitative. Ethnography is an important branch of the interpretative paradigm, concerned with participant observation – where the observer is not »a fly on the wall«, but becomes a participant in the activity which she/he is studying. To make sure that he is not the »fly on the wall« Fritz Wallner is a great traveller and interpreter of the different kind of cultures: a man who lives his ideas.

About action research

Action research in education has blossomed in the last ten years. Inevitably different people define it in different ways, but the universally agreed characteristic, is that it is research designed to improve action. Sometimes this is expressed as »to enhance the quality of action«. Theory is created not as an end of itself, but in order to advance practice...This intention often results in action research being cyclical, because striving for improvement is seen by many teachers as an ongoing professional commitment.

Because action research entails an intention to change action involving people, it is seen by those who practice it to demand not only a strong ethic of respect for persons, but also to demand democratic involvement of the people on whom it impinges. The concept of the »critical friend« has been developed by action researchers, meaning someone who responds to the invitation to invest some time and effort into critically examining one's action research findings, and who agrees to work within the ethical framework of the enquiry – which defines matters such as the ownership of data.

Kersten Reich

Towards a Constructivist View of Action Levels in Learning Processes – a Plead against Naïve Realism

The constructivist realism as developed by Friedrich Wallner is no naïve realism based on a simple copy theory. Like the interactive constructivism[1], which I follow, the constructivist realism also opts for a context related and culturalist view. We never just learn images in a situation which then can be programmed into us by instructions like into a computer. Even when learning by heart, we need to refer to a learning context which makes knowledge appear relevant and meaningful as well as significant to us and our acting (e.g. the act of learning by heart).[2] In the following contribution I would like to describe three action levels of learning[3] that can cause mutual strangification, a circumstance which can be well described by Wallner's theory of strangification. At the same time, this contribution shall point out why a sensuous and »real« starting position is necessary, yet, not sufficient for the constructivist part of learning.

What are the contexts of action that particularly foster an easy, efficient, extensive, and solid learning? Learning theories facing this question will immediately connect it to another question: What are the action levels like, that can be assumed and may be planned in order to stimulate successful learning? At least since Rousseau published his novel on education, *Emile*, education theorists have been discussing the question, if it is better to learn in an actual situation, in a practice from which learning tasks may emerge in a sort of »natural way«, or if it proves more advantageous to summarize and prepare things beforehand in such manner that the learner may quickly learn as much as possible in an artificially created situation as, for example, represented by school.

What point of view will a constructivist theory of learning assume when dealing with this problem today? I will try to analyze this question by offering a simplifying distinction of three action levels to be taken during the act of teaching or learning with regard to actual perception, sensory experiences or more abstract

1 Cf. to http://konstruktivismus.uni-koeln.de

2 Cf. hereto e.g. John Dewey in: »Democracy and Education« (1985, 146 ff.); Dewey established in many works that cognitions can not be observed in an isolated way, but always presuppose a sphere of experience. This means an important basic attitude for learning: It can not only ask for contents and its conveyance, but also needs to pay attention to the action-related significance for the learner and the communication connected therewith as a frame of action.

3 Cf. Reich, K.: Konstruktivistische Didaktik. Neuwied u.a. (Luchterhand) 2004^2.

generalization. By doing this, I am going to introduce some distinctions that may help teachers and learners to critically observe and question themselves as to the level of acting they enter at a time.

Levels I will define as observer's constructions, i.e. perspectives we take when looking at a learning process. A level is thus meant to describe a field of actions placed in a similar observation sphere or context and showing common features which enable us to identify a structure, some kind of order, or special patterns that can be compared. For a survey of the levels that I am going to introduce, refer to diagram 1 (below).

Learning and teaching action levels	Communication (dialogues)	Objects	Contents	Relationships (behavior)
immediate subjective experience (being there)	S – O	I see/perceive, so I know	appear as quasi-images	appear as quasi-images
conventional experience (regulated dialogues)	S – IC – O	I see/perceive, as others see/perceive, so I know	are set up conventionally from outside and confined to a limited range of knowledge	are set up conventionally from outside and confined to a particular behavior
discourses (open dialogues)	S – IC 1 IC 2 IC 3 etc. – O	I see/perceive, as is seen/perceived differently, so I know	are agreed upon openly as possibilities within a variety of knowledge according to viability criteria	are agreed upon openly as possibilities out of varying forms of behavior according to viability criteria

S = subject; O = object; IC = interpretive community

Diagram 1: Three levels of learning

a) Immediate subjective experience

When reflecting on the self-observations of a teacher or a learner, s/he first of all appears to be a subject facing reality *for herself/himself*. This reality seems to represent itself in the subject: In a given situation, s/he experiences objects in the world, things, events and other subjects in an *immediate subjective* way and *immediately* visualizes them. It is part of the realistic intuitions that we rather trust an actually experienced reality than one that has only been theoretically described, e.g. by being put in mere words, by being dreamed or pretended. This kind of realism always appears solid to us because since childhood we have been encouraged to make use of our senses in order to verify how real or certain things are »in reality«. We are supposed to permanently distinguish on an objective, relational and contents level what »really« happens in order to delimitate this reality from what has been only imagined, was based on deceptions or was meant but is not really significant. The claim of a subjectively perceived immediate experience of reality, i.e. a reality which is *real* to us, is meant to help us to distinguish actions which we are forced to carry out due to accurate perception and reasonable understanding and also help us to delimitate them from those that we can or should refrain from due to insufficient certainty or deception.

Yet, in such realistic expectations we experience day by day that we are placed in reality together with other people who all have a gradually different perception or ability of conception of this reality. How do we react to these subjective differences within a supposed objective immediate experience that actually should be equal to everybody? Our confidence in an objective perception seems to be solely based on looking very closely and exactly at objects, taking them up in an unfractured way and mirroring them in us in order to come close to reality and to what true reality is.

Within immediate subjective experience we are close to our individual perception and therefore close to the interface between ourselves and the world *out there*. This is what philosophers described as a subject-object-relationship (S – O). I see the world, I perceive something, and I immediately seem to know what *is*. According to Hegel, this is the basic step into consciousness. He called this step sense certainty.[4] However, this is a very subjective point of view; we assume that we can see a thing in private and that the world is exclusively at our disposal. If we claimed this, we would have to bear problematic consequences: Nobody will see anything except for what s/he sees the way s/he sees it, s/he will remain all on her/his own and will not understand anything but her/his individual immediate subjective experience that seems to be very limited if we take a look from outside.

If we took this subjectivity for granted, everything would end up being interchangeable. But when we critically view our action, is there any such interchangeability? To insist in such privacy or pure subjectivism is impossible when living within a cultural community. However, the private as well as the subjective can describe a borderline-condition of communication, conceding the subject to have *her/his* immediate subjective experience and perception, while at the same time demanding from her/him to communicate with *others* about how to interpret her/his singular experience in the context of generalizations. Thus, s/he is now able to state the fact that in this particular culture this or that or another phenomenon will be perceived predominantly in this particular way, but nevertheless I, as a special individual within this culture, do see something else in addition. Nowa-

4 I use the term *sense certainty* (»sinnliche Gewissheit«) in my German publications to describe this level of acting.

days, I am granted to claim such subjectivity within certain limits which are regulated by communicative agreements on common interests– as, for example, language and other conventions.[5]

The constructivist approach stands in contrast to all copy or correspondence theories of knowledge. The subject-object-relationship (S – O) as a mere copy relationship is nothing but an illusion. For the act of perceiving (containing anything that has been perceived in terms of culture already) always implies claims, expectations, habits, preferences, sensations that enter into those perceptions and ideas. This is regulated by convention beforehand as well as during the act of perceiving. So I may see a table and I feel that it is beautiful. But how do I know about the table? It is due to cultural habit and to a world developed and transmitted within a culture, due to my situation in life-world and to language, due to preconditions placed far beyond my capacity of perceiving. Perception first of all is a means, a method of acquiring various contents of a culture. In a singular moment perception is even more, it is immediate subjective experience (what Dewey named *primary experience*) in the abundance of impressions, feelings, associations. The beauty of a table, however, I do not know until I have been initiated into the subtle cultural game of differences that produce different perceptions of tables as constructed distinctions.[6] This is why immediate subjective experience represents an important action level with learning: It grants a subjective sphere of experience for individual examination of facts and statements in order to create their viability in the actual experience.

If the comparison between subjective experience and the objectivation of life-world is supposed to take place from a mere realistic perspective and if it is expected that the fight will be decided only in favour of one's own perception against everything else, then constructivist epistemology sets in to disillusion our expectations. What can we put forward in particular against such realism and mere subjectivism as it can always be detected in learning theories? I am going to state some reasons:

---

5 Though undermined during recent decades, judging according to the criteria of normal/abnormal does, still, serve as a conventional barrier between what may be and what may not be approved.

6 Bourdieu writes in his famous book *Distinction: A Social Critique of the Judgement of Taste:* »Taste classifies, and it classifies the classifier. Social subjects, classified by their classifications, distinguish themselves by the distinctions they make, between the beautiful and the ugly, the distinguished and the vulgar, in which their position in the objective classifications is expressed or betrayed.« Thus the language game about the table and the beauty is a construction of distinctions that makes distinctions. It shows limitations of the subjective experience, but it is a necessary step to give the subject a distinction it can work on.

- A realism that wants to make us believe that reality can be easily copied or mirrored, is unable to make us understand why human cultures have reacted so differently to the supposed pure nature out there. Why weren't we all supplied with the same understanding by images? In the succession and coexistence of cultures we need to admit that there are not only different versions of world creation within different cultures, but, in present times, also within one culture.
- Even the hard sciences were unable to establish a world image in which they achieved a concluding agreement on facts. At most, they managed to agree a little bit more in joint discourses for a certain time on a methodical level than, for instance, the cultural sciences which need to admit a larger spectrum of indeterminacy from the very beginning.[7] Yet, the venture of an unambiguous reconstruction also follows a methodical narrowness which constantly produces risks in other areas as a consequent effect.[8]
- Today, we can no longer fail to notice the postmodern offences inflicted on science. Nelson Goodman, for instance, talks about the loss of the one world also leading to the loss of the one correct version of world.[9] Nowadays, we need to engage into the idea that several »correct versions« of world exist successively and simultaneously. It does not matter which construction of world we look at, we will always discover and invent different, but at the same time – each for itself – correct (viable) solutions within them. Putnam has stated his conclusion from this understanding when examining Goodman as follows: Each construction of world can be formalized and each of the thereby developed formalisms represents a completely legitimate parlance; yet, Goodman would say (and Putnam would agree) that none of them can claim to be in such a way *as the things are independent of experience*. There is more than just one true description of reality. (cf. Putnam 1993, 254)

Immediate subjective experience, as a first level with learning, now appears conflicting against the background of this problematization:

---

7 Some very restricted areas show a consensus, which, nevertheless, is regulated by conventions. Cf. thereto for instance from an interactive-constructivist perspective, e.g. the pedagogically relevant analysis on time by Hasenfratz (2003).

8 These effects have clearly emerged during the 20th century. The stronger scientific-technical progress was developed, the higher grew the risks, which were caused by it, as well as the perception of the risks (e.g. the risks of nuclear energy, nuclear weapons and other weapon technologies, gene technology, complex ecological crises; they also include the possibilities of mass murder and the destruction of life which show a scientific-technical background).

9 This loss is explicitly elaborated on and described from the perspectives of very different post-metaphysical theories of the 20th century. I also speak of movements of offended reason which, amongst others, lead to a genesis of constructivist thinking, cf. Reich (1998 a, b).

(a) It is consistently part of our human experiences that we need to – and also can – rely on immediate subjective experience, our own perceptions. In doing so, we experience the differences of theory and practice and consider it to be a realistic and viable attitude to believe in theoretical predictions and statements only then if there are practical clues of verification, that is, if we can find, see, and touch objects in our own experience, our perception and if, thereupon, these objects pervade our conscience as images and can therefore be counted as real. This also includes, for instance, experiences in which we see something as an eye-witness which we can report on. We are particularly scared if something has been hidden or concealed from us so far and is now revealed to us in a situation. When being amazed or terrified, we are very close to *the real* and change our view of reality. This includes all experiences which we make when we allow an immediate subjective experience to produce an as comprehensive as possible effect on us, without having ourselves pinned down too rashly to specific patterns of interpretation or previous experiences. In such moments we are open for assuming new perspectives on events and also to oppose the singularity of experience against generalization because we rather trust our subjective feelings than the conventional requirements from outside.

(b) At the same time we consistently need to concede that by now the so called »pure« reality has been long since interwoven with human constructions, which – as prerequisites – determine what we had until just now thought as pure perception. Regardless what event, we are always unable to completely step out of what we have become. Our socialization has aroused feelings like disgust, shame and doubt, our patterns of interpretation allow only specific perspectives, and our environment determines us on specific preferences of perception and impulses. Although we think that, due to our immediate subjective experience and perception, we have our very own view on what we perceive, we readily fail to notice how many other opinions have already become part of our judgment.

Learners and learning theories that refer to immediate subjective experience will, from a constructivist view, be unable to relinquish critically observing the supposed realistic images which are produced subjectively in situations of perception against the background of their cultural/social use and context. Yet, constructivism is not claiming that objects or situations could not be comprehended in a particularly close and direct sensuously manner. In his pragmatic approach, John Dewey has already established that, regarding learning, immediate images are granted a particular dignity: Learners are supposed to make as many direct experiences as possible in order to increase their awareness for the use of objects within their life-world by *experience*.[10] Yet, Dewey also pointed out that this would

10 More precisely, this does not mean immediate images in the sense of an unambiguous reflection, but images which are created by a subject for itself in a concrete, direct,

never produce »pure« images[11], because man defines the significance of immediate subjective experience within his understanding and explanations only by its use and context. Insofar, nobody will be able to sufficiently learn something if s/he just tries to remember objects of seemingly immediate subjective experience.

A concrete image focuses on what is there. I take a walk and see a tree. I can have various immediate subjective experiences with this tree. I can touch it, climb it, rip off branches, grind leaves between my fingers. Yet, if I want to explain such experiences in a symbolic way to myself or others, my immediate subjective experience (in terms of an inner image) is of no use to me. I have to start describing, producing images in my mind's eye which are more than just a copy, create words, detect meanings. As soon as I start to talk, the tree has changed in something different. It is no longer the one image that it seemed to be until right now. According to brain researchers, it is, anyhow, not the pictured tree, because, as the brain researcher will explain to me, as a human being I already enter presupposing prerequisites into the image. These help to produce a human image which may appear to me as a real image, but would produce a completely different image for another category.[12] Insofar, images always have to be discussed against the background of generalizable possibilities and prerequisites within the act of copying.

Yet, particularly with learning, we consistently place a large emphasis on images. Until today, this form of naturalism is particularly common with pedagogics and didactics. Teachers are preferably ushered into a position where they offer to the learners such supposed images which associate and locate an object with the designated denotation in order to build up a realistic world picture. Particularly during the first school years this tends to be a popular method. Object lessons serve to show a pictorial world which is claimed to be the real world – this is supposed to produce a realistic basis for a cultural understanding. Yet, unfortunately this also produces an illusionary world in which people believe that they are able to produce an unambiguous world with simple images by means of perception.

Perception itself disposes of no criterion for the cultural evaluation of the contexts of the world. Insofar, perception may deceive us exactly when living in a quasi-world (as symbolized by the film »The Trueman-Show«, for instance). Perception is only of help with the cultural evaluation of the world if we notice the contradictions between the promised, expected, standardized world and our concrete (perceptible) experiences made within this world. Yet, the promises, expec-

---

sensuous situation in which it is then enabled to compare this creation immediately with the experience in the situation (verification of reality and experience).

11 As an introduction hereto, cf. Dewey (1985); Neubert (1998).

12 With regard to such biological understanding, brain researchers tend to deduct a realistic and naturalist point of view by failing to take notice of the cultural integration and conveyance and by reducing everything to biological aspects. As introduction hereto, cf. e.g. Edelman/Tononi (2000, in particular 140 ff., 207 ff.).

tations will often easily seduce us to only perceive what others want us to perceive, i.e. we will judge according to desired and undesired perception.

Standardization by means of desired images is quite large: correct spelling, nice handwriting, a correct image, the exact denotation, an unambiguous use of signs and symbols, the correct experience. Therefore, the first years in school are, for instance, the time in life when children start to explain to their parents that the image of the world they have been provided with so far is not correct because the teacher has provided them with a completely new one. Already before attending school, we not only develop a certain egocentrism of reality construction alongside the makeup of symbolic abilities, as elaborated by Piaget, but also tend to show an animistic disposition of world explanation. This is where the belief in the image is based and rooted so deeply that, despite a constructivist epistemology, it can only scarcely be forsaken later on. It seems as if the senses themselves have been called up to understand reality. Yet, we need to understand beforehand that senses do not dispose of criteria that are necessary to see what other prerequisites have already entered into this understanding. Senses take reality the way it is right now. Whether landscape or architecture, toy or tool, traffic or virtual media, the existence of a world which can be immediately experienced in a subjective way, always forces perception into those images that are perceived and whose reality seduces us to believe in their actuality and truth.[13] In animism, for instance, additional logical connections may be created, emerging from such perceptions. We see lightning in the sky and hear massive thunder and now we can also establish a personified originator who is marked as the producer of this inapprehensible. If we trust in images, we soon run the risk of an exaggerated generalization because we are seduced by the image to believe in the simple logic of seeing, in animistic or other projections, or in simplification. This is particularly valid if these images are presented by teachers because they are normally perceived as someone knowing more, respectively knowing things better.

Constructivist educationalists should handle images with care. In order to make visible the constructions which have already entered the concept of reality, they would need to – with reference to Friedrich Wallner's terminology – strangificate every naïve realism. On one hand, we need to yield to the impulse to create our own experiences with learning comprehensively and, by means of concrete, sensuous, objective experiences, acquire images that arouse the imaginary. Yet on the other hand, the teacher will have to intervene and relativize in order to

13 With reference to the media, which increasingly replace natural realities by artificial realities and therefore provide perception with simulated impulses as base material, Baudrillard states that our today's world represents an age of simulation which we will only be able to escape if we allow ourselves to be seduced to another (real) world which puts a stronger emphasis on the non-simulated. Yet, this direction seems to be quite improbable, as the artificial, the constructed, which returns as reality to our perceptions, is growing, cf. further Reich/Wild/Zimmermann (2004).

fight the illusion that such an unambiguous world may be built up as a copy model. In particular, he will have to re-orientate herself/himself on a linguistic level and avoid saying: »Look, this is exactly how the world *is*«, but rather say: »What images do you see, what is familiar to you and what is unfamiliar, how have people in former times perceived it and what has changed until today, what different interpretations are there?« This, nevertheless, does not rule out to causally ask for re-construable contexts in unambiguous copy sequences: »In a given sequence of actions, which could be the first and which the last image?« – this is a popular causal question in order to reproduce logical sequences of action. Yet, it only describes this one causality which, again, is generally very limited in its significance.

Taking a closer look at learning processes, we can establish that, in a strict sense, there are no immediate images with respect to the contents of learning. Contents are constructed and made by man in order to predicate something about realities, but partly also in order to describe the unreal. It is possible to give an account of the contents, yet it is impossible to copy it in a strict literal sense. Content is not a sensuously tangible object, but it leads a discourse *on* or offers an interpretation *about* objects. If I ask you to read this text and tell me what actually happened in reality, I give inaccurate directions. I can only tell what has been described, but not what the event actually was like in the end. A text is no direct eye-witness, at most, it can be written by an eye-witness and it always contains less than what has happened in a given situation or has been experience. Contents in learning – irrespective of its form – can not be understood as a concrete image, because it is always an interpretation, governs my perception, and offers sense and perspectives.

b) Conventional experience

It is an interpretive community that has joined subject and object as a mediator (S – IC – O) and that, in accordance with norms demanded by the actual way of life, will influence and guide my perception by establishing contexts and spaces for interpretation. In former times, depending on social classes for example, there used to be strongly judging norms, while now norms and values are becoming more open, more ambivalent.[14] So today I may very easily happen to have arguments with others, whose judgment differs from mine. Each of us may then insist on her/his subjective perception and play it off against the others. Thus someone may state: »I do see it the way it is. I see what's happening. I can definitely de-

14 This is, for example, shown in Giddens' (1991) approach describing the transition from modernity to a reflexive self-identity that is referring to risks similar to those pointed out by Beck (1992) in his »Risk Society«. Zygmunt Bauman (e.g. 1989, 1992, 1997) describes these aspects in his essays in a very instructive way.

scribe what I am perceiving.« Judging in terms of subjectivity, we could not at all deny that. However, such subjectivity, resulting in a mutual lack of understanding, is nowadays regarded as a hypertrophied subjective demand and is also an illusion, as within a culture nobody could be able to fend all for herself/himself.

Thus, in learning we are confronted with a double perception: on the one hand there is immediate experience perceived subjectively, each subject being allowed to have his very personal experiences (= individual view). On the other hand, those perceived experiences have been rendered controversial, for they never can be completely pure, completely free or undetermined, because they already contain culturally established perspectives and norms conventionally regulating our perception and coordinating it with other people's perception so that our mutual acts may be coordinated (= social view).

In teaching and in learning, therefore, perceptions almost always have been regulated by convention, i.e. the dialogues taking place between teacher and learner are subject to the norms established by interpretive communities having decided beforehand on the correctness, the truth, the honesty of justification and validity.

Conventional contents tends to appear especially in those educational subjects in which the members of a community, regardless of the many potential or actual differences between them, have come to a long-term agreement on which technical language to use, which scientific or technical rules to obey, and what particular conventions to share. Such rules and conventions are being interpreted as laws, as universal norms, as valid methods. Deviations from those norms will have to be tolerated to enable the development of innovations; however, any deviation will have to be plausibly explained as logical with regard to the rules existing. I will resume the meaning as well as the risk of conventional learning as follows:[15]

- The meaning is, first of all, that we can hardly find reasons for denying the cultural necessity of learning a language, of acquiring grammatical structures and keeping to the rules of orthography, of learning the numbers and mathematical functions, of knowing how to handle money, time, norms and prescriptions, or of knowing the capitals of various countries, the predominant practices, routines, or institutions existing – that is, to jointly reconstruct everything that has been established as a meaning, as a sense, as a rule, in such way that as many as possible members of a culture may deal with it in a viable manner and also have to in order to get on in their life-world.

15 To apply this to all of the members of a culture will, however, remain an ideal, as there will be deviations. In postmodernism there is an increase in possibilities of deviations as well as in globalized knowledge.

- The risk is that by establishing conventions we will automatically land ourselves with a meaning that will narrow our perspectives that will nail us down to habits, will limit the range of creative solutions and may easily tempt us to feel that there is almost nothing new to be found. This would mean that the world could not be designed in an essentially different way anymore.

c) Discourses (open dialogues)

Interactive constructivism will deny neither efficiency nor benefit of conventions. However, it consistently points out the idea that conventions can and should claim validity only with regard to a particular viability, that will have to be cleared up with the learner continuously participating and that will be established for a limited period of time only, so that we may remain open to realizing present problems as well as future solutions. This is why conventional claims for truth and correctness, especially with regard to learning, will have to remain relative. To recognize this relativity in learning, it seems to be important that with learning we frequently appeal to and arrive at a discursive action level, which will enable the learner to critically examine, for him as well as together with others, the immediate subjective experience he has gained and the conventions given to him beforehand.

What do we understand by a discourse? In the narrow sense of the word it simply refers to a »speech« or an »argument« people have in dialogues. The Greeks already dealt with the concept of the disputation as a way of exchanging, examining, and valuing thoughts. On another level, discourses today also refer to scientific schools. Thus for example we will talk of the »discourse of psychoanalysis« or of the »philosophical discourse of postmodernism« to refer to a more or less clearly defined field of exchanging ideas in science. In interactive constructivism the term is defined in a still more complex way[16]: Here *discourse* means any kind of symbolic order of intentional processes of understanding. At the same time the term refers to reasons or rules on the basis of which this order claims validity. It is being observed within an interpretive community for particular intentions and a limited period of time. This meaning of the word *discourse* is more complex than »speech and argument«, because, instead of just describing contents and relationships by words and speech, we also ask for the rules taken for granted, for the observations already made, for the cultural perspectives and contexts, which together constitute the background on which contents and relationships appear and, also, what this means with regard to interpretation.

The aim of learning by open dialogue (discursive learning) is to allow the learner to look at the preconditions and rules of what is offered to her/him through immediate subjective experience, as contents and codes of behavior through con-

16 For more detailed description cf. Reich (1998 b, chapter 4).

vention, and as better judgment through discourse. Sooner or later the learner must find out and decide for her/himself what will fit her/him best and how to transform it into her/his situation of life. To this may add particularly a discursive view of learning. How can we encourage such learning in and through discourse? In a discourse the conveying of contents and relationships always involves open dialogue. Thus, as a result from different views by various interpretive communities, there may be numerous, contradictory, or ambivalent justifications of the subject-object-interrelation (S – IC 1 – IC 2 – IC 3 – etc. – O).

At this point there may often occur a conflict with the conventional level of learning and teaching action. Such conflicts cannot be avoided altogether and should be taken as reasons for questioning the respective conventions with regard to their validity promised as a result of former discursive justification. To achieve that aim by methods appropriate to the learner and to the requirements s/he can meet as a member of a particular age group, is to be considered as one of the difficult tasks in teaching.

One of the conventions about learning will say, for example, that in order to enable everybody to learn effectively, there has to be silence in the room. Being silent has been embodied in a discourse of discipline, which will be observed out of habit. As a matter of fact, in former learning scenarios which were centered on the teacher, it was absolutely essential for the learners to keep their mouths shut. However, in altered teaching methods the teacher as well may be urged to keep his mouth shut.[17] Then, due to the learner's activities, the noise level will rise. Now teacher and learners will have to find out together, to what extent the implicit convention may still be considered as valid, or in what way it has to be transformed. In a joint discourse, arguments for and against will be stated and a new convention will be declared valid for this particular group and for a limited period of time. Simultaneously the rules according to which the discourse will proceed, must also be reflected upon: Is it adequate to have majority decisions, or will the group need to protect individual learners who, due to the noise, cannot concentrate sufficiently? Offering his advice, the teacher will play an active part in the discursive process. Evaluations may help to specify the claims shared by all members of the group as well as conflicting points of view, thus achieving at best a solution sufficiently viable for all members of the group.

A discursive concept is a concept which not only describes objects that can be sensuously experienced, reproduces contents and imitates behavior. A discursive concept will demand more from learning: Looking at the level of immediate subjective experience, it is particularly the use of experiments that may promote teaching by question instead of by result. John Dewey showed this very clearly and claimed it a fundamental approach in education. To be curious about objects, to behave exploringly, ready to take a detour or even a wrong way in achieving

---

17 As an example cf. Finkel (2000).

knowledge, to behave in a particular situation by referring to experiences already gained before, to express oneself by using extended means, allowing presentation in more than only a rational, language-dominated way: those are fundamental claims forming the preconditions for discursive understanding.

While learning, we will quite often face the question what learners are actually supposed to learn. Why is some material considered to be important while some other seems to be unimportant? Who is to lay down the aims, contents, methods, and the standards for tests and exams? Learning theories favoring the copy or correspondence view of knowledge will remain completely uncritical of those questions and, in submission to what is considered to be an authority, will take over what seems to be forced on them by prescription as a quasi-image from outside. An uncritical learning theory abides by majority decisions and instructions appearing to be indisputable. Mostly, they are assumptions settled by experts and bureaucracy, hiding, however, to the learner the preconditions according to which they were selected. The learner will learn in a way which is considered as a custom. He will achieve apparent expertise without gaining any sufficient knowledge of the methods telling him what and when and why he should learn. A more complex competence taking into account contents and relationships may not be acquired by the learner until s/he is enabled to learn in a way as it is provided by discursive learning theories. It is then that s/he will ask her/himself as well as others what rules and preconditions resulted in favoring these particular contents and behaviors while neglecting others. By and by s/he will be able to establish a critical, reflecting conscience and to examine by way of her/his personal experiences the viability of contents and behaviors with respect to her/his individual situation of life: »The others may say so, but will it fit me, too?«

Some specific characteristics apply to relationships, when they become the objects of discursive reflection. Behavior in discursive relationships does not follow logic of contents but refers to a special logic of relationships. Here it is of decisive importance that teacher and learner develop their communicative competence. Unlike causal and linear attributions, as they are often to be found in scientific or technological processes, relationships will follow different laws. The interplay of contents and relationships will influence the roles taken by teachers and learners.

Looking at the action levels of learning in an overall context, we need to concede that they actually only document a certain logic of learning in a simple form which has to be enriched by other perspectives. Here, the interactive constructivism refers, for instance, to the perspectives of construction, reconstruction, and deconstruction for acting, it refers to the observer, the participant, and the agents as differentiation of roles of acting, and it also refers to the symbolic, the imaginary, and the real as reflections of the description level – just to name some important terms. Regarding the action levels as described here, a reflection on them clearly shows that, from a constructivist perspective, every form of naïve realism has to be abandoned. Only by deducting on a discursive level we can disclose what we look for as a prerequisite in immediate subjective experience. It may have been this temptation which caused Friedrich Wallner to call his theory a constructivist realism, yet, I also think that I can gather from his works that he – as well as I – will, due to the constructivist approach, disapprove of a naïve copy theory as well as of a more subtle derivation theory based on a supposed unambiguous *reality*. Also, from the perspective of his theory, he will emphasize that it is particularly the strangification between these levels, which develops when we alternate between them that can lead us to a deeper knowledge on our versions of reality.

Reference

Bauman, Z. (1989). *Modernity and the Holocaust*. London: Routledge.

Bauman, Z. (1992). *Intimations of Postmodernity*. London: Routledge.

Bauman, Z. (1997). *Postmodernism and its Discontent*. New York: New York University Press.

Beck, U. (1992). *Risk Society*. London: Sage.

Dewey, J. (1985). Democracy and Education. In: *The Middle Works 1899 – 1924, Vol 9*, Carbondale and Edwardsville: Southern Illinois University Press.

Edelman, G.M./Tononi, G. (2000). *Consciousness. How Matter becomes Imagination*. London: Penguin.

Finkel, D.L. (2000). *Teaching with your Mouth Shut*. Portsmouth, NH: Boynton/Cook Publishers.

Giddens, A. (1991). *Modernity and Self Identity*. London: Polity Press.

Giddens, A. (1991). *The Consequences of Modernity*. Stanford: University Press.

Hasenfratz, M. (2003). Wege zur Zeit. In S.v. Neubert & K. Reich (ed.), *Reihe Interaktionistischer Konstruktivismus. Bd. 2*. Münster: Waxmann.

Neubert, S. (1998). *Erkenntnis, Verhalten und Kommunikation. John Deweys Philosophie des »Experience« in interaktionistisch-konstruktivistischer Interpretation*. Münster: Waxmann.

Putnam, H. (1993). *Von einem realistischen Standpunkt. Schriften zur Sprache und Wirklichkeit*. Reinbek: Rowohlt.

Reich, K. (1998a). *Die Ordnung der Blicke. Band 1: Beobachtung und die Unschärfen der Erkenntnis*. Neuwied u.a.: Luchterhand.

Reich, K. (1998b). *Die Ordnung der Blicke. Band 2: Beziehungen und Lebenswelt*. Neuwied u.a.: Luchterhand.

Reich, K. (2004). *Konstruktivistische Didaktik* (2. edition). Neuwied u.a.: Luchterhand.

Reich, K./Wild, R./Zimmermann, L. (2004). Simulation als Kommunikation. In S.v. Neubert & K. Reich (ed.), *Reihe Interaktionistischer Konstruktivismus, Bd. 3*. Münster: Waxmann.

Hans Rudi Fischer

Rationality, Reasoning and Paralogical Thinking

Rationality, rule-following, and logical inference

Logic plays a fundamental role in the specification of humans as rational beings. Traditional logic has been dealing with rules of inference since ancient times, and consequently with the operational basis for the manufacturing of knowledge, i.e. of true statements. »Laws« of logic must govern the order according to which humans think, speak, and reach conclusions which are judged to be rational. This understanding of rationality is tied to logic and its »rules of thought«. Since the time of Aristotle logicians have been trying to separate the valid forms of syllogistic inference from the invalid ones in order to pave the rational, the royal, road leading human reason(ing) to true knowledge.

In dealing with mental illness those guiding differences are of particular interest which constitute, and historically rigidify, mechanisms of the inclusion or exclusion of rationality. With reference to the distinction mentally ill vs. mentally sound any deviation from the »laws of inference« of logic has from times immemorial been taken to be a criterion of exclusion from rational discourse. »Mentally disturbed«, insane, people seem to lack the kind of logical sense of order which we call rationality: here irrationality seems to reign in the form of a logic in disarray. The order of psychiatry shares the view of philosophical logic that the »laws of thought« embody fundamental principles of rationality and, consequently, speaks of »disturbed«, of »paralogical« thinking. The distinction between logical and paralogical thinking (paralogismos, Greek: false, incorrect, inference) focusses on the procedures enabling the human mind to draw inferences.

If, however, inferring can be understood to be the rule-governed progression from A to B, from the One to the Other, then all the processes classified as processes of understanding necessarily involve rule-bound inference. What I want to show is that human rationality not only cannot be reduced to the use of logical, apriori valid, patterns of inference (syllogisms) but that it is, in most cases, not even tied to this particular form of »logical laws«.The charge of irrationality which has been levelled against the logically Other for thousands of years might thus be revealed to be profoundly irrational because it rests upon the belief in the validity, completeness and universality of logic, a belief that cannot rationally be justified. If it can be shown that we all draw our inferences in precisely the same way as those people who are alleged to be »mad« then »paralogical« inference can no longer be maintained as a rational criterion of irrationality.

Charles Sanders Peirce (1839-1914), the founder of pragmatism, spent four decades on the investigation of induction and deduction, models of thinking well established in logic and the philosophy of science, and supplemented them by an inferential procedure which he called abduction. In this article I want to elucidate the role and the function of this mode of inference in order to exploit it for the understanding of hermeneutical processes – with particular emphasis on »irrational« ways of thinking and communicating. I find abduction, i.e. abductive reasoning, so extremely interesting because although on the basis of logical rationality, it is obviously paralogical and irrational, it nevertheless to my mind appears to be the psychologically most relevant form of thinking of all. I shall, therefore, interpret paralogical thinking against the horizon of abductive modes of inference because, in this way, I can avail myself of the opportunity to discover, or invent, rationality in the irrational, i.e. grasp a sort of rationality deviating from logic. I want to establish a hermeneutical logic which does not exclude »deranged thinking« as irrational but embraces it as another form of discursivity which is fundamentally intelligible.

It is these very paralogical patterns of thinking which are encountered in myth and poetry just as well as in dreams, in science, and in the realities of our ordinary thoughts. And such violations of logically valid inferences do not only belong to the core of all creativity and innovation, they are, paradoxically enough, a necessary requirement for any endeavour to reconcile life and logic. In this way I want to contribute to the demystification of the myth of an exclusively logic-dependent rationality and show that all our actual thinking is permeated by such paralogical figures of thought as have generally been ascribed to magical and mythological thinking and have also been, and still largely are, considered to be characteristic of so-called schizophrenic thinking.

Exotic thinking or logical correctness

Michel Foucault's book *Les mots et le choses* was inspired by an »encyclopedia« which shakes the very foundations of our thinking and works an »exotic magic« that seems to conjure up in front of our eyes the very bounds of the unthinkable. Foucault quotes a Chinese encyclopedia itself »quoted« by Jorge Luis Borges, in which

»[...] the animals are grouped as follows: a) animals belonging to the emperor, b) embalmed animals, c) tamed animals, d) suckling pigs, e) sirens, f) animals of fable, g) stray dogs, h) members of this group that display mad behaviour, k) that are depicted with the finest brush made out of camel hair, l) and so on, m) that have broken the water jug...« (qu. from Foucault, 1974, p1. 17)

How are the Same and the Other treated here that it irritates our thinking in such a massive way, making us consider such an »encyclopedia« unthinkable and deranged? This fictitious encyclopedia, invented by the Argentine writer Jorge Luis Borges, demonstrates the fundamental arbitrariness of all taxonomies because any sign may be semantically connected with any other sign in a system of signs, because the criterion of the »same« is measured by/against what must have been established by the observer prior to his observation and description. We have here the fictional example of a kind of thinking which, according to the orders and standards of the logicians, must be categorized as »paralogical«.

Foucault specifies similarity as the fundamental category of epistemology until the end of the 16th century. Thinking in similarities is for him the basic principle of the organization of knowledge before the dawn of the classical »age of representation« (17th century, Descartes) which begins to establish, in a series of steps, the modes of thinking based on identities and differences. What was designated as paralogical or palaeological thinking in our century was the normal kind of knowledge organization for pre-classical thinking up to the 17th century – if one accepts Foucault's archaeology. Foucault calls the thinking in similarities which, in his view, is kept alive today only by the arts, »homo-semanticism« (p.82), and he sees the insane and the poet as occupying two extreme opposite poles in the range of similarities: The madman »perceives nothing but similarities and signs of similarity. All signs to him are similar and all similarities have the value of signs. At the other extreme of the cultural space ... there is the poet who re-discovers the hidden relations between things as well as their familiar similarities underneath all their labelled and predictable ordinary differences.« (p.81)

Borges' fictitious example of »exotic« thinking is at the same time an example of a defamiliarizing transformation (as by Fritz Wallner analysed and utilized). Viewing and describing phenomena and things through the spectacles (the concept) of another taxonomy or grammar constitute an act of defamiliarization: the supposedly familiar appears strange. To discover strangeness and different ways of thinking, it is unnecessary to appeal to other cultures or faraway times, it is enough to look at the grammars existing side by side and working in parallel within a group of people in communication. I shall quote a simple example taken from the language game relating to fruits. The grammar of the ordinary language game here tends to stick to visible »similarities«, to the visual, to »surfaces«, and it labels certain fruits as berries and others as nuts. Berries comprise strawberries, raspberries, blackberries, currants etc. Nuts comprise peanuts, cocoanuts, hazelnuts etc. If we, however, play the appropriate language game of the botanists, then we encounter a completely different organization which thoroughly abstracts, and accordingly deviates, from the visible similarities of the ordinary language game. With the berries we do indeed find the predictable raspberry but also such unpredictable fruits like lemon, banana or cucumber. The situation with the nuts is no less »exotic« because, for the botanist, they comprise not only the predictable peanut but also unpredictable fruits like the strawberry (a »syncarp«, i.e. a compound nut fruit) or the edible chestnut.

So the exotic character and the fictionality of Borghes' example are immediately relativized by the fact that we can formulate the following fully legitimate equations on the basis of the taxonomies of the botanist:

A strawberry is a nut.
A banana is a berry.

Zoology could easily supply other relational orderings that appear similarly bizarre from a common-sense perspective. It must be noted here that statements like »A banana is a berry« constitute inferences drawn on the basis of a specific kind of logic (a grammar of description) which is consistent in itself and rule-bound. On the basis of the logic of his criteria (his rules, his grammar) for the use of the concept of ›berry‹ the botanist is able to explain exactly why a banana belongs with the berries. In this he must rely on implicit premises which may be shown to be »grammatical regulations« in the sense of established »measuring methods« employed to survey and organize reality. The metaphor of a »measuring method« which is occasionally used by Wittgenstein may here be replaced by the metaphor of a »method of thinking« or »law of thought«. The botanist's statement that a banana is a berry is, therefore, not the result of faulty reasoning; it is simply the outcome of a different way of thinking which deviates from everyday thought.

Wittgenstein keeps returning to questions of this kind in his philosophy of logic. In what sense are logical laws as »laws of thought" absolutely and universally valid, or to what extent are they conventional, culturally shaped standards of »correct thinking«? In the context of his discussion of Gottlob Frege's critique of psychologism Wittgenstein notes the following which I want to quote in full:

»In seinem Vorwort zu ›Grundgesetze der Arithmetik‹ spricht Frege davon, daß die logischen Gesetze keine psychologischen Sätze. Das heißt, wir können die Wahrheit der logischen Sätze nicht durch eine psychologische Untersuchung herausfinden – sie hängen nicht von dem ab, was wir denken. Frege stellt dort die Frage, was wir den sagen würden, wenn wir auf Menschen stießen, die im Gegensatz zu unseren logischen Sätzen urteilen. Was würden wir denn sagen, wenn wir auf Menschen stießen, die unsere logischen Gesetze nicht a priori anerkennen, sondern durch einen langwierigen Induktionsprozeß zu ihnen gelangen? Oder wenn wir gar Menschen fänden, die unsere logischen Gesetze überhaupt nicht anerkennen und logische Sätze aufstellen, die den unseren entgegengesetzt sind? Frege schreibt: ›ich würde sagen: Hier haben wir eine neue Art von Verrücktheit‹ – während der psychologische Logiker nur sagen könnte: ›Dies ist eine neuartige Logik.‹« (Wittgenstein 1970, p.243f.)

Something that does not obey the laws of logic is, consequently, declared to be »deranged«, deficient, and relegated to pathology. Foucault's discourse analysis with regard to madness has brought such processes to light. The mere possibility of thinking in a different way is held to be unthinkable. Here I am in favour of the view of the »psychological logician« that deranged thinking (and speaking) should not be conceived of as a sort of faulty thinking but as a different mode of thinking. Only in this way can it be understood as being fundamentally connectable with the discourse of its community.

Different thinking follows different rules, i.e. a different grammar. Wittgenstein, in his middle period, step by step deconstructs the belief in the absolute validity of logic, begins to speak of logics in the plural, and finally replaces the concept of logic by the concept of grammar as that kind of logic which regulates and structures ordinary thinking and speaking. Inspired by this idea of a different grammar or logic that is potentially coherent and consistent in itself, I shall now turn to the classical psychiatric paradigm concerning »deranged logic«.

Exotic thinking: Are Indians stags and strawberries nuts?

In the 1940ies (1944) the Dutch psychiatrist Eilhard von Domarus investigated the thinking of patients with a diagnosis of schizophrenia and specified the causal core of the schizophrenic »thinking disorder« as a certain deviation from deductive-syllogistic inference. The results of the analyses carried out by Von Domarus met with intensive critical interest in psychiatric research for some time but are no longer of great relevance today. Although I shall try to show that the Von-Domarus-Principle is false on logical grounds, it seems to hold a key to the understanding of »schizophrenic thinking«.

Von Domarus reports that a patient, diagnosed as schizophrenic, believed in the »identity« of Jesus, a cigar box and sexuality. An instance of »exotic« thinking or an instance of poetry? A closer examination of the case yielded the »missing link« between the three concepts for the patient, namely the property of »encirclement«. The head of Jesus was encircled by a halo, the cigar box by a revenue band, the woman by the leer of a male (op.cit., p.108 f.). For the schizophrenic patient – in contrast to »normally« thinking people – the »objects« (Jesus, cigar box...) have something in common which connects them. That is to say, there »exists« a universe of discourse in which the concepts in question »meet« in such a way as to fall into the same class. So the patient recognizes a hidden relation between obviously extremely disparate things which remains invisible to the normal observer.

Von Domarus assumes that the usual pattern of our thinking corresponds to the Modus Barbara the best-known instance of which has to do with the immortal Socrates:

Major Premise:	All humans are mortal.
Minor Premise:	Socrates is human.
Conclusion:	Socrates is mortal.

Von Domarus' argument will be quoted extensively because it is of special relevance for »schizophrenic thinking«.

In its most precise form our logical thinking follows the so-called Mode of Barbara. If, in the figure, area A designates »All men are mortal« and area B »Socrates is a man«, then we conclude correctly that »Socrates is mortal«.

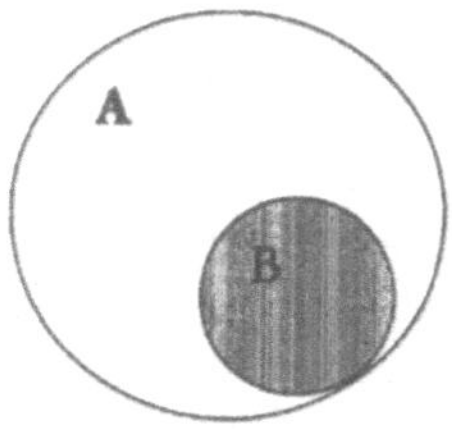

Figure 1

From the figure it follows at once that the last statement yields no new knowledge. To the concept »man« belongs by implication also the man Socrates, and hence, simply by definition, as it were, Socrates is mortal. Experience shows that the conclusion is justified only if the major premise implicitly contains the minor premise. If thinking does not take this into consideration, we arrive at what seems to be contrary to, or other than, normal thinking, or to be paralogical (op.cit., p.109f.).

In the eyes of the anti-psychologistic logician Von Domarus' explanation »Experience shows that the conclusion is justified only…« is a psychologistic misunderstanding of logic. How humans actually think is – as the earlier quotation from Frege politely indicates – of interest only to psychological logicians. Logic has nothing to do with experience – and that is why its practitioners fight psychologism in logic –, the conclusion of a valid syllogism follows with necessity, »mechanically«, as it were, from the premises, and it guarantees truth even if no human being ever actually reasoned that way. Thus a standard is laid down for what we call »thinking« (in the sense of consistent, rational, etc. reasoning). And here experience will, in principle, always come too late to serve as a legitimating instance because what is admissible as »justification« of a conclusion and what is not was established a priori. The logician who is tied to an absolutist conception of logic has, therefore, no choice but to classify deviant taxonomies and divergent kinds of order as »deranged«; a »new kind of logic« based on different rules is for him unthinkable.

But let us first specify in greater detail how logicians and paralogicians differ. An arbitrarily selected illustration, supported by the following figure, will elucidate the nature of paralogical thinking.

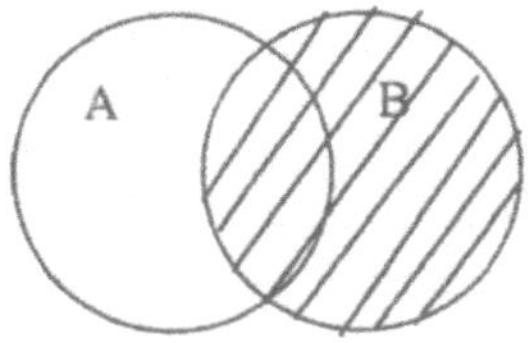

Figure 2

If A means »Certain Indians are swift« and B means »Stags are swift«, the area of intersection of A and B symbolizes the common element of swiftness.

It follows for the paralogical thinker that »Certain Indians are stags«, and he will act as his conclusion directs him to do. A glance at the figure reveals a further most important point. Because everything which lies outside the common intersection of A and B, the law of contradiction is excluded from paralogical thinking and its paragrammatical language [....] The difference between logical and paralogical thinking may be stated: whereas the logician accepts only the Mode of Barbara, or one of its modifications, as basis for valid conclusions, the paralogician concludes identity from the similar nature of adjectives.« (op.cit., p.110f.)

The formal structure of such paralogical thinking has become part of the history of the study of schizophrenic thinking as the Von-Domarus-Principle and has proved to be very stimulating and influential there. This Von-Domarus-Principle essentially states that many schizophrenics deduce the identity of two things (subjects) from the identity of at least one predicate (adjective) which they have in common. So the »Modus Stag« represents a logical delinquency that violates fundamental logical »laws of thought«.

Let us now, for simplicity's sake, translate Von Domarus' example which contains quantified particular statements (»certain....«; quantifier »some«) into universal statements (all), which will not change its paralogical structure. Then the example reads:

Modus Stag:

Stags are swift.	(MaP)
Indians are swift.	(SaP)
Indians are stags.	(SaM) conclusion

This syllogism rests on premises that normal discourse might accept as true, nevertheless the inference is – even for the non-logician – obviously invalid because it leads to a false conclusion: Indians are stags. Logicians speak of a »fallacia consequentis or non sequitur«, a fallacy with reference to the conclusion. The recognizably false result (conclusion) is the criterion here that there is something wrong with the syllogism.

In order to temper the blatant exotic nature of this inference let us recall the above-quoted »correct« inference in the context of botanical taxonomy: strawberries are nuts. The reason why the inference is invalid and why its potential »truth« is accidental can be proved quite well by the logic of concepts which deals with the extension of concepts – I shall come to that in the next section. The invalidity of the inference can be made clearer for the non-logician when the concepts are substituted by abbreviations (appearing in brackets after the statements); in this way we can get rid of the meaning of the words and their connotations and stick to the formal pespective of the logician.

The invalid Modus Stag:

All M are P.
S is P
―――――――――
Ergo: S is M.

The validity of Modus Barbara also »shows itself« in abbreviations:

All M are P.
S is M.
―――――――――
Ergo: S is P.

It must be admitted that the validity of this inference and the truth of its conclusion are due to the abstraction from all content (i.e. from the dimension which has also been termed sense, intension, or connotation) and the exclusive focus on form (i.e. the extension, the set of referents, the denotation).

At this stage I shall merely mention the triviality that the diagnosis of a deviation must always be performed from a separate and independent position. That is to say that the chosen logical standard of evaluation will determine whether something is paralogical or not. Gregory Bateson, who has occupied himself with the thinking of schizophrenics for many years, had become acquainted with the ideas of vonDomarus in the late forties and made them his own. In his – meanwhile famous – double-bind theory (Bateson et al. 1956) Bateson refers to the Von–Domarus –Principle as an indication of the fact that schizophrenic utterances are replete with metaphors which are, however, not »labeled«, i.e. not used, as such by the schizophrenic. As an instance of such a »distorted syllogism« Bateson offers what he later calls the Modus Grass (which appears frequently in his later work).

Men die.
Grass die.

Men are grass.
(cf. Bateson 1981, p.275)

Now the conclusion »Men are grass« might very well be understood metaphorically in the same way as »Indians are stags«. Recall the names of Indian chieftains like »Great Stag« that appear in the stories about the »Wild West«. In this context, Bateson speaks of a »syllogism of metaphor«. He variously uses Peirce's concept of abduction, in particular for the clarification of the pragmatic (communicative) effect of metaphor, and he interprets this pattern of inference as a fundamental strategy of knowledge. In a letter in 1980 he links the Peircean concept of abduction with the syllogism »Modus Grass«.

The Von-Domarus-Principle ties the paralogical structure of schizophrenic thinking to the syllogism »Modus Grass«, and so I want to show in the following that such modes of inference correspond to what Peirce called abduction, a mode of inference that had been forgotten by logic for over two thousand years and that represents a pervasive everyday manner of organizing thinking. It is therefore not a practicable criterion of irrationality, on the contrary, it excludes a figure of thinking which exhibits a different form of rationality.

Abductive inference

In Peirce's semiotic theory of cognition abduction plays a decisive role because only by abduction can we add to our knowledge of the world. In the context of this article I can give only a very reduced analysis and presentation of this subtle theory. Before visualising abductive reasoning by means of Venn diagrams in order to make visible what the paralogical consists in and what its knowledge-creating power is, I shall clarify Peirce's logic of abduction.

Peirce introduces the new kind of inference as »reasoning a posteriori«, thus setting it apart from deduction a priori, and he replaces the three classical terms, major premise, minor premise, and conclusion, by his own terms: rule, case, and result. In this way, the sequential order in which the premises and the conclusion are known may be taken into account. Thus each of the three statements of the classic syllogism could in principle take any of the three positions, whether they are rule, case or conclusion. The minor premise (the second premise of the classic syllogism), for example, may become the inferred conclusion, as is the case in abduction.The major premise which contains the predicate may naturally also be formulated as a rule (law):

All humans are mortal. If X is human, X is mortal.

Let me present here the most famous of all syllogisms, the Modus Barbara, the deductive model of inference of the first figure, the best-known instance of which has to do with the immortal Socrates:

Major Premise	(rule):	All humans are mortal.	(MaP)
Minor Premise	(case):	Socrates is human.	(SaM)
Conclusion	(result):	Socrates is mortal.	(SaP)

The categorical syllogism relates three concepts, S (subject), P (predicate), and M (middle), in three statements (major premise, minor premise, conclusion). In order to examine their validity I have added these terms to the statements and included in brackets the abbreviations indicating the characteristic position of the concepts in the first figure (MP, SM, SP).

In Peirce's view, the goal of all inferential thinking is to discover something we do not know and thus enlarge our knowledge by considering something we do know. In view of what has been said, the inferential procedures presented here are of different quality with regard to the way in which they increase our knowledge. In Peirce's terminology, the three forms of inference are the following:

Forms of Inference

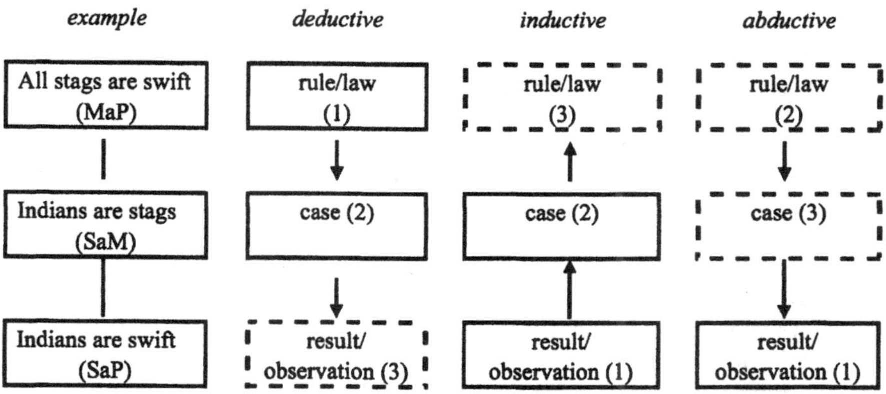

Boxes with continuous lines contain premises/hypotheses that are presupposed as given/true. Boxes with dotted lines contain hypotheses that are inferred.

Figure 3

In logic as well as in the philosophy of science a valid deduction is considered to be truth-conserving; if the premises are true, the conclusion must be true, too. The price to be paid for this necessary truth, however, is that the information content of the conclusion is already implicitly contained in the premises. The »mortality of Socrates", the conclusion supplied by Modus Barbara, is nothing new, it was completely contained in the premises. Deduction, therefore, is not synthetic (content-increasing), does not lead to new knowledge. It is analytically true (redundant) and has, therefore, been considered to be merely an »explanatory statement" in the more recent discussion. Deductive thinking proceeds from the general (the rule), through the subsumption of the singular case under the rule, to the assertion of the particular (the result), as the arrows in figure 1 indicate.

Peirce developed his theory of induction over several decades, so I can only present a brief summary of its essentials. In the case of induction the premises (the initial basis) are observational statements and an inferred conclusion (e.g. a hypothetical rule: All M are P) is considered to be content-increasing but not truth-conserving because the inference is only a hypothesis that cannot be proved with ultimate certainty. Induction – the converse of deduction – progresses from the particular to the general. Therefore the arrows point »from the bottom to the top«.

The abductive mode of inference involves two steps. In a first step a »phenomenon« to be explained or understood is presented (1), in Peirce's terminology, a »result«, which is the derived conclusion in the classical schema; then a second step introduces an available or newly constructed hypothesis (rule/law) (2) by means of which the case (3) is abduced. Peirce has examined these three modes of inference in great detail and shown convincingly that all three operate together in our thinking in different ways. Here I shall concentrate on abduction only.

What is the function of abductive inference? For Peirce it is »[...] the process of forming an explanatory hypothesis. It is the only logical operation which introduces any new idea; for induction does nothing but determine a value, and deduction merely evolves the necessary consequences of a pure hypothesis. Deduction proves that something must be; induction shows that something actually is operative; abduction merely suggests that something may be.« (CP 5.171, cf 1991a, p.333) Abduction may thus be conceived of as a principle that allows us to reconstruct how conceptual order is achieved through the imposition of a hypothesis (in the form of a minimal theory, an idea, a rule or a law-like hypothesis) – which inaugurates constructivist thinking. Here I can only hint at the great variability of this schema; it enables us to bridge the traditional gap between the arts and the sciences because it can be used as a model both of explanation and of understanding.

Presented as an inverted modus ponens – as in Peirce's writings – the abductive schema looks like this:

Abductive reasoning as an inverted modus ponens:
from effects to causes (causal explanation)

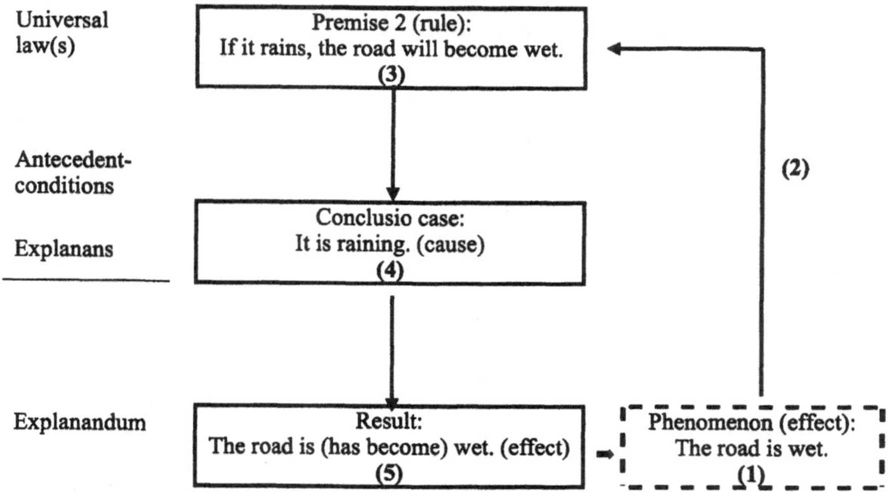

Figure 4

This schema becomes a (nomologically-deductive) explanatory principle if the first premise (the result) contains an unexplained surprising fact (perception, observation) – for Peirce the beginning of all scientific querying – which is then explained causally as the effect of a cause. In this context, Peirce also speaks of »reasoning [...] from consequent to antecedent« (CP 6.469, 1.74), of reasoning from effects to causes – a fallacy in (traditional) logic (a fallacia consequentis).

The causal formulation of the explanation of the phenomenon that the road is wet would run as follows: The road is wet because it is raining (because it has rained). The rain is the cause inferred from the effect (the consequent). Abduction, i.e. inferring causes from effects, represents an explanatory principle which, though logically invalid, may still be confirmed inductively. The (potential) confirmation of such hypotheses (logical inferences or theories) says nothing about reality (ontology) in the sense of a representation or mapping, all it says is that the hypotheses are functioning. Therefore, the structures of our logic(s) or our theories do not mirror the structures of things nor are they derived (deduced) from them. With the primary act of the formulation of such a hypothesis a paradigm, a rule, a method of measurement is provisionally laid down by means of which we then »measure« or »compare« what we conceive of as »nature«. Only in a second act arise the notions of »correct/incorrect«, fitting/non-fitting, rule-conforming/rule-breaking etc. The actual constructive act consists in the apriori specification of a »measuring method« by the cognizing subject (the scientific community) because the world cannot determine for us directly what kind of measuring method or paradigm we must use. And just as the measuring method must be specified before measuring can take place, so induction must be directed/governed/controlled by a hypothesis that has been constructed abductively beforehand. The world, or nature, thus functions as a selection mechanism, as a constraint, which determines whether our hypotheses fit or fail. In the latter case the scientific community is forced to change the theories, paradigms or conceptual systems in such ways as will allow the derivation of viable hypotheses that enlarge our knowledge of the world in the constructivist sense. Viable hypotheses, therefore, do not admit of positive statements about how the world really is but only of negative ones to the effect that other hypotheses do not work. We can, on the other hand, also draw the conclusion that, for a reality different from ours, we would need other »standards«, other systems of categories etc. to be able to orientate ourselves in it because the ones we have would not work.

If an abductive inference establishes itself in the scientific community as a new paradigm (a new explanation of a certain phenomenon, like Kepler's hypothesis of the elliptical orbit of the planet Mars), then the logic of the corresponding conceptual system has changed.

The construction of meaning in a semiotic system/system of signs: Abductive inference as the interpretation of signs, or as intentionalist explanation

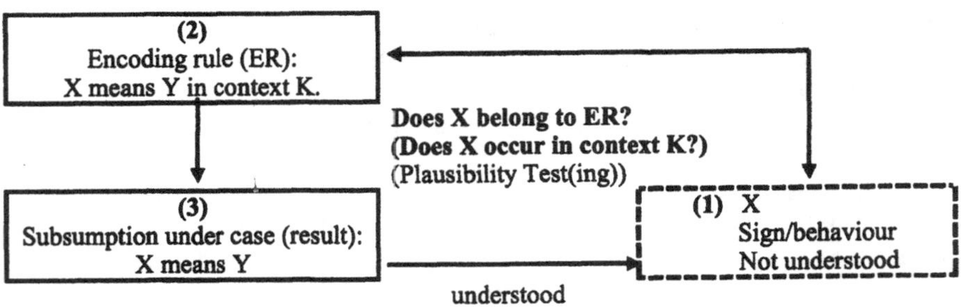

Figure 5

If we replace the surprising fact by the incomprehensible behaviour of a person, then an abductive inference may help us to construct an intentionalist explanation through motives (reasons) that makes the behaviour intelligible. All intentionalist or functionalist explanations in psychotherapy thus become interpretable as hypothetical constructions with abduction as their modus operandi.

(1) Observation: Person A shows behaviour V in context K, utters x, etc.
(2) Hypothetical rule: A behaviour x in context K has the meaning/function (f).
(3) Case/conclusion: A's behaviour V has the meaning (f) (is motivated by f).

If we consider the mechanism on the semiotic plane, a sign is introduced as an unexplained result to which, by way of the construction of an encoding rule, or the application of a familiar encoding rule, meaning is or can be assigned (contexts, frames, etc. being of significance, too) (cf Keller 1995, U. Eco 1985).

Abduction, as a cognitive operation, creates the framework which makes it possible to attribute a singular meaning to signs. The interpretation of signs – as the schema shows – is always abductive, or in other words: the fundamental constructive principle of all semiotic interpretation is the finding or inventing of a hypothesis (abduction), i.e. the act of semiotic understanding on the part of a hearer can consist only in the attribution of meaning through a – his/her – frame of reference (encoding rule). Therefore, abductive inference is the basic principle of all hermeneutical procedures.

We can now say by way of summary that the hearer always makes abductive inferences when trying to understand signs. As speakers in communication we always make deductive inferences (Keller 1995). Deductive inference in the form of a practical syllogism may also be used for the reconstruction of goal-directed rational behaviour. The Finnish philosopher and student of Wittgenstein's, G. H. von Wright, has introduced this approach into the logic of actions (1963/1977). The syllogism may be represented as follows:

I want to reach goal Y.	Premise
I assume that saying (doing) X will lead to Y (be understood as Y).	Rule
Therefore I do (say) X.	Conclusion

cf. Wright 1963/77; Fischer 1987; Keller 1995

Transferring this idea to our schema we can represent mutual communicative understanding on the basis of intersubjectively shared rules (i.e the same grammar) in the following way:

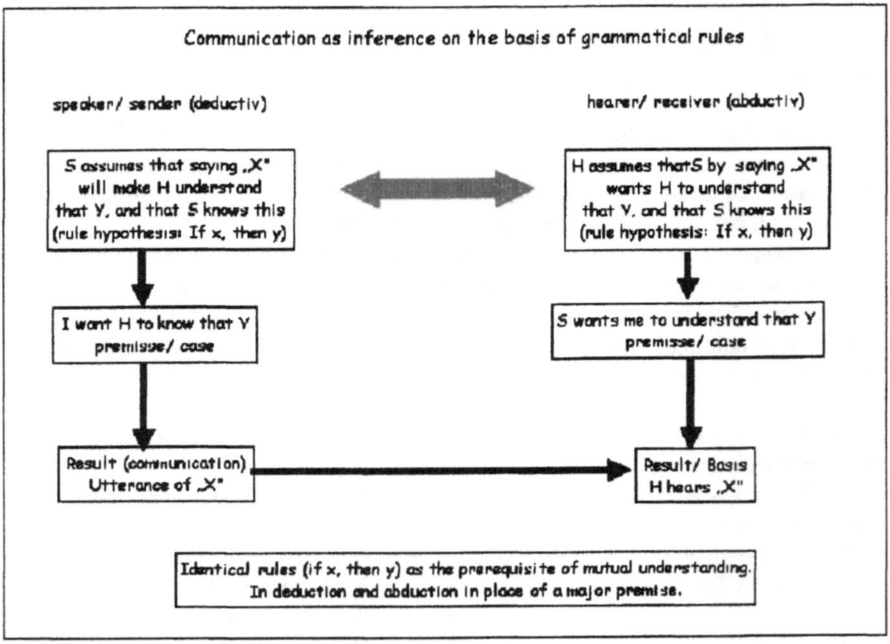

Figure 6

This goes to show that mutual understanding will only be achieved if both participants use the same rule hypothesis (in the schema: if x, then y) and therefore play the same language game. This schema shows in a simplified manner how worlds can fall apart if the hearer »decodes« the signs of the speaker on the basis of a different grammar (culture, context), although and precisely because both participants are using the same signs. Let us now turn to the suggestion that the grammar of the »insane« has been changed and that they therefore think and infer, speak and understand in different ways.

Paralogical thinking as abductive reasoning

In his analysis of paralogical thinking Von Domarus had presupposed that reasoning according to Modus Barbara, i.e. according to a deductive syllogism, was normal reasoning, »normal« meaning something like rational and healthy. As synthetic inferences are content-enlarging only if they go beyond the information contained in the premises by predicating something of the subject in the conclusion that is not contained in the premises, our thinking cannot and must not remain exclusively deductive if we ever want to extend our knowledge by a mere iota.

If we take Peirce's theory seriously, then the hiatus between logic and life can only be bridged by abductive modes of inference because both inductive and deductive inferential procedures evidently do not add to content and, therefore, cannot lead to new knowledge. It is the central insight of abduction theory that there can be no induction without a hypothesis that has been inferred, i.e. constructed abductively beforehand. Seen from this angle, all changes in thinking, everything new, any addition to what we know, are brought about by violations of established »laws of thought«, taxonomies and logics. The Von-Domarus-Principle maintains that the structure of paralogical inference consists in inferring the similarity or identity of subjects from the similarity or identity of predicates (adjectives).

I want to show now that this kind of paralogical thinking is, in fact, abductive reasoning, in order to fathom the sort of rationality possibly residing in irrationality and the kinds of linkage (comprehensibility) to deranged thinking that might exist. In this way I shall try to demonstrate how the extensional and the intensional meaning of concepts may be shifted by means of abductive reasoning, and that this is precisely where and why paralogical inference is knowledge-enlarging.

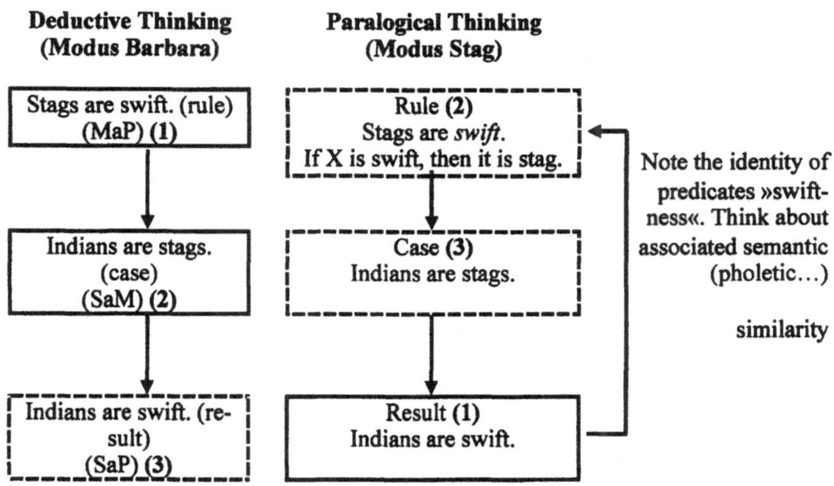

Concerning the structure, this is an abductive inference which is used with every interpretation (diagnosis). Herby the two sentences (1+2) are the product of hypothetic inference, only the result is given.

Figure 7

Compared with Modus Barbara, »Modus Stag« thus reveals itself as an abductive inference. The abductive form of inference synthetically (i.e. content-enlargingly) derives the identity of subjects from the »similarity« of predicates.

In what follows I shall try to give a more precise account of this »content-enlargement« in order to show how the extensional and the intensional meaning of concepts may change. It is quite likely, therefore, that the hypothesis will become a self-fulfilling prophecy because non-fitting perceptions, i.e. perceptions that do not inductively confirm the hypothesis, will penetrate to the observer's field of awareness only with great difficulty. It has thus become clear how reality is constructed through a system of concepts, i.e. how we create the world we live in by means of abduction.

Some way back metaphorical thinking was introduced. Without entering into a theoretical account of metaphor here (cf. Eco 1985) I simply want to show by means of a diagram that the function of metaphor may also be reconstructed as a kind of abductive inference. One might possibly use this sort of abductive inferential procedure to generate metaphors. And I think that this is what Bateson thought of as a metaphorical syllogism. We are thus getting closer to the main point I want to work out with regard to »deranged« thinking, namely a new semantics of concepts.

Metaphors as abductive reasoning

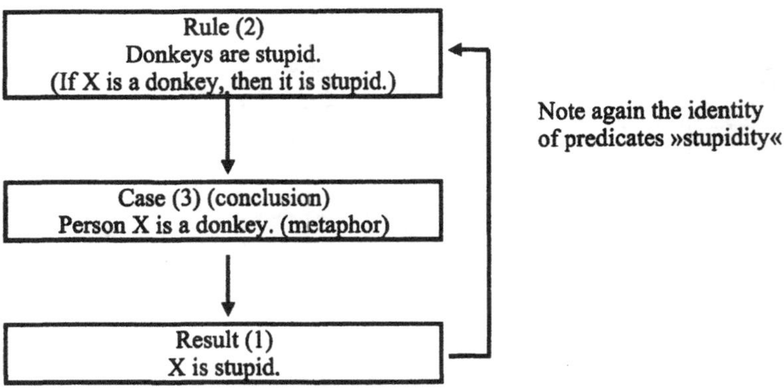

Figure 8

From a semiotic point of view an abduction is the incorporation of a sign into a coding system (mini-theories, hypotheses) whose specific logic supplies the frame within which the phenomena turned signs become meaningful. From here the idea of abduction takes us either to the primarily processual thinking of Freud and psychoanalysis in general, or to Lacan's structuralist theory of the unconscious. So there are many interesting roads leading from logic into psychology and back which I cannot follow here. I can't show here why an abductive inference is invalid (cf. Fischer 2000).

With the introduction of the traditional logical distinction between intensional and extensional meaning it can be made quite clear that we have here a change of meaning. Extensional meaning (set of referents, also called denotation) comprises the class of objects to which the concept may be correctly applied. The intensional meaning (also called conceptual content, connotation or sense) of a term comprises the properties ascribed to an entity that determine its subsumption under a specific concept. In other words, the intension of a concept is the criterion by which it may be decided whether an entity belongs to its extension (set of referents) or not. For the clarification of the problem of how the meaning, i.e. the information, contained in the conclusion of abductive inferences changes, I want to make use of Peirce's own analyses. He considered the idea that conclusions which enlarge our knowledge must involve a change of the information content of the concepts used, in his reflections on the informational aspects of induction and hypothesis construction (abduction). An extensive presentation of his analyses is not possible here, so I shall simply refer to some of his important insights.

The difference between inductive and hypothetical (abductive) inferences is, from an informational perspective, that inductive inferences enlarge the extensional range of the predicate in the conclusion without its intension becoming smaller. Abduction or hypothesis, however, according to Peirce, enlarge the intension of the subject concept in the conclusion, without its extension, its set of referents, becoming smaller. This is in contradiction to the logical principles that maintain that any intensional enlargement of a concept implies the reduction of its extension and vice versa. There is some plausibility here because the set of referents associated with a concept will obviously diminish if its intension becomes highly specified. And conversely, the less specified a concept is the greater will be its set of referents, its extension. Thus the concept »thing« is extremely poorly defined intensionally so that very many »entities« will necessarily fall under it, i.e. belong to its extension. Now consider the abductive inference of Modus Stag with regard to this aspect.

1) All Stags are swift	(MaP, Rule)
2) Indians are swift	(SaP, Result)
3) Indians are Stags	(SaM, Case)

The identical predicate (P) of the two premises is replaced by the term M in the conclusion which is characterized not only by P but by additional properties (features). This is to say that S is not only P but also M. The subject Indians (S) in our conclusion is not only swift (P), as asserted in premise 2, but also a stag (stag-like) (M). And M (»stag«), according to the premises, extensionally represents the same object domain as P (swiftness). As, however, in an abduction, P assumes the function of the middle term, as »swiftness« is the standard (means) of comparison and the concept »stag« (M in the valid syllogism) becomes the predicate in the conclusion, the subject is ascribed stagness as an additional predicate. If we interpret this inference abductively, the concept »Indian« is intensionally enriched in the conclusion or, in other words, the sense of the term Indian (its intensional meaning) is changed. Understanding all this in terms of established logic would imply the classification of paralogical thinking as faulty thinking, as the »deranged logic« of orthodox psychiatry and the logicians.

Just as measuring requires a measuring standard, so our understanding of rationality presupposes that everybody draws inferences in the same way, i.e. follows the same rules. Logic is therefore not arbitrary in the sense that it may be changed according to personal whim. And this is just what is shown by the paralogical thought of a schizophrenic: he has become unintelligible. So here we are up against a rigid must of both logic and grammar. As long as I want to be undestood, I must obey the rules of grammar and logic. If I follow grammatical rules that are different from the established ones, then nobody will understand what I am saying and the question may arise whether I am following any rules at all: »Die Schritte, welche man nicht in Frage zieht, sind logische Schlüsse, ...nicht weil sie wahr sind, sondern, dies ist es, was wir denken, schließen, nennen.« (Wittgenstein, BGM S. 96)

With recourse to Wittgenstein's late philosophy of grammar (logic) which I have dealt with extensively elsewhere (Fischer 1987), I should like to summarize the relationship between rationality and rule-following in the following way: Language exists only where rules are at work and the same holds for what we call thinking. Wittgenstein's analyses demonstrate that local rule systems like language games are a conditio sine qua non of rationality. What is described as reasonable or rational appears to be the consequence of rules or of processes organised in a rule-like way, and not the reverse (Hayek 1980; Keller 1990; Fischer 1999a, b).

Rule-following is a kind of practice that can only be accounted for progressively, in a feedforward loop, i.e. pragmatically, because any retro-gressive account becomes caught in a vicious circle. Rationality, therefore, is not the foundation of rule systems; we follow the rules blindly – as Wittgenstein says (1953, Philos. Investigations § 219) – as soon as we have learned to talk and think. Rationality is conceivable only on the basis of rule-following. And so the possibility emerges to give up a concept of rationality that is dogmatically tied to logic, and to discover rationality in the irrational.

Making an inference in a way deviating from logic, as is the case with the abductive Modus Stag, therefore counts as »fallacious« from the logician's point of view. If, however, the hypothesis is correct that rule-following is the foundation of all rational thought, then the question poses itself whether para-logical inference follows rules which are different from the established ones. If this is accepted, para-logical thinking can be made intelligible in principle. In other words, and this is the decisive point for me, there is a transition from fallacious thinking to a different kind of thinking. And it is precisely this sort of transition that cannot be managed with and in traditional logic because it consists essentially in the violation of its rules. Traditional logic excommunicates paralogical approaches and, as a culturally established order of correct thought, banishes them to the realm of the irrational. From this perspective the Modus Stag, as a typical pattern of »paralogical thinking«, does indeed – like all abductive inferences! – violate logical laws, but it might also be interpreted as a creative transformation of the semantic content of the concept »Indian« and the whole conceptual system (language game) – as it always happens, by the way, in the course of »paradigm changes« –, so that it might be rescued from the ghetto of the fundamentally incomprehensible and meaningless.

As a different kind of thinking and speaking is necessarily connected with different behaviours and different actions, the rationality of a certain kind of thinking is not decided logic-internally but by the ways in which it is connected with the actions of individuals and supports the orientation of individuals in their interactional contexts. In other words: There is no absolute standard of judgment for the rationality of any kind of thought and action but only a relational one. Abductively inferred hypotheses help to construct new, i.e. different standards. And such standards are – just like the laws of logic – not true and false in themselves but simply more or less useful in realising specific interests and purposes. So, in the long run, pragmatic – and not purely logical – criteria decide whether paralogical thinking allows for viable action that may prove its mettle inductively.

Pure logic is inadequate to judge the rationality or irrationality of an utterance or an action because paralogical (abductive) inferences or hypotheses may, in fact, be rational (i.e. correct). Their rationality, however, is different from the rationality chained to Aristotelian logic. Peirce, consequently, assigns rationality to paralogical abduction if it serves to control human actions:

»An abduction is a method of forming a general prediction without any positive assurance that it will succeed either in the special case or usually, its justification being that it is the only possible hope of regulating our future conduct rationally, and that induction from past experience gives us strong encouragement to hope that it will be successful in the future.« (CP 2.270)

To the extent that such abductive inferences open up new knowledge and/or change the semantics of a conceptual system, they prove to invent or construct relations, transitions and connections which did not (have to) exist before or could not be seen or perceived at all.

If abductively constructed hypotheses are corroborated inductively then the pre-empirical rules (logic) of a conceptual system are transformed or adjusted, – as is the case with all »scientific revolutions«. Such creative abductions must be seen as adjustments of theories, logics, standards and norms of thought, in fact, of our total conceptual universe (world picture), they change our mental map(s) more or less fundamentally.

With regard to the rationality of individual thought »paralogical thinking« will certainly de-viate from conventional logic, but as long as it is not chaotic and just follows other rules it may, in principle, be brought back into the framework of intelligibility. The concepts used are then not without sense but are used in a different way and therefore have a transformed new meaning. There is connectability here for a hermeneutically operating psychotherapy (Fischer 1990a, 1999a).

The rationality of such paralogical thinking may reveal itself in its usefulness and functions for the individuals in question as it may provide orientation in their discursive and non-discursive environments. Basically this is also the core of the theory of schizophrenia developed by Bateson and the Palo Alto Group. Deranged thought and action is, accordingly, a learned approach to solving problems in the context of disturbed family interactions and therefore relational in terms of that context. The rationality and functionality of such thinking is, therefore, not detectable in the individual but can only be discovered in the interactional context (the family, as a rule) in which it acquired its function. A deviation from logical norms of thought may reveal an adaptation to the discursive and non-discursive environment and consequently a paralogical kind of rationality which proves the relativity of logic as well as its plurality. A closer look thus makes it deeply irrational to rely totally and exclusively on the rationality of logic.

References

Apel, Karl-Otto (1975). *Der Denkweg von Charles Sanders Peirce. Eine Einführung in den amerikanischen Pragmatismus*. Frankfurt/Main: Suhrkamp.

Arieti, S. (1955). *Interpretation of Schizophrenia*. London: Crosby, Lockwood, Staples.

Bateson, Gregory (1980). Syllogisms in grass. Letter, in: *The London Review of Books. 2. Jg. Nr. 1, 24. Jan. 1980*. p.2.

Bateson, Gregory (1981). *Ökologie des Geistes*, Frankfurt/Main: Suhrkamp.

Bateson, Gregory (1982). *Geist und Natur. Eine notwendige Einheit*, Frankfurt/Main: Suhrkamp.

Bateson, Gregory (1991). *A sacred unity. Further Steps to an Ecology of Mind* (ed. by Rodney E. Donaldson). New York.

Bateson, Gregory und Bateson, Mary Catherine (1993). *Wo Engel zögern. Unterwegs zu einer Epistemologie des Heiligen*. Frankfurt/Main: Suhrkamp.

Bateson, Gregory, Jackson, Don D., Haley, Jay & Weakland, John H. (1956). Toward a theory of schizophrenia, *Behavioral Science 1*: 251-64 [German in: Bateson 1981, 270-301].

Bühler, Karl Ernst und Hans Rudi Fischer (1984). Regelbegriff und Rationalität. In R. Haller (ed.), *Ästhetik, Akten des Internationalen Wittgenstein-Symposiums 1983* (p.246-249). Wien.

Domarus von, Eilhardt (1964). The Specific Laws of Logic in Schizophrenia, in J.S. Kasanin (ed.), *Language and Thought in Schizophrenia* (pp.104-114). New York: W.W.Norton.

Eco, Umberto (1985). *Semiotik und Philosophie der Sprache*. München: Fink.

Eco, Umberto und Sebeok, Thomas A. (Hrsg) (1985) *Der Zirkel oder Im Zeichen der Drei. Dupin, Holmes, Peirce*. München: Fink.

Fischer, Hans Rudi (1987). Sprache und Lebensform. Wittgenstein über Freud und die Geisteskrankheit. In *Monographien zur philosophischen Forschung. Bd. 242* (p.367). Frankfurt: Athenäum. [2. edition: Heidelberg, Carl-Auer.]

Fischer, Hans Rudi (1989). Rezension zu Hans Radermacher, »Kant, Swedenborg, Borges«, in: *Conceptus, Zeitschrift für Philosophie, Bd. 60*, 111-113.

Fischer, Hans Rudi (1989b). Wittgenstein und der Wahnsinn. Zu einer anderen Philosophie des Anderen der Vernunft. In: *SPUREN. Zeitschrift für Kunst und Gesellschaft. Hamburg. Heft 29, Aug. 1989*. 35-39.

Fischer, Hans Rudi (1990a). Sprachspiele und Geschichten. Zur Rolle der Sprache in der Psychotherapie. In: *Familiendynamik, 3* (pp.190-211). Stuttgart: Klett-Cotta..

Fischer, Hans Rudi (1990b). Madness and Method. In Rudolf Haller (ed.), *Ludwig Wittgenstein. A Reevaluation. Proceedings of the Intern. Wittgenstein-Symposium 1989*. Hölder-Pichler-Tempsky: Wien.

Fischer, Hans Rudi (1994). Is there any logic in madness? Linguistic reflections on an interpersonal theory of mental illness. In: *Wittgenstein Studien 1/94, 10-1-94*, Springer.

Fischer, Hans Rudi (1998). Vom Sehen zum Erkennen. Erkennen als konstruieren von Wirklichkeit. In: *Bewußtsein, Wahrnehmung, Nervensystem* (pp.215-231). In Gion Condrau, Gerhard Langer, W. J. Meinhold (eds.). Zürich: Walter.

Fischer, Hans Rudi (1999a). Rationalität als offene Ordnung. Zur Logik und Evolution neuer Sprachspiele: In Hans J. Schneider, Matthias Kroß (eds.), *Mit Sprache spielen. Die Ordnungen und das Offene nach Wittgenstein* (pp.149-168). Berlin, Akademie Verlag.

Fischer, Hans Rudi (1999b). Rationalität, Logik und Wirklichkeit. Zu einem konstruktivistischen Verständnis der Logik. In Gebhard Rusch (ed.), *Wissen und Erfahrung. Festschrift für Ernst von Glasersfeld*. Carl-Auer-Systeme.

von Hayek, Friedrich A (1980). *Recht, Gesetzgebung und Freiheit. Band 1. Regeln und Ordnung: e. neueste Darstellung des liberalen Prinzipien der Gerechtigkeit und der politischen Ökonomie*. München: Verlag Moderne Industrie.

Heidegger, Martin (1972). *Frühe Schriften*. Frankfurt/Main: Klostermann.

Heims, Steve Joshua (1993). *Constructing a social science for postwar America: The Cybernetics Group 1946-1953*. Cambridge: MIT Press.

Kant, Immanuel (1798/1977). Anthropologie in pragmatischer Hinsicht. In: *I. Kant, Werkausgabe. Schriften zur Anthropologie, Geschichtsphilosophie, Politik und Pädagogik, Band XII*. Frankfurt/Main: Suhrkamp.

Keller, Rudi (1995). *Zeichentheorie*.Tübingen und Basel: FranckeVerlag.

Keller, Rudi (1995). *Zeichentheorie: zu einer Theorie semiotischen Wissens*. Tübingen, Basel: Francke

Peirce, Charles Sanders (1931-35, 1958). *Collected Papers of Charles Sanders Peirce*. Bd. I-VI (1931-34) ed by Ch. Hartshorne and P. Weiss. Vol. VII-VIII (1958) ed. By A.W. Burks. Cambridge, Massachusetts/London.

Peirce, Charles Sanders (1975). *Charles Sanders Peirce: Contributions to The Nation. Parte One: 1869-1893*. Compiled and Annotated by Kenneth Laine Ketner and James Edward Cook. Lubbock, Texas, Texas Tech Press.

Peirce, Charles Sanders (1982-93). *Writings of Charles S. Peirce. A chronological Edition*. Ed. By M.H. Fisch et al. Vol I-V. Abekürzt als W (plus Bandzahl). Bloomington: Indiana University Press.

Peirce, Charles Sanders (1983). *Phänomen und Logik der Zeichen* (edited and translated by Helmut Pape). Frankfurt/Main: Suhrkamp.

Peirce, Charles Sanders (1991a). *Naturordnung und Zeichenprozeß. Schriften über Semiotik und Naturphilosophie* (edited and translated by Helmut Pape). Frankfurt/Main: Suhrkamp.

Peirce, Charles Sanders (1991b). *Schriften zum Pragmatismus und Pragmatizismus* (ed. by Karl-Otto Apel). Frankfurt/Main: Suhrkamp.

Peirce, Charles Sanders (1986). *Semiotische Schriften Bd. 1-3* (ed. and translated by Christian Kloesel and Helmut Pape). Frankfurt/Main: Suhrkamp. Quoted as SS + Volume number and page.

Richter, Ansgar (1995). *Der Begriff der Abduktion bei Charles Sanders Peirce*. Frankfurt/Main, Berlin, New York, Paris, Wien: Peter Lang.

Riemer, Ines (1988). *Konzeption und Begründung der Induktion. Eine Untersuchung zur methodologie von Charles S. Peirce*. Würzburg: Königshausen und Neumann.

Ruckstuhl, Urs (1981). *Schizophrenieforschung: Die theoretischen und empirischen Beiträge der Experimentellen Psychologie*. Weinheim und Basel: Beltz.

Schönrich, Gerhard (1990). *Zeichenhandeln. Untersuchungen zum Begriff einer semiotischen Vernunft im Ausgang von Ch.S. Peirce*. Frankfurt/Main: Suhrkamp.

Sebeok, Thomas A. und Umiker-Sebeok, Jean (1982). *»Du kennst meine Methode«. Charles S. Peirce und Sherlock Holmes*. Frankfurt/Main: Suhrkamp.

Sebeok, Thomas A. und Umiker-Sebeok, Jean (1985). *»Sie kennen ja meine Methode« ein Vergleich von Charles S. Peirce und Sherlock Holmes*. In: Eco u. Sebeok (pp.28-87). München: Fink.

Wittgenstein, Ludwig (1969). *Schriften 1. Tractatus logico-philosophicus, Tagebücher 1914-1916, Philosophische Untersuchungen*. Frankfurt/Main: Suhrkamp.

Wittgenstein, Ludwig (1970). *Schriften 7. Vorlesungen über die Grundlagen der Mathematik*. Frankfurt/Main: Suhrkamp. (Quoted as VGM + page)

Wittgenstein, Ludwig (1977). *Vermischte Bemerkungen*. Frankfurt/Main: Suhrkamp.

Wittgenstein, Ludwig (1980). *Lectures, Cambridge 1932-35*. Oxford: Basil Blackwell.

Wright von, Gh. H. (1984). *Erklären und Verstehen* (2. edition). Königstein: Athenäum.

Vincent Shen

Reasonableness, Strangification and Quality Control in Psychotherapy

Rationality, reasonableness and quality control

When thinking about the problem of quality control in psychotherapy, I would like, first of all, to distinguish between rationality and reasonableness. I make this distinction for two reasons. First, although it is true that all qualitative research and therapeutic treatment refer to »reasonableness«, yet the aspect of »control« in the term »quality control« implies certain element of rationality. Second, since »therapy« is an act of taking care which brings the patient back to a life of sanity, this kind of caring should be an act of reasonableness rather than that of rationality. I tend to think that a life of sanity is a life of reasonableness. Here we have a contrasting situation of »reasonableness« with »rationality«. Let me first of all explain what I mean by »rationality« and »reasonableness«.

Rationality is a function of human reason which directs and organizes our knowledge and action by referring to a rigorous efficiency which is best illustrated by science. On its rational side, science should organize theories according to logico-mathematical structures. On its empirical side, science should control its relation with the reality through systematic experimentation. The interaction of these two aspects must be submitted to the control of validity in checking the correspondence between the rational side and the empirical side and thereby assure us of their coherence and unity.

On the other hand, reasonableness is a function of reason in which we refer always to the dimension of totality in our knowledge and action. On its cognitive side, reasonableness concerns the dimension of meaning. The model of this cognitive activity could be found in the understanding and interpretation of a text. In psychotherapy, a symptom or a group of symptoms, as meaningfully organized signs expressing mental illness, could be read in a dynamic way as meaningful text appealing to human understanding. I propose therefore a dynamic reading of symptoms with a hermeneutic process taking the patient as center of concern. Seen from hermeneutic point of view, understanding and interpretation are typically human activity. They could be extended to any form of relationship human beings entertain with the dimension of totality of their existence.

In understanding the meaning of a text, a reader has to refer, not only to its linguistic meanings, but also to the totality of his own subjectivity as constituted of all his experiences and his life story, and the totality of his relationship with Being or Reality Itself. On its practical side, all actions related to human subjectivity, his life story and personal or collective involvement in meaning constitution are subject to the function of reasonableness. Besides the totality of one's subjectivity and life story, reasonableness refers also to the totality of Being or Reality Itself and one's situation in it. It concerns with the totality of Being and is therefore not limited to human subjectivity, human experience and human meaningfulness. It refers to the totality of Reality so as to reveal the ontological dimension of our meaning constitution. On this level, reasonableness could be seen as the effort of reason itself to attain a comprehensive understanding of itself.

Reasonableness is therefore caught within the tension between the reference to the totality of human subjectivity (his life story) and the reference to the totality of Being. In contrast to modern Western science and analytic philosophy which gravitate on rationality, Chinese philosophy puts emphasis on reasonableness by unceasing reference to the dimension of totality, either that of human existence or that of Reality Itself. For example, Confucianism would refer to the totality of human existence, whereas Daoism would refer to the totality of Reality Itself to rid of any human-centered tendency. Reasonableness, as the function of reason that refers to the totality of human subjectivity (his life story) and the totality of Being (Reality Itself), is the effort of reason to enhance itself to its highest level of possibility so as to achieve its own self-understanding.

Reality itself, life-world and constructed reality

Now, let me proceed to another distinction that I would make to show a reasonable vision of Reality. Concerning this, in basing on Fritz Wallner's distinction between Wirklichkeit(Reality Itself) and Realität(Constructed Reality), I have proposed to mediate these two realms by Life-world. Therefore we have a conceptual framework constituted of the triple concepts of »Reality Itself«-»Life-world«-»Constructed Reality«. Life-world is important for us because we are living in it, practicing culture and science within it, and also constructing it with all kinds of activities of intervention. For me, the Life-world is to be considered partially as resulted from human construction, and partially as emerging spontaneously from the dynamism of Reality Itself. Understood in this sense, Life-world(Lebenswelt) is serving as mediation between Reality Itself(Wircklichkeit) and Constructed Reality (Realität).[1]

My basic consideration here is based upon the fact that modern European science and technology today have effected the unhappy consequence that ecological disequilibrium, pollution, other environmental problems and mental illness become more and more serious in the self-enclosured Constructed Reality. To

1 This distinction is made by Fritz Wallner. Here I understand »mediation« in its dialectic sense, that is, a dynamic and interactive way of going between and going beyond.

avoid this from by an approach of deeper meaning, human being should change his ways of constructing his knowledge and building up his Life-world, not merely according to the logico-structural constraint of language or according to any man-made procedures/rules of constructions, but more according to the rhythm of Nature and the natural make-up of human beings. The Life-world must be seen as partly constructed by human beings, partly constructing itself spontaneously with the rhythm of nature. [2]

People have a natural expectation that the future construction of the Life-world should go to the better and not to the worse. But what is the criterion for distinguishing the better construction from the worse one? The inspiration from Chinese philosophy such as Confucianism and Daoism tells me that the criterion lies in the principle that human construction of Life-world should participate the creative rhythm of Nature, not to dominate it. Therefore we should distinguish *participative construction* from *dominative construction*. Human construction of the Life-world should be a participative one, not a dominative one. Since there might be better as well as worse constructions of the Life-world, depending on whether the construction is participative or dominative, Life-world should not be identified with the Umwelt. Life-world is to be considered partially as human construction, partially as emerging itself spontaneously from the dynamism of Reality Itself. That's why I have modified the theory of two types of reality in Constructive Realism into a theory of three types of reality: Reality Itself, Constructed Reality and Life-world as mediating the two.

For a better notion of psychotherapy, I should say that a life of sanity consists in the construction of a meaningful life world according to the rhythm of Reality Itself and Human existence. The purely dominative character of all artificial constructions and the distortion of or losing contact with Reality Itself and Human existence are two main reasons for mental illness. This is why we wittiness more and more mental illness together with the deterioration of natural environment. To be reasonable, we need an ontological vision consisting of three levels of reality: Reality Itself, Constructed Reality and Life-word serving as the mediation between them.

Manifestation, interpretation and construction

Now, I would like to make a third distinction between »manifestation«, »interpretation« and »construction«, in which interpretation serve as the mediation between

2 In modern western science, nature is defined as the totality of phenomena to be explained and predicted by natural laws, and in modern technology nature is seen as the totality of material resources to be manipulated and transformed by technical process.

manifestation and construction. This distinction is important for relating our vision of Reality to the totality of human existence or human life story.

Phenomenologically speaking, Reality Itself appears as manifestation, without which there is no phenomenon at all. The colorful objects before our eyes are manifestations, the symptoms of a certain kind of diseases, either physical or mental, are also manifestations. Without manifestation, we would have no objects or true knowledge of objects. Without manifestation, we know no other persons or other selves either. The reason why that we know there is some other person, is because of the fact that we perceive, feel or in touch with some body. Even if sensation is a very important mode of manifestation, it is not the only mode, and neither does it offer us complete information about what appears. Our experience shows that there are some objects captured by our attention, but this does not exclude the fact that much more other things appearing in out eyes and are transmitted to our retinas without even being noticed by us. In the case of psychotherapy, we should say that, although in the diagnosis the therapist could try his best to observe the symptoms of a patient, this would not mean that he could grasp all the manifestations of the mental illness in question merely through these observed symptoms.

In some sense, we can say that manifestation comes from the generosity of Reality Itself that overwhelms all our interpretation and construction of it. Yet, all manifestations, before their going through any construction, both linguistic and scientific, were already mediated by interpretation. Interpretation is a way of seeing something as something. »To see as« is the hermeneutic structure of cognition in interpretation. For example, when an act of lifting a hand appears in our perception, it could be interpreted as calling a taxi, as a gesture of greeting or as an act of voting...etc., before we could say it out and construct it as a scientific object.

In the case of psychotherapy, an abnormality in corporeal behavior or a disorder in linguistic behavior could be interpreted as a symptom of hysteria. As phenomenon showing itself off, there is no discrimination between normality or abnormality. But now, through a special way of seeing, it could be diagnosed as abnormal or in disorder. Interpretation could be linguistic, merely tending toward language or merely symbolically and culturally formed attitude. In any case, interpretation is a process of symbolic mediation by which a phenomenon could be articulated and constructed as an object of discourse and science. Interpretation happens in the Life-world, which, as we said, is the mediation between Reality Itself and Constructed Reality.

Construction and scientific rationality

Now, phenomenon, after being interpreted, tends to be constructed by our language and procedures of research. In construction there is the intervention of language, empirical and theoretical, and it is here that scientific rationality intervenes. Since the main rational instrument of science is theoretical language, its progress depends much on the construction and development of theories. Theories are presented either through steps of generalization, and are then extended to new domains of experience through the process of experimentation. It is also very important to control the validity of these theories by the procedures of experimentation consisting of identifying a specific phenomenon in order to effect a corroboration or falsification of the theory in question. Experimentation is therefore not only the way by which science extends its theories to new domains of experience, it is also a way of controlling the validity of theories.

Since these procedures are quite operational in nature, science, on its practical side, also has a deep involvement in action. It changes the construction of language meaning as well as that of the states of affairs through its operational character. On the one hand, the operation of formal reasoning and calculation in the logical structure of theories will transform the meaning of language into an abstract and structural setting. On the other hand, the operation of experimentation intervenes also into the construction and organization of the states of affairs in specific context of space and time. The construction of science could become a quite autonomous enterprise and loosing contact with Reality Itself and Life-world. In this sense, science could find itself in an ontological situation itself leading to mental illness, because all construction enclosured within itself without contact with Reality Itself or with Life-world is the beginning of all mental illness.

Generally speaking, the practical side of scientific rationality could be analyzed by the mutual relationship between means and end. Under the constraint of logical reasoning and calculation, this kind of rationality could be entitled, in the first instance, as »strategic rationality«, when in calculation it envisages logical connections between possible actions. In other word, it analyses an action of grand scale into smaller but feasible actions and then relates them step by step to put together by systematic logical connection. Western modern science could also be characterized, in a second instance, as possessing a certain »instrumental rationality«, when in experimentation or in application to technology it makes the decision as to whether one action is rational or not only according to the criteria of efficiency, that is, the efficiency of utilizing a certain means by which we can attain the envisaged end. Science, as an autonomous enterprise or as strategic and instrumental rationality, is tentative to enclose its enterprise within itself and to loose contact with Reality Itself and the Life-world so as to become a purely artificial construction and therefore leads to mental illness.

Yet, science could also be looked in another way round. I myself would consider science, in an ideal mode and not in its actual Western modern mode, as a human interpretative construction of the environment, and it should be a participative construction of reality. In order to do this, we need first of all information from the environment. I see the need of empirical data in science as a need of information from the environment. Or, better said, it is needed by the fact that we should go outside of ourselves and gather information from the reality.

Most scientists, since the time of classical empiricism of John Locke and David Hume, sustain the position that, in order to know reality, the first thing we need is empirical data, either as ideas (John Lock) or as impressions (David Hume) from sensations. For them, the term »empirical data« refers therefore to its literal meaning as the given in our sensible experience. Hume used the term »impression« to emphasize the passively impressed contents of sensation, compared with which concepts were but confused or blurred impressions. A Twentieth Century's successor to this term is the »sense data« proposed by G. E. More and Betrand Russell, which refers to the immediate objects of perceptual awareness, such as color patches and shapes. Apart from the questions such as how could there be private mental objects having all the physical objects appears to be, their individuation, their duration, and their relation to physical surface of objects we perceive, the empiricists' ideas, impressions and sense data seem tending to say that the objectivity of Reality Itself could manifest only in a passive way. Objectivity means passivity. But today, since the operational character of science becomes more and more evident, it is also clear now that there is no pure passivity in the formation of empirical data.

On the contrary, empirical data are human construction on the level of controlled experimentation. Empirical data are results of the scientist active intervention into a specific area of experience. For example, the empirical data that a brain scientist collects, records and analyzes in the laboratory, as I see it, are all active interventions through very sophisticated computerized technology. If understood in the passive sense of empirical data, there will be no data at all for the brain research. Therefore, we can say that the »empirical data« is nothing but our sensible construction of information from the environment; the final end of this construction must consist in manifesting the Reality Itself rather than construction for construction's own sake. If there is any passivity at all, it is only to show that the scientist should go out of himself towards an intersubjectively controllable field of constructed reality based upon Reality Itself. In other words, he should go out of his own subjective construction or imaginative invention in order to render a phenomenon intelligible in a intersubjectively controllable way. In saying this, I would understand the empirical data as *the first step of strangification in empirical construction*, that is, the scientist's act of going out of himself and of searching for information about *the other*, the reality under examination. Whether the intersubjectively controllable should be limited to experimental methods operated on mere sensible objects is a debatable question. Here the controlling procedure might have the danger of distorting the manifestation of the real nature of the object in question. Scientist should always notice this danger.

For me the use of controlling procedure is to proceed in such a way that it lets the object manifest its own nature rather than under the control of instruments and measures. Empirical data in this perspective is caught up within two things, manifestation and construction. Empirical data are meant for the manifestation of some aspects of Reality Itself, but they cannot manifest Reality Itself except in a constructed way. Besides, manifestation and construction is mediated by the function of interpretation. On the Level of ontology, we have Life-world as mediating Reality Itself and Constructed Reality. On the level of epistemology, we have *interpretation* as mediating *manifestation* and *construction*.

Let me take the example of our mental activities related to propositional attitude, such as seeing, perceiving, thinking, believing, knowing, judging, inferring, concluding, doubting, hoping, fearing, expecting…etc., which are related to the truth of some propositions, such as in the cases where we can say that »I see the apple is red«, or »I hope there are cookies in the jar«…etc. In these cases, there are already linguistic intervention, such as *apple, red cookies, jar* ...etc. and are thereby already linguistic constructions of some sort. Here we can always find a kind of construction through linguistic interpretation. In the case of non-propositional attitudes, such as being in pain, thirsty, itching, hunger...etc., although sometimes without using words, we are also, by these sensations or feelings, informed of our mental state. They are considered by me as manifestations. But this manifestation is always tending to be elaborated by some linguistic interpretations. Whenever there is intervention of linguistic factors, there is interpretation. Language manifests state of affairs, but it manifests them in being already a kind of interpretation. For example, when I feel painful, it is not only manifesting a kind of non-propositional attitudes. The term »pain« also gives a linguistic interpretation to the whole physiological and psychological process of feeling pain.

Temporality, historicity and story

Now let me come to the triple distinction of human existence: Temporality, Historicity and Story. Before this, we need to return to our concept of symptom as manifestation and its understandability within the life story of each person. We said that mental illness manifests itself through symptoms. Symptoms are meaningful because they signify the mental illness in question. The symptoms manifesting the mental illness and lived by the patient might have their appearance in bodily and behavioral phenomena in a certain spatial, temporal context, showing a certain structural pattern and etiological relations. Although symptoms are never exhaustive of all potential manifestation of a mental illness, and our observation could not be exhaustive of all potential symptoms, still they are susceptible of phenomenological descriptions, as Karl Jaspers has pointed out, and the structural pattern of the bodily and behavioral phenomena are susceptible of genetic-structural method, as Minkowski and von Gebsattel have pointed out, and finally, the spatial, temporal and etiological context could be analyzed by using the categorical analysis as emphasized by Israeli, Strauss and Binswanger.

Further, signs and symptoms are to be interpreted with reference to the patient's life story and his social-cultural-historical context. The vicissitudes of events that happen in one's life constitute the story of one's own life. It is important in the process of psychotherapy, to listen to the story(ies) told by a patient and his significant others, such as his friends, parents, lovers...etc. In listening, it is important to first bracket any psychotherapeutic and philosophical theories, just listen attentively in order to let manifest the patient's historical world. The capacity and art of listening are therefore very important for therapeutic practitioner. Although the story told is already a linguistic construction by the patient or his significant others, the art of listening consists in returning from the constructed story back to its Life-world(social-cultural-historical) context in which the meaning of the symptoms is to be interpreted.

Again, we could say that all stories happen in a certain mode of existence, and this could be situated in a certain ontological context. About this, Heidegger would say that human existence is characterized ontologically by Sorge (Care), which, when directed to things, is called »worry« or »preoccupation«, whereas when applied to a person, is called »concern« or »solicitude«. Heidegger points out clearly that Care is more original than Worry or Concern. Different from Heidegger, Binswanger proposes Liebe (Love) as a more original mode of existence that happens in the encounter between human persons. In understanding Binswanger's idea that Love is a more original mode of existence, I do not take Love as already a derivative expression of desire. My understanding of the Asian spiritual tradition, such as the Confucian concept of ren仁, which means the ontological innerconnectiveness of human person with other persons, with nature, Heaven and the Ultimate Reality, or the Daoist idea of Motherly Care which is an inexhaustible and creative generosity from the Dao, and the Buddhist idea of Compassion coming from the innermost Buddha nature of every sentient being, all these bring us to a understanding of Love which is more original than Sorge and desire, and should not be taken as already a derivative expression of them.

In comparison with this original Love or original generosity, we should say that Care(Sorge) is but a mode of existence which concerns only with the realization of one's own being, whereas Love and generosity concern with the other and could realize itself only when the goodness of the other is realized. Sorge could be self-fish and leads to self-enclosure, and thereby cause mental illness. Love begins with an original act of generosity with which one goes always outside of one's self to the benefit of the other. But, even if Sorge could be exclusive of Love, Love is not exclusive of Sorge. On the contrary, in Love there could be Sorge, a Sorge which is already transformed by the original generosity of Love. This is the sound way to mental sanity.

To give an ethical and philosophical foundation to a sound way to mental sanity, I sustain an ontology of dynamic relation, in which strangification, generosity and love are the most important virtues. Strangification means the act of going outside of one's self and go to the stranger, the other. In strangification there is first of all an act of defamiliarization by going outside of oneself. Then there should be appropriation of other's language or language understandable to others. Finally, one could re-contextualize oneself in the other's or the stranger's context, and could pronounce thereby one's own scientific findings, cultural values, religious believes in language/expressions/belief system understandable to others. The most important capacity of a psychotherapist is therefore the capacity of language appropriation, strangifcation and unselfish concern and care.

Instead of thinking as Heidegger did, who considered Sorge, caring for one's own being, as the most original mode of human existence, I would consider Love or generous caring for others as the most original mode of human existence. Desire is already the unconscious dynamism of this most original mode of existence, whereas generosity and unselfish love and care are its conscious expression and ethical promotion. In human existence, the process of going out of one's self and go to the other constitute the process of human temporality, in which there is always a kind of Ausser-sich, of going outside of one's own and going to the other, which unifies our possibilities of existence in the future, our already-is of the past and our making present or the presencing of the always passing moments of now.

Now, from this ec-static temporality we could derive a certain kind of historicity, consisting of all the happenings within the stretching-along between the birth and death of a unique person or community. The action and passion, the aggression and the affection caused by the vicissitude of each person constitute his historicity, or what Dilthey called the connectedness of life (Zusammenhang des Lebens), conceived as an ordered sequence of experiences (Erlebnisse) in time.

It is from the historicity of each one that there could be story of each one to be told. Story, that is, events put into a specific arrangement of plot in which one person both acts and suffers, is told and retold either in an oral manner or written manner. This is to say that a story is a linguistic construction, a construction on the existential interpretation of historicity for communication or sharing with others. In the process of curing, it is most important to listen to the stories told by the patient or his significant others, even more important than psychotherapeutic theories. Sometimes we have even to put all theories into bracket so as to listen to the stories of the patient and his significant others. In listening to these personal stories, not only could psychotherapist bring then the story told back to the Erlebnisse or even the Zusammenhang des Lebens of the patient, but also in this way could the therapist show his professional care of the patient in the context of the patient, that is, through an act of defamiliarization and recontextulization.

Words of conclusion

In conclusion, I would emphasize again that psychotherapy is a process of taking care which brings the mentally ill back to reasonableness. The process of psychotherapy itself must be reasonable rather than rational. This being said, the so call quality control in psychotherapy should rather be understood as the self-control of psychotherapist within the range and to the demand of reasonableness. This would be in need of two visions and some related qualities of the psychotherapists. First, an ontological vision consisting of Reality Itself, Life-world and Constructed Reality. A life of sanity consists in the participative construction of a meaningful Life-world according to the rhythm of Reality Itself, whereas dominative construction and with it the distortion of or losing contact with Reality Itself would lead unfortunately to mental illness.

Second, a vision of human existence consisting of temporality, historicity and story. Although a story is a linguistic construction on the existential interpretation of historicity, it is most important for a reasonable psychotherapist to have the capacity to listen carefully and concernedly the stories told by the patient or his significant others.

I do not propose to itemize and structuralize the quality control, but I would say that with these the above two visions in mind, the most important qualities of a reasonable psychotherapist and his professional training will be »openness and conformity to Reality Itself«, »participatory construction instead of dominative construction«, »language appropriation«, »strangification«, and »concernedly listening and unselfish caring«.

Cor van Dijkum

Constructive Realism: Looking Back and Forward

1. Looking back

1.1 The start

It seems a long time ago since I met Fritz Wallner and was inspired by his talk about constructive realism. It was the start of a number of publications, first of all as a try-out to test and elaborate his intriguing ideas about constructing reality without denying the existence of reality. In our booklet *Constructive Realism in Discussion* (Dijkum & Wallner, 1991) we went into the depth of quite fundamental discussions about the nature of reality and the way human beings cope with it. The world was not given to man by God and Nature, but in a long and painful struggle, man could construct and reconstruct his environment and try to overcome the misery that reality sometimes brought to mankind. As was heroically proclaimed by the Vienna Circle (1929) that was made possible by practicing science, the miracle that came into human history at first as the natural sciences and in more recent periods as the social sciences.

In my opinion constructive realism had to start with this scientific optimism. But we had to go beyond the hard work of Schlick, Von Neumann, Carnap to lay ground for the logic of science. And thereafter we had to go further than Popper (1934, 1967) in his pain to improve the positivism of the Vienna Circle, because he brought into the world of the social sciences a regressed logic that simplified the relation between the scientific practice and the real world too much. With this logic of simple falsificationism[1] social scientists could only (a) enumerate and falsify trivial facts of human life, (b) fell back into ideologies, (c) and certainly could not construct new facts in the world.

1.2. Logical foundations

Anyway, with modern life and science we had to (re)construct advanced logic and philosophy to understand the way science constructs a new world. In our booklet that was for example done for mathematics by van Dalen. He showed referring to Dutch mathematician Brouwer who in his time opposed the doctrine of Hilbert[2],

1 Of course this is a shortcut for an analysis with many more arguments. See for example: Dijkum (1991).

2 The logical base of Popper's simplified falsificationism.

that mathematics was more than finite formal logic. In understanding the world of never ending numbers the mathematical intuition constructed concepts such as continuum, recursion and incompleteness. In this framework a mathematician was a creative subject that constructed a world of fascinating numbers, such as irrationals, transcendental, transfinite numbers, the measurement of a circle, fractals, and so on.

Constructive realism discussed thereby that instruments of modern science dedicated to finite logic at the same time seem showed the borders of that finite logic. This freed the way for constructive realism to use computers in a creative way. That was understood by Wallner and Peschl when they refer to the future playground of psychologists: cognitive science. In this new domain computers were used as a metaphor for the human brain, and epistemology was integrated with neuro- and computerscience.

In my article I underpinned that in a logical way by referring to the metamathematical investigations of Gödel and Turing. Gödel (1931) proved that the idea of Hilbert (and Popper) that everything in mathematics could be completely deduced from a finite set of axioms was doomed to fail. Even the simplest part of mathematics, that was arithmetic, was incomplete. Arithmetic statements could be formulated for which neither the correctness nor the incorrectness could be proved in a finite way. It was foresaid by this investigation that computers could produce results that were not understandable within the framework the results were produced. In another way Turing (1939) proved that computers (Turing machines) could not calculate whether they were calculating. Computers were unguided projectiles. Or in philosophical terms: they were not able to reflect on themselves. Also the logician Tarski (1933) struggled with the problem how it was possible that apparently true statements could be formulated in a logical framework, but could not be proved within the same framework. According to him a hierarchy of never ending logical frameworks made this possible, the next level was the metareflection of the lower level.

1.3 Surprisingly modern science

The idea that computers as finite devices could show the borders of finite calculations was at an amazing way demonstrated in our late century by computer simulations. Until the sixties of the 19th century it was thought, in spite of the logical investigations of Gödel, Turing and Tarski, that computers were precisely controlled devices. What went in was transformed in a controlled way to what went out, and as a consequence the same input would always lead to the same output. But when the meteorologist Lorenz in 1963 made a model of the atmosphere he was surprised. With ›the same input‹ a totally different output could be the result. At first he thought that it was because of a tiny difference in input. But specifying more decimals brought still the same problem, in some regions of values an arbitrary small difference resulted in a totally different output.

Mathematicians were intrigued by those results, and examined the equations by which an input was transformed to an output. Characteristics of the equations of Lorenz were they dealt with an evolution in time: a starting value of a variable as input resulted step by step (in time) in changing values of an output variable. An example is the way an initial population grows year by year when there is a positive difference between birthrate and death rate. As a mathematical consequence one has to work with differential equations. Essential was that the differential equations Lorenz and other worked with were non-linear differential equations, a little bit more complicated than linear equations[3]. A fundamental investigation of such equations showed that they could not be solved analytically and moreover that it could be demonstrated that with some values of the parameters of such equations an arbitrary difference in starting value resulted in substantial differences in the values of output variables.

According to the Dutch mathematician Verhulst (1966) such computer simulations, gave rise to a revolution in mathematics. Perfectly deterministic machines produced results that were completely unpredictable according to the algorithm that produced it. As ›a Baron von Munchhausen‹ computer programs seems to be able to escape from their own algorithm. Completely deterministic programs produced order at one hand and incomprehensible chaos, from the viewpoint of the algorithm, on the other hand. However at the same time it was agreed with Turing that the computer program itself could not decide whether it escaped from itself. For that, another computer program had to jump in, or better a human being as a medium that was able to jump to the other computer program.

In such a way the interaction between human beings and computer hard- and software gave rise to a completely new program of research in the natural sciences. In this program a wonderful new world of chaos and order showed up. For example, in Meteorology it was discussed that »a butterfly in Brazil could cause a typhoon in Japan«. With this metaphor it was understood why arbitrary small disturbances in the atmosphere sometimes could cause major events. Or in geodesy in which the problem was solved, by reference to fractals, how you could measure the length of a coast whereby ever shortening your path of measurement (from bays, to rocks, to stones, to gravel, to grain of sand) gave rise to infinities. Or in biology in which the growth of populations, or the spread of a disease, in some situations, was at last understood as a fundamental unpredictable process. Or in the medical sciences in which the rhythm the heart, the pattern's of EEG of the brain could be described as the typical outcome of a non linear process. With this it was hoped that such understanding makes it possible to cure, or better prevent,

3 A well known example from demography (Verhulst 1838) is that of saturated growth of a population

disturbing events as heart a-rhythm or epilepsy. Anyway, in the natural sciences the use of computers constructed a whole new landscape of never before observed phenomena.

1. 4 Constructivistic reflections

The question rises whether these phenomena already exist in nature and modern science discovered them or whether instruments of modern science brought these phenomena into existence. Following the scholastic of the old Vienna Circle one can perhaps solve this philosophical problem by supposing that there is no meaningfully distinction between ›discovering‹ on one hand and ›bringing into existence‹ on the other hand. When there is an infinite number of an outcome possible of a non-linear process, the observation of that process is at that moment a (finite) selection of those possibilities. Moreover because such a selection has to jump out of the set of observations until that moment, it brings into existence for the observer a new set of observations and consequently a new set of related phenomena. One could consider this as construction of reality, because of the capability of the observer to jump out of the logical framework with which the old world was understood. This can be sharpened by application of Wallner's idea that we live with ›cognitive reality‹ as our world, and with an outside world as ›environment‹ and external source of possible observations.

For the construction of cognitive reality the languages we use is of utmost importance. That was understood by Löfgren when he introduced with the physicist Bohr »the nondetachability of language«, that is the idea that we can isolate and communicate sentences as finite strings of symbols, but we can not detach us from processes of interpretation. Language is a complementaristic phenomenon in which we partially isolate interpretations but not completely, and as a consequence a subject is always needed for communication and the intersubjective construction of reality. De Zeeuw extented this idea by supposing that language was not only a matter of uttering sentences, but also involving a human actor interacting with other actors in constructing cognitive reality. Also these acts in the range between bodily gestures and the architectural environment in which one is communicating seem to have a syntax and a semantic and are symbolically interpreted. In this respect language is extended with symbols of acts, or to be considered as Wittgenstein did, as a language game. In all these considerations authors of the booklet brought in fascinating stuff for modern science.

1.5 The past of the social sciences

According to De Comte (1840) the rational enterprise of science made it possible to support the integral development of humanity. Sociology was a kind of social physics, but the complexity of the human interaction with society was at a different level (than of the natural sciences) and that was why sociology was aiming higher. In the 19th century past of psychology notions of mental side of human action were introduced by the German philosopher and mathematician Herbart. And hopefully Fechner (see: Boring 1988) introduced thereafter a difference equation to grasp the dynamics of the way a human being reacted in a subjective way to a stimulus from outside.

For constructive realism such onsets to understand the dynamics of human (inter)action are sufficient for a start of a constructive program of research. It was aiming at the same goal the Vienna Circle reading ›How can man construct and reconstruct his environment and try to overcome the misery that reality sometimes brought to mankind?‹ Moreover, for my ideas of constructive realism it was interesting that as well Fechner as well followers of Comte, introduced the need to use differential equations to describe the dynamics of human (inter)action.

From this it was a small step to the idea that linear differential equations were too simple to grasp the way human beings (inter)act. As an example: when I take twice the medicines my GP prescribes, my pain will normally not be twice less. Or another example: I usually will not use twice more words when you use twice more words. More abstractly and put into other words: the feedback I give to another being, or to myself, will usually not be simply multiplied by the same number as the feedback I received is multiplied. With the idea of feedback, linear or not linear, one can build simulation models of (inter)actions, for example such as are developed in systems dynamics[4].

With such inspirations I started years ago a program of research with colleagues in the social science in which computer simulation was used to describe, understand and handle the predictability and unpredictability of linear and non linear human (inter)action. Concerning the social sciences we were amazed by the number of authors that implicitly included the idea of feedback in their theory, but not in their methods of research[5]. On the other side we were stimulated by researchers from the natural sciences who were intrigued by the way human beings try to create order in apparently chaos. How can you use chaos to create (partial) order? Or touching the essence of human existence: how can you organize patterns of order and chaos to establish your own identity? The constructive concept of selforganizing systems showed up, and we read the works of Maturana, Varela, Haken (1982) and Prigogine (1977). With the aid of computer simulations of the selforganizing models Prigogine and Haken provided we tried to get the essence

4 In Dijkum & Mens-Verhulst (2002) the idea of feedback, linear and non linear, is more systematically elaborated.

5 The theory was dynamic, involving feedback loops and development of time patterns. The methods of research were however static and only capable of grasping time independent relations in data (see: Dijkum, Mens-Verhulst, Lam & Kuijk 2002).

of this concept, and moreover try to apply it to our empirical research of non-linear behaviour of human beings.

As such our program to use simulation to describe, understand and handle human behaviour was a success. We did a lot of interesting empirical research in the domain of psychology and sociology that was related with theoretical investigations in the domain of epistemology, methodology and computer science. We published many articles in journals and books and Internet, and presented papers at a number of interesting conferences in very different domains. We also showed how human actors handled patterns of chaos and order in their efforts to construct solutions for their problems[6].

However, looking to our ambitions and hope for the social sciences we were disappointed. It was fighting a losing battle against the dominating way of doing research in the social sciences. The simple falsifications that Popper[7] brought into the world of the social sciences appeared to be an obstacle. As already was observed by Holzkamp (1972) in the seventies of our past century, and still discussed by critics of the social sciences, the majority of social researchers are locked in the stereotypes of what social research should be. At one hand you have dominating quantitative researchers that only believe in significant results of descent experiments or surveys, merely use static linear models that calculate hundreds of correlations, feed rapports with series of multivariate analyses, or statistical stuff that only peer reviewers can value[8]. The reported results in their scientific journals are however valid and reliable according to their methodology of simple falsificationism. The only handicap is that they are most of the time trivial and concerning the way they get the results (their methodology) difficult to understand for an outsider.

On the other hand, as a mirror, you have the qualitative researchers as a tolerated minority. They believe in participant observation and qualitative interpretations and try to describe unique and incomparable experiences of individuals. They do not want to count, certainly not to simulate, and feed their rapport with literal quotations of interviews, subjective own interpretations and theories in fashion. They have of course, as quantitative researchers do, their own journals and peer reviewing system establishing what already is established. The reported results are valid according to their own qualitative methodology, most of the time nice to read, but also often quite trivial and filled by stereotypes and do not really enter new knowledge.

---

6 An illustrative example is showed in Mens-Verhulst, Dijkum, Lam & van Kuijk 2003.

7 Reading Popper well brings a far more sophisticated version of the idea of falsification. The problem is that Popper himself did sometimes exaggerate, and moreover that followers of Popper in the social science did not read Popper well.

8 Or not, but when it is heavy stuff, they will not admit it. Anecdotes can illustrate that in a nice way.

This situation would not be a problem when resources (money, positions in the research and education organizations, access to scientific media, etc.) were not exclusively set aside for the ›quantitative researchers‹ and their peer protected colleagues, and for a small part of it for qualitative researchers and their incrowd. Alas, this is exactly the case. That can be illustrated by a overwhelming number of case studies, for example concerning: acceptation and rejection of articles in dominating scientific journals; granting of proposals of research; courses in universities that are accepted and not accepted by educational authorities[9]; the content of published research rapport in scientific journals; the acceptation of journals by established groups of researchers[10]; the way how the social science citation index protect a group of established conservative researchers.

One could wonder why an obviously outdated methodology such as simplified falsficationism regulates in such a strict way the production of the social sciences. Why do most of my colleagues in the social science do such boring research with so many trivial results? Well the reason could be quite simple, they are educated with simple falsificationism (and of course do not read Popper and Lakatos well, and certainly not authors like Turing, Tarski, Gödel and Wallner), and earn their salary in the way they did in the past. Why should they change? Certainly not, because our society has a place for such pretended scientific activities. Social sciences support ideologies with research that the society needs to maintain order amid possible chaos. To use the social sciences to support the creation of harmony in our social systems could be for the benefit for the whole of our society, as was understood by Comte (1830-1842):

»Sociology studies the balance of mutual relations of elements within a social whole. There must always be a [...] spontaneous harmony between the whole and the parts of the social system. It is evident that not only must political institutions and social manners, on

9 For example the social sciences in the Netherlands give priority in their program of education to the standard statistical methods such as can be found in the Statistical Package of the Social Sciences (SPSS). There is nothing wrong with this, but courses in computer simulation, as scientific legitimate and equally valued by students, are at the last place and as a consequence because of restrictions in resources and time not to be found in the curricula.

10 Concerning simulation there are at the moment three examples of excellent journals that are not well accepted in the social sciences: Journal of Artificial Societies and Social Simulation, Non Linear Dynamics in the Life Sciences and Kybernetes. All Journals were not at first to be found in the Social Science Citation Index. However, the first Journal is accepted, but still with a low impactfactor. The second one proved by calculating their impactfactor that it was higher than many of the well accepted Journals. The third one is only to be found in the Science Citation Index, a long time a reason why an article published in this Journal was not accepted by established social science researchers.

the one hand, and manners and ideas on the other, be always mutually connected; but further that this consolidated whole must always be connected, by its nature, with the corresponding state of the integral development of humanity [...].«

But when elements of a social whole are groups who try to dominate and voluntary or involuntary suppress the interests of other groups as happen at an amazing scale in our modern world, ideologies will taken over the reason of the mutual balance between the interest of different social groups. The social sciences by Comte and others meant to be the instrument to create a fair play between individuals, groups and nations will be reversed to the opposite. And let us be realistic, what will show up, as the result of social research is most of the time the prejudice of the common sense of the day. One only has to refer to the survey industry, in the Netherlands coming with telephonic interviewing to a plague of everybody happening to be at home to realize that something else is manifesting than scientific reasoning. It is in our modern society understood by firms and policy makers that the simplicity of social research is a wonderful instrument to maintain images to support their power plays. What Popper fought is apparently coming back stronger as it was because some of the arguments of Popper became a doctrine and an ideology itself.

2. Looking forward

2.1 The future of the social sciences

It is clear that the social sciences are not a progressive force for the society as such. Therefore the courage and mutual cooperation is needed of individuals that take science serious. Of course worldwide there are a number of groups that try in a constructive way to create other practices of sciences than supporting established images of the world.

In my practice I found several individuals and groups that are enthused by the potential of computer simulation to create new and inspiring images of possibilities in the world. It is no coincidence that among those other scientists people are to be found that are quite known with the practice of science. I can refer to members of the Research Committee Sociocybernetics (RC51) of the International Sociological Association that originally are moved by Wiener's concept of feedback, but in a next move are inspired by and struggling with the ideas of self-organizing systems of Foerster, Maturana and Luhmann. Thereby I can refer my colleague van der Zouwen who went into the depths of the art and science of interviewing and analyzed the process of interviewing with the aid of the feedback concept. Against the stereotype of the dominating practice that the process of posing questions has to be standardized as much as possible, he made a plea to enlarge the freedom of the interviewer to pose a question in an intelligent way. Ashby's law of variety learned that against the sometimes unpredictable reaction of the respondent the interviewer has to create room for an unpredictable question to be found in the variety of his repertory of questions[11].

On the other hand I found enthusiasm for computer simulation in young upcoming social researchers. It is wonderful that one of my research projects was supported by two intelligent PhDs, but because we could not find sufficient financing of our ›exotic research‹, and they considered other careers in social sciences as too boring, they went to software firms and were lost for the social sciences. It was a complaint for many talented students of social sciences in the Netherlands[12].

Leaving the Netherlands, it is encouraging that worldwide in RC51 a number of young colleagues are as well moved by feedback idea and selforganizing systems, as well by the wonders of computer simulation. Moreover, their interest is intensely connected to their worries about societal problems in their countries. That is a good base for research projects that are relevant for science and society with the advantage that those projects are not stuck into simple falsificationism. At the moment RC51 is satisfied with the idea that by organizing conferences two generations of scientist, the old and wise generation quite known with the dominating practice, and the young and clever generation not yet distorted by that practice, can exchange information and learn from each other. In the future it is the hope that momentum is gained to organize and finance that practice.

Being back in the Netherlands another signal for hope is showing up in the new generation. Because the spread of PCs and enthusiasm of young people for computer games hype is unfolding: gaming as an academic activity of software programmers and developers of games. With this, fantasy is coming back into the mind of young social scientists, and computer simulation is an evident accepted activity. Also here is the advantage that those youngsters are not yet spoiled by the dominating practice of the social sciences. Concerning history also here is the hope that this new generation will find an old generation interested in ›Simulation and Gaming‹ [13] and mutual cooperate.

2.2 A topic for constructive realistic reflection

In all those research projects one element is of utmost importance. To let succeed those projects different disciplines has to work together, for example software engineers with psychologists, psychologists with sociologists, economists has to turn

---

11 He reported his research in his farewell speech as retired professor, unfortunately only in Duch available.

12 As a consequence professors recruted many students from foreign countries.

13 There is even a Jounal *Simulation and Gaming*.

in, and all those specialists cannot do without logic and mathematics. It is then the question how all these different disciplines with very different theories and languages can communicate with each other. One skill one has to enter is the skill of facilitating the communication between different individuals in a group with different scientific cultures. It is the skill of applied social psychology, and as such developed as a part of group decision support.

However, another skill is more typically the domain of philosophy. That is certainly demonstrated by Wallner when he entered the concept of strangification in his discourse. In his opinion (ontological) strangification is involved when a discipline apply his system of thinking to a very different discipline. A meanwhile classic example is the application of the concept of actor to software, nowadays known in the field of computer simulation as agent (simulation). Another example is the use of the Gestalt concept into the natural sciences, nowadays practiced in system dynamics as a holistic system view. There many more examples of the influence a discipline has with its concepts on another discipline. Some of these strangifications are a success, other a problem. Wallner introduced as an association of an unsuccessful strangification the concept of alienation. In my opinion the way Popper tried to impose Hilbert's finite logic to the social science is such an example of not productive strangification e.g. for the society a form of alienation. For disciplines working together on a topic of research it is an immense problem how concepts of one discipline can be made useful for another discipline, and vice versa. It is a wonderful task for a philosopher to guide this process, and strangification is one of the successful concepts of constructive realism that can be used in his or her practice.

Reference

Boring, E.G. (1988). Gustav Theodoor Fechner. In J. R. Newmann (eds.), *The world of mathematics*. Washington: Tempus.

Carnap, R., Hahn, H., & Neurath, O. (1929). *Wissenschaftliche Weltauffassung*. Wien.

Comte, A. (1830/42). *Cours de Philosophie Positive*. Paris: Bachelier.

Dalen D. van (1981). *Brouwer's Cambridge Lectures on Intuitionism*. Cambridge: Cambridge University Press.

Dijkum C. van, & Wallner F. (1991).(Eds.). *Constructive Realism in Discussion*. Amsterdam: Sokrates Science Publisher.

Dijkum, C. van (1991). Towards a New Methodology: from Popper to Social Cybernetics. In Mutual Uses of Cybernetics and Science, special issue of *Systemica*, Vol. 8 (edited by R. Glanville & G. de Zeeuw). Amsterdam: Thesis Publishers.

Dijkum, C. van (1997). From Cybernetics to the Science of Complexity. In *Kybernetes*, 6/7, 725-738.

Dijkum C.van, Mens-Verhulst J. van (2002). Sociocybernetics Going beyond the Logic of the Social Sciences. In *International Review of Sociology*, Vol. 2, 2, 193-201.

Dijkum, C. van, Mens-Verhulst J. van, Kuijk E. van, & Lam N. (2002). System Dynamic Experiments with Non-linearity and a Rate of Learning. In *Journal of Artificial Societies and Social Simulation*, Volume 5, Issue 3.

Gödel, K. (1931). Uber formal unentscheidbare Sätze der Principia Mathematica und verwandte Systeme. *Monatshefte für Mathematik und Physik*, vol. 37, pp.349-360.

Haken, H. (1982). *Evolution of Order and Chaos in Physics, Chemistry and Biology*. New York: Springer Verlag.

Holzkamp, K. (1972). *Kritische Psychologie*. Frankfurt: Fischer.

Lakatos, I. (1978). Popper on Demarcation and Induction. In G. Currie & J. Worral (ed), The Methodology of Scientific Research Programmes. In *Criticism and the Growth of Knowledge*. Cambridge.

Lorenz, E. (1963). Deterministic Nonperiodic Flow. In *Journal of Atmospheric Sciences, 20*, pp.130-141.

Mens-Verhulst, J. van, Dijkum, C., Kuijk, E. van, & Lam, N. (2003). The self-regulation of fatigue and associated complaints: an exploratory simulation. In *Patient Education and Counseling* Volume 49, Issue 1, 2003, pp.53-57.

Prigogine, I. (1977). *Self-organization in Nonequilibrium Systems*. New York: Willey.

Popper, K. R. (1934, 1959). *The Logic of Scientific Discovery*. London: Hutchinson. (The original German version *Logik der Forschung* was published in Vienna in 1934).

Popper, K.R. (1967). *The Open Society and Its Enemies*. London: Routledge and Kegan Paul.

Tarski, A. (1933). Der Wahrheitsbegriff in den formalisierten Sprache. In *Studia Philosophica*, vol. 1, pp.261-405.

Turing, A. M. (1939). Systems of logic based on ordinals. In *Proceedings London Mathematical Society*, serie 2, vol. 45, pp.161-228.

Verhulst, P.-F. (1838). Notice sur la loi que la population suit dans son accroissement. In *Correspondance Mathematique et Physique, publiee parA. Quetelet* 10, 113.

Verhulst, F. (1996). *Nonlinear Differential Equations and Dynamical Systems*. Berlin: Springer.

Vienna Circle (1929). *Wissenschaftliche Weltauffassung: Programmschrift des Wiener Kreises*. Vienna.

Wiener, N. (1948). *Cybernetics, or Control and Communication in the Animal and the Machine*. Cambridge MA: MIT Press.

Wiener, N. (1950/1954). *The Human use of Human Beings; Cybernetics and Society*. Boston: Houghton Mifflin.

Zouwen, H. van der , Dijkum, C. van (2001). Towards a Methodology for the Empirical Testing of Complex Social Models. In F. Geyer & H. van der Zouwen (eds), *Sociocybernetics: Complexity, Autopoiesis, and Observation of Social Systems* (pp.223-241). Westport: Greenwood Publishers.

Kwang-Kuo Hwang

The Necessity of Indigenous Psychology: The Perspective of Constructive Realism

I have devoted myself to the development of Chinese indigenous psychology since the early 1980s, which has also caused me to pay close attention to the indigenization movement of psychology in other areas of the world. By the early 1990s, I realized that many of the ontological, epistemological, and methodological disputes that have occurred in the progress of the indigenization movement are essentially philosophical problems, and that it is necessary to find a solid philosophy to provide persuasive answers to the controversial issues related to the emergence of indigenous psychology. Eventually, I determined that the philosophy of constructive realism, advocated by Fritz Wallner (1994) of Vienna University, can be used to serve such a function. It enables social scientists to understand not only the reason non-Western countries began to develop indigenous psychologies, but also provides a strategy for developing the field. Nevertheless, constructive realism is basically a philosophy developed by a Western thinker. It may still be insufficient for solving the arduous problems encountered by non-Western scholars in developing indigenous psychologies.

In this article, I first introduce my supplements to the main ideas of constructive realism for the sake of distinguishing two types of knowledge: that used in the lifeworld, and that of the scientific microworld. Then I use Li's (1988, 1992) worldview equilibrium model to illustrate the specific features of knowledge used by Chinese people in their lifeworlds. Finally, I use a body-mind-spirit model proposed by Chen and Bhikkhu (2003) to explain how people in Chinese culture may use these two types of knowledge in different stages of life. In this way, I explain why it is necessary to develop indigenous psychology in non-Western countries.

1. Two types of knowledge in scientific microworlds and people's lifeworlds

Constructive realism classifies reality into three categories: reality itself (*wirklichkeit*), lifeworlds, and microworlds (Wallner, 1994). *Reality itself* is something that cannot be understood by human beings. Human beings can understand only the worlds they have constructed with language, which include *lifeworlds* constructed by cultural groups in their long-tem history of development, and *microworlds* constructed by individual scientists.

The separation of the knowable world into lifeworlds and microworlds is very helpful for social scientists in coping with the challenges encountered by indigenous psychologists, although it is insufficient for answering all related questions. Therefore, I will review the previous discourses on the difference between the types of knowledge constructed in the lifeworld and the scientific microworld (Hwang, 2000), and compare them from five aspects, namely, the constructor, ways of thinking, types of rationality, patterns of construction, and functions of worldview (see Table 1).

	Lifeworld	Microworld
Constructor	Cultural group	Single scientist
Ways of thinking	Originative thinking	Technique thinking
Types of rationality	Substantive rationality	Formal rationality
Patterns of construction	Participative constructive	Dominative construction
Functions of worldview	Meaning of life	Recognition of world

Table 1: Two Types of Knowledge in Lifeworld and Microworld

In order to acquire systematic knowledge about the external world, human beings have constructed a variety of microworlds about religion, ethics, aesthetics, and science. In consideration of our main theme, I focus only on the microworld of scientific knowledge.

The microworld of scientific knowledge is constructed by a single scientist, while the language and knowledge used by people in their lifeworlds are constructed by a group of people living with the same cultural background for a long period of time. In the originating centuries of a particular culture, people concentrate themselves on observing the external world and contemplating the nature of every object in their lifeworlds. They attempt to get rid of their own will and intention, and try their best to make each thing manifest itself in the language they create to represent it. Heiderger labeled this way of thinking *originative thinking* or *essential thinking* (1966). In contrast, the language used by scientists to construct microworlds of scientific knowledge is intentionally created to reach a specific goal. The language has a compulsory and aggressive character that demands the most gain with the least cost, and is a product of *technical thinking* or *metaphysical thinking* from Heiderger's perspective.

From the perspective of insiders living in a given society, collective consciousness and social representations are all rational (Durkheim, 1912/1965). But there is a fundamental difference between the rationality used for constructing a microworld and that used in a lifeworld. In their lifeworlds, people emphasize the importance of *substantive rationality,* which refers to the value of ends or results judged from a particular position. It is completely different from the *formal rationality* used by Western scientists to construct scientific microworlds after the European Renaissance. Formal rationality emphasizes the importance of goals or results and provides no clear-cut means and procedures for reaching them. Only a few persons who are familiar with the special means and procedures can use them to pursue worthy goals. Substantive rationality pays attention only to value-natural facts and the calculability of means and procedures that can be used by everyone to pursue their personal goals (Brubaker, 1984).

Scientists construct their microworlds with Cartesian dualism through *dominative construction* (Shen, 1994). They construct these microworlds about various aspects of the external world that concern human beings in order to attain the goal of controlling and utilizing nature. These microworlds are neither permanent nor absolutely certain; each has its own specific goal. When the goal loses importance, or when people are faced with new problems, scientists must construct new microworlds to address these problems. In contrast, people construct knowledge in their lifeworlds by *participative construction*, especially in premodern civilizations. Anthropologist Levy-Bruhl (1910/1966) indicated that the cultural systems of primitive people are constituted on the law of mystical participation, which conceptualizes human beings and nature as parts of an inseparable entity that can be viewed as a consciousness of cosmic holism (Taylor, 1871/1929).

The worldviews of the lifeworld and the microworld are essentially different. As people of a given culture contemplate the nature of the universe and the situation of humankind, they gradually formulate their worldviews with original thinking in the course of their history. Walsh and Middleton (1984) indicated that a worldview thus formulated usually answers four broad categories of questions: Who am I? What is my situation of life? Why do I suffer? How do I find salvation? Generally speaking, a worldview describes not only human nature but also the relationship between an individual and the external environment, as well as the individual's historical situation in the world. In addition, it provides a diagnosis for problems and prescribes a recipe for their solution.

The worldview in a microworld does not serve such a function. In his lexicon theory, Kuhn (1987) indicated that the scientific lexicon is composed of a set of terms with structure and content. Scientists use terms in the lexicon to make propositions in theory for describing the nature of the world. Theory and lexicon are inseparable. The microworld of a theory cannot be understood without its specific lexicon. Different theories are understood with their various lexicons. When a theory is changed, its lexicon will change with it. Each lexicon contains a method to recognize the world. Members of the same scientific community must master the same lexicon, understand the meanings of each term, and share the same worldview in order to communicate with one another. In order to think about the same problem and engage in related research in the same scientific community, they must share the same worldview. However, the worldview of a microworld provides no answers to problems related to the meaning of life. It is essentially different from the worldview of a lifeworld.

The contrast between the two types of knowledge in microworlds and life-worlds enables social scientists to understand why non-western countries must develop an indigenous psychology. These two types of knowledge have different meanings for people from western and non-western countries. In western countries, scientific microworlds were developed from within the civilization after the 14th century Renaissance. However, in non-western countries, research methodology and the philosophical foundation for constructing scientific microworlds are transplanted from outside the civilization. They are essentially heterogeneous and different from the knowledge inherited from internal cultural traditions, with an obvious discontinuity between the two types of knowledge (Hwang, 1999).

2. The worldview model of equilibrium

Anthropologist Li Yi-Yuan (1988, 1992) analyzed the folk religions, legends, and myths prevailing in Chinese society and constructed a Chinese worldview model of equilibrium using the method of structuralism. The word *equilibrium* used in Li's model comes from the Confucian classic the *Golden Mean*, in which the term was used to mean »to reach balance and harmony." Li proposed that the most fundamental operating rule in traditional Chinese cosmology is to seek balance and harmony between humans and nature, humans and society, and humans and ego. The most ideal and perfect states in traditional culture all aim at such a state of balance and harmony. In order to reach these ideal states, it is necessary to maintain balance and harmony within each of the three systems. The worldview model of equilibrium is comprised of balance and harmony within each of the three systems. It is represented in the following chart.

The state of harmony and equilibrium	1. The system of *tian* or natural order	Sub-system of tempo-ral relations
		Sub-system of spa-tial relations
	2. The system of *ren* or individual organisms	Sub-system of inter-nal harmony
		Sub-system of exter-nal harmony
	3. The system of *shehui* or society	Sub-system of worldly relations
		Sub-system of other-worldly relations

Table 2: Li's Worldview Model of Equilibrium
(Adapted from Li, 1992, p.130)

According to Li, the first level of harmony is harmony with nature. The idea of harmony with nature is consistent with the idea of unification with heaven in traditional China. It can be expressed in two aspects: time and space. In Chinese folk belief, harmony of temporality is manifest in the explanation of one's fortune in life in coordination with cosmic time. Four pairs of signs represent the time, date, month and year in which a person was born. The two characters of each pair are adopted from ten celestial stems and twelve terrestrial branches, and are usually called *eight characters*. The eight characters that represent one's birth time may determine one's life experience or fate (*ming*). To many Chinese people, fate is determined at birth. In coordination with cosmic time, an individual's life experience will take on various changes as a consequence of good or bad luck. In the traditional system of Chinese belief, fate is unchangeable, while luck can be changed with the aid of various forces. Seeking harmony with temporality is revealed in this changeable fortune.

The second aspect of maintaining balance with nature is spatial arrangement. Ideas of spatial harmony are constructed on the concepts of *yin* and *yang*, five primary elements (*wu-hsin*), and eight trigrams (*ba-gua*). The combination of these factors constitutes a belief in geomancy (*feng-shui*). The traditional belief in the harmony of temporality and spatiality can be said to be the most important framework for Chinese for understanding the existence and function of the universe. It can also be viewed as the fundamental rule for explaining why human beings exist in the universe.

Li's second level is maintaining harmony within the individual. Li (1992) divided this type of harmony into two parts: internal substantial harmony and external formal harmony. The former explains the harmony within the human body mainly by the dynamic equilibrium between the two opposing forces of *yin* and *yang*. Based on these concepts, a very complicated system of Chinese medicine and food has been developed. If an individual's body is basically cold, that person should consume more hot foods to keep in balance, while a person whose body is basically hot should consume more cold foods. If the body overheats, more cold food or medicine will be needed to keep the balance, and vice versa. The foods people should eat changes with the weather. More hot foods should be eaten in the winter, and more cold foods should be consumed in the summer to maintain the balance of cold and hot within the body.

The harmony of the external form is mainly represented in the use of one's name. To individuals in most cultures, their names are just signs or symbols. But in the traditional Chinese theory of naming, names entail a transforming force for the individual. Two aspects represent a person's name. The first is related to the five primary elements, the second is the number of strokes required to write one's name. Both show an individual's search for balance in external forms.

The third level of harmony should exist in a person's social relationships. This type of harmony is the steadfast goal of the Confucian value system, which is the ethical foundation of social order. Traditional Confucian ethics emphasize the importance of two aspects: the arrangement of relationships among family members, and heredity and the continuance of the family system. The former entails a synchronic harmony in the lifeworld. Its value is manifest in such ideals as »benevolent father and filial son«, and »righteous husband and submissive wife«. The latter is a diachronic harmony in the social order. Both the dead and the living members of a family or clan are seen as a unit. Real harmony can be reached only when both of them are balanced and harmonious. There is a popular expression that illustrates the need to balance both aspects: Of the three major offenses against filial piety, not producing an heir is the greatest one. The ceremony of ancestor worship in folk society also displays the earnest Chinese desire for balance with the supernatural.

Li's worldview model of equilibrium represents the contents of substantive rationality in Chinese cultural tradition. The concepts of person, body, disease, and ethics contained in his conceptual framework can be viewed as participative construction in Chinese culture, and can be further analyzed with the symbolic approach of cultural psychology. This type of approach is a second-degree interpretation constructed by researchers at a cultural level. It is different from the first-degree interpretation provided by people for their own actions. Psychologically, ordinary Chinese may habitually use this set of worldviews to explain, deal with or solve their problems in their lifeworlds. But they may have their own explanations for their actions. Under the impact of Western culture, many Chinese may give up their traditional worldview and adopt modern science to deal with the problems of daily life. The kind of influence cultural traditions have on people's actions is the research focus of indigenous psychology in non-Western societies.

3. The body-mind-spirit model

With an understanding of the holistic structure of Chinese cultural tradition, we may use the body-mind-spirit model of spiritual care proposed by Bhikkhu and Chen (2003) to discuss the applicability of these two types of knowledge in different stages of one's life. The body-mind-spirit model distinguishes three aspects of object self when one is introspective about one's own existence:

1. Physical self: This is one's self-consciousness focused on the functionings of self originating from one's physical needs: Examples include eating when hungry, warming oneself up when cold, resting when tired, pursuing benefit, and avoiding harm. All these physical needs may make one aware of one's own existence as an organism.
2. Psychological self: This is one's awareness of one's own psychological functioning. It originates from the process that occurs when an individual attempts to acquire social or material resources from the outer world for the sake of satisfying various physical or psychological needs. An individual has to learn various types of knowledge in order to control the outer world effectively, thus the person may acquire a sense of self-efficacy.
3. Spiritual self: Being a human being who is able to think, feel, act, and experience various domains of life, this aspect of self enables one to get a comprehensive understanding of one's entire life, including one's personality, values, beliefs, and motives.

These three aspects of self correspond to the three levels of the body-mind-spirit model proposed by Chen and Bhikkhu (2003). According to the model, an individual is only aware of biological existence at the newborn stage. At this stage, a person's primary motive is to satisfy various needs originating from the physical body. Other psychological functions remain in a state of underdevelopment. Therefore, the body is located on the outer most circle of self, as shown in Fig.1.1. The maturation of mental functions enables learning of various kinds of knowledge in order to control the outer world and maintain a state of equilibrium in adolescence (Fig.1.2). Once a person enters the adult stage, mind and body are fully developed, and it is expected that the functioning of physical and psychological activities is under the guidance of the person's values and beliefs. One's spiritual self, psychological self, and physical self may coordinate with one another, so that one feels that one's potentials are fully developed with a sense of self-efficacy.

In the sunset stage of life, biological desires originating from the physical self slowly weaken. The need for spiritual cultivation may increase gradually. An individual tends to spend more and more time with spiritual work and thinking about issues related to life and death. In the last stage of life, the physical self may fade gradually, while the spiritual self becomes more and more apparent and dominates the outermost circle of life.

4. The usage of two types of knowledge

Considering the Chinese cultural tradition and the two types of knowledge described previously in terms of the body-mind-spirit model, social scientists can understand not only the meaning of modernization to non-western countries, but also the reason non-western countries have to develop indigenous psychologies. Let us take the case of Chinese culture as an example. During the progress of their history, Chinese people have developed a variety of sciences including Chinese medicine, architecture, flood control, astronomy, and a calendar system. However, Chinese sciences are essentially different from the modern science developed by the West.

After publishing a series of his works on *The History of Chinese Technology and Civilization* (Needham, 1954-1987), Needham (1970) indicated that Chinese people had developed their epistemology of knowledge on the basis of their concept of *dao* by using the primitive mode of things to promote welfare of human beings. It is indeed a science of organism, which is essentially different from the Western science of mechanism, which is constructed on the basis of logical reasoning with an abstraction from »matter« to »form«. According to the worldview model of equilibrium (Li, 1992), the Chinese science of organism was developed on the presumption of maintaining harmony with the nature, just like the concepts of disease and health or geomancy. As indicated in Table 1, this type of knowledge has been developed by Chinese people in their long history and can be used to solve many problems in people's lifeworlds, although it is essentially different from the scientific microworlds constructed by modern scientists.

As a consequence of close contact with Western culture since the end of 19th century, an important implication of modernization for Chinese society is the adoption of a Western system of education. Chinese adolescents now have to learn various kinds of scientific knowledge in schools. They may enter various social organizations after graduation and use their knowledge to do a variety of production work. The process can be understood in terms of the progress from Figure 1-2 to Figure 1-3. In other words, the body-mind-spirit model enables social scientists to explain how an individual acquires a sense of self-efficacy by practicing what was learned in school so as to control the external world effectively in a social institution.

With this claim, I do not mean that the Eastern cultural tradition will disappear as a consequence of modernization. In fact, cultural traditions are stored in language. When children learn their mother tongue, they learn their own cultural tradition at the same time. However, only a few cultural experts are able to construct a systematic knowledge or a microworld of knowledge about a particular aspect of their own culture. Most ordinary people have only common sense knowledge about their culture that enables them to use their cultural heritage to deal with various problems in different stages of life.

5. Conclusion

In conclusion, this discussion enables social scientists to understand why psychologists in non-western countries have to develop indigenous psychologies. From the perspective of social change, modernization is an inevitable trend for almost all countries of the world. Most universities and research institutes in non-western countries have adopted a western system of education, and professors mostly conduct research on the basis of western philosophy of science in attempt to construct various microworlds of science. It is no different for psychologists. When non-western psychologists do research on the mentality and behavior of local people, they may find that people are indeed a mixture of local and foreign cultures. In order for non-western social scientists to develop indigenous psychologies, it is necessary for them to understand the meaning of modernization, and to adopt western philosophy of science so as to be able to construct scientific microworlds about their own cultural traditions, and use these microworlds as a guide for conducting research in indigenous psychology in the local society.

Based on such a belief, I constructed the Face and Favor model of Chinese social behavior (Hwang, 1987), used it to analyze Chinese cultural traditions (Hwang, 1995), and then constructed a series of theoretical models on Confucian relationalism (Hwang, 2000, 2001). In attempt to integrate all my pervious works, I am now working on a new book entitled »Constructive Realism and Confucian Relationalism: Philosophical Reflection, Theoretical Construction and Empirical Research«. In that book, I will discuss how to use constructive realism as a philosophical foundation for developing indigenous psychology. I hope that my approach may lead to a new direction for this field.

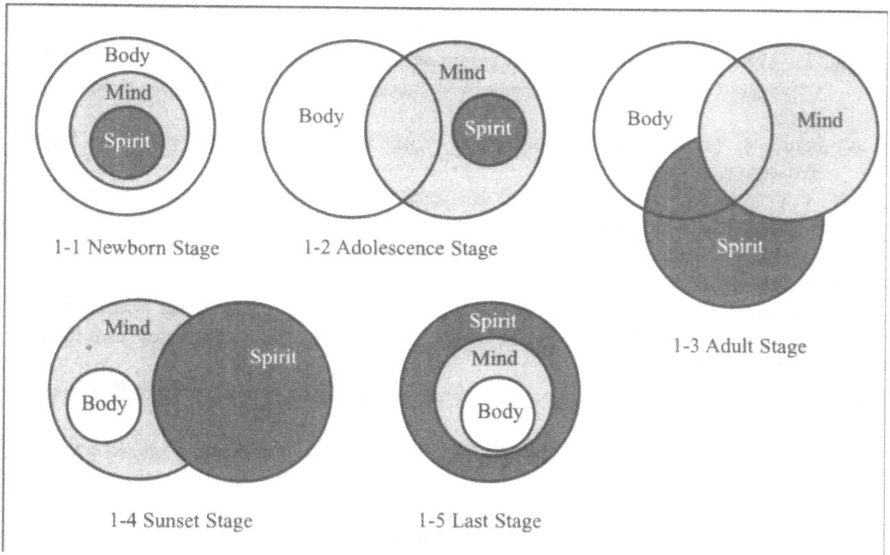

Figure 1: A Body-Mind-Spirit Model of Spiritual Care
(Adopted from Chen & Bhikku, 2003)

References

Brubaker. R. (1984). *The Limits of Rationality: An Essay on the Social and Moral Thought of Max Weber*. London: Geroge Allen & Unwin.

Chen, Chin-Yu and Bhikkhu, Hui-min (2003). *A Model of Spiritual Care for Hospice.* Paper presented in Conference on Functions of Religion in Psychological Rehabilitation after Disaster. Taipei: National Taiwan University.

Durkheim, E. (1912/1965). *The Elementary Forms of Religious Life.* New York: Free Press.

Heiderger, M. (1966). *Discourse on thinking.* New York: Harper and Row.

Hwang, K. K. (1987). Face and Favor: the Chinese power game. *American Journal of Sociology*, 92(4), 994-974.

Hwang, K. K.(1999). Filial piety and loyalty: The types of social identification in Confucianism. *Asian Journal of Social Psychology*,2,129-149.

Hwang, K. K. (1995). *Knowledge and action: A social-psychological interpretation of Chinese cultural tradition* (In Chinese). Taipei: Sin-Li.

Hwang, K.K. (2000). The discontinuity hypothesis of modernity and constructive realism: The philosophical basis of indigenous psychology (in Chinese). In *Hong Kong Journal of Social Sciences, 19*, 1-32.

Hwang, K.K. (2000). Chinese relationalism: Theoretical construction and methodological considerations. In *Journal for the Theory of Social Behavior, 30(2)*, 155-178.

Hwang, K.K. (2001). The deep structure of Confucianism: A social psychological approach. In *Asian Philosophy, 11(3)*, 179-204.

Kuhn, T. (1987). What are scientific revolutions? In L. Kruger, L. J. Datson, & M. Heidelberger (Eds.), *The Probabilistic Revolution* (pp.7-22). Cambridge, Mass.: MIT Press.

Levy-Bruhl, L. (1910/1966). *How Natives Think*, Trans. by L. A. Clare. New York: Washington Square Press.

Li, Y. Y. (1988). Ancestor worship and the psychological stability of family members in Taiwan. In K. Yoshimatsu and W. S. Tseng (Eds.), *Asian Family Mental Health* (pp.26-33). Tokyo: Psychiatric Research Institute of Tokyo.

Li, Y. Y. (1992). In search of equilibrium and harmony: On the basic value orientation of traditional Chinese peasants. In C. Nakane & C. Chiao (Eds.), *Home Bound: Studies in East Asian Society* (pp.127-148). Hong Kong: The Center for East Asian Cultural Studies.

Needham, J.(1954-1987). *Science and Civilization in China*, 6 vols. Cambridge: Cambridge University Press.

Needham, J.(1970/1978). *Clerks and Craftman in China and the West: Lectures and Addresses on the History of Science and Technology*. Cambridge: Cambridge University Press.

Shen, V. (1994). *Confucianism, Taoism and Constructive Realism*. Bruck: WUV-Universitäsverlag.

Taylor, E. B. (1871). *Primitive Culture*. Fifth edition, 1929 printing. London.

Wallner, F. (1994). *Constructive realism: aspects of new epistemological movement*. Wien: W. Braumuller.

Walsh, B. J., Middleton, J. R. (1984). *The Transforming Vision: Shaping a Christian World View*. Downers Grove, IL: Inter-Varsity Press.

Michael Weiss & Linda Roethlisberger

Medusa's Mirror strangified. Linking CR with PsyQ®

1. Strangification: Self-reflection as scientific method

Constructive Realism (CR) is a philosophy of science that does not want to dictate to scientists how to define or to practice science (see Wallner, 1992a: 19f). Its intention is to enable scientists to reflect on themselves and their work. In short: CR offers a service for selfreflection in science (see Pellert, in: Wallner, 1992a: 83f). What do we understand by ›service for self-reflection‹? CR wants to motivate scientists to leave their familiar terrain/their discipline in order to switch along with their familiar methodological constructs into new and unfamiliar contexts (see Wallner, 1992a: 95). By doing so, they will gain new knowledge about themselves and their ways of practising science. In metaphorical terms, a scientist travels into a strange country with a strange culture. There the scientist becomes concious of the familiar within the unfamiliar: he or she starts to reflect on himself/herself and his/her personal and scientific settings (see Greiner, in: Greiner and Wallner, 2003: 83f).

CR calls this method *strangification*: the method of strangification represents a method of selfreflection, in so far as it reveals new perspectives about the scientist and his/her (scientific) context (see Greiner, in: Greiner and Wallner, 2003: 59). As a consequence strangification implies therapeutical elements: Strangification does not want a scientist to run along linear lines with the aim to get to know parts of the world better (see Wallner, 2002: 210f). On the contrary, it enables him/her to take a halt to reflect on himself/herself as well as the taken way. The method of selfreflection as a service of CR consists in a wide range of selfimages and potentialities for acting (see Pellert, in: Wallner, 1992a: 83f). As a result he/she can tread new and unknown paths.

2. Selfreflection: knowledge as mediation

Knowledge produced by strangification has nothing to do with the discovery *of truth* or the so-called ›given world‹. ›Knowing‹ in CR means inventing realities (see Weiss, 2004: 20f). »Reality is understood as the domain which is the result of a processes of constructions.« (see Wallner, 1992a: 94) There is no immediate insight in the given world. The given world cannot be seen as it really *is* (see Wallner, 2002: 242f). In CR there does not exist a relation between the given world and reality (see Wallner, 1992a: 41). The only way to gain knowledge lies in strangification and strangification is mediation (see Wallner, 1992a: 95).

2.1 Medusa's mirror

As a result of this process of strangification, the new context now serves as a kind of mirror. It is open to scientists to reflect themselves and their realities. Metaphorically speaking, the new context can be compared to the Medusa's mirror: nobody was able to look at this Greek mythological monster's face without beeing transformed into stone and consequently die (see Le Van, 1996). It looked as if each attempt to kill her was going to fail until Perseus entered the stage. To his advantage he gained the support of Athene and her shield. Using it as a mirror, she caught the monster's reflection. Consequently Perseus had no need to look into Medusa's face directly; so it was easy for him to behead her.

Where can we find the connection between this legend and the method of strangification? Therefore it is important to refer to Medusa as a godess representing the world of nature (see Le Van, 1996). She symbolizes the earth with its elements and its everlasting rhythme of emerging and ceasing. Nobody is able to see the world as it is, nobody can know the given world. Only with the help of a mirror it can be harnessed. In relation to this aspect CR too claims that there does not exist an immediated insight into the given world (see Wallner, 2002: 242f). The myth stands for a switch of contexts as well: Athene's shield can be used as a mirror for mediation; due to the method of reflection it now becomes possible to work with the immediate. But it is not possible to compare the immediate with the mediated world as there is no way to look into Medusa's face directly.

Anyway, there is no need to see how far the immediate is identical with the mediated. Attempts of this kind would lead to permanent uncertainty (see Puntel, 1993: 142f). It is fare more important that reflection reveals something. The domain of selfknowledge clearly shows that there is no direct relation between immediacy and mediation: With my eyes I can see, but I am not able to look into my face. Only with the help of a mirror this becomes possible. Selfknowledge creates the need of a new context making strangification (of myself) possible. Once again the mirror-metapher symbolizes the following: selfknowledge means to reflect oneself on something else. Consequently there is a need for contexts to carry out selfreflection. But which contexts can be of use? Basically each context, like each mirror can be applied in order to see oneself in it.

For the defeat of Medusa, Perseus used a shield; he could also have used a pocketmirror for doing so. In other words: if you want to fly you can use a Concord or a Paraglider. The decisive moment is that *something* must be used – human beings are not able to fly without anything, they have to apply some tools. A tool like a Paraglider or Concord for flying should be called *medium*.

2.2 MEDIAL REFLECTION

A mirror is a *medium* making it possible to look myself into the face. In this way all sorts of contexts are *media* helping to realize selfreflection. Selfreflection without a *medium* is not possible – there is no immediate selfreflection (see Wallner, 2002: 242f). Selfreflection is a form of ›medial self-knowledge‹ (in German: ›Mediale Selbsterkenntnis‹) (Weiss, 2004: 46) therefore this process will be called MEDIAL REFLECTION in the following.

3. Mirrors of self-reflection

MEDIAL REFLECTION is a method, which enables anyone to reflect on himself/herself. Based on the method of strangification, the variety of contexts in which MEDIAL REFLECTION can be practised should now be pointed out.

The question ›What does this mean to me?‹ can be asked about anything imaginable and is accompanied by the expectation of a useful answer. But you need not assume that the answer to such a question gives information about the nature of the thing, the situation or the statement. What it does is to provide information about the person who answers (see Wittgenstein, 1996: 66f). The answer of the question ›What does the Medusa-myth mean to me?‹ says less about the myth itself, but more about my interpretation and attitudes towards it. In short: the answer to that question provides knowledge about me and my beliefs (see Wallner, 1992a: 95). Another example should illustrate this issue: ›What does spirituality mean to me?‹: My answer to that question makes my attitudes towards this topic obvious. Now we assume that somebody let us call him ›X‹, answers this question with: ›To me, spirituality means: life after death‹. This would mean that ›X‹ believes in a life after death. X's belief in life after death got transparent through the question about spirituality. ›X‹ could also ask ›What does money mean to me?‹; and answer: ›Money means something negative to me‹. This statement does not give any information about money as an object of exchange. It far more reveals X's attitudes/believes towards money. (It will probably not be easy for X to get a lot of money due to the fact that he places little value on it.)

3.1 ›Therapeutical‹ implications on MEDIAL REFLECTION

Up to now this exposition should have shown that really everything, even the smallest sandcorn, can be used to reflect oneself on it (see Wallner, 1992a: 95). In this way, an endless variety of contexts and media for selfreflection arises. The result is a growing realization of believes. What happens, if I do not like some of my beliefs at all? What, if some of my beliefs are more obstructive than constructive?

Before answering, it has to be said that personal beliefs, attitudes and settings can be called ›structurings of phenomena‹ (in German: ›Strukturierungen von Phänomenen‹) (Wallner, 2002: 31). This means, phenomena are edited in a specific way. The process of editing can be called *formulating beliefs*. Let us go back to the assumption of money as something negative: it may be possible that ›X‹ wants to gain prosperity. But his attitude concerning money does not allow him to get wealthy. Now there are two possibilities: either ›X‹ disclaims prosperity or he changes his attitude. A change in attitude would mean that ›X‹ restructures one of his beliefs. Successful restructuring means that a personal, though problematic attitude has been changed by MEDIAL REFLECTION. ›X‹ will now answer the question ›What does money mean to me?‹ differently. In this way the method of MEDIAL REFLECTION and therefore the method of strangification can be defined as ›therapeutical‹ methods: they supply the potentionalities for personal transformation and individual development.

4. PsyQ®: a possible context for MEDIAL REFLECTION

The so-called PsyQ® method was developed by Linda Roethlisberger, the head of TRILOGOS – a Swiss institute dealing with developement of personality and consciousness training (see www.trilogos.ch or: Roethlisberger, 1999, 2000; Gissrau, 2002: 48f). One of the main issues of this specific training is individual development, by selfreflection. With the help of Roethlisberger's method we will now examine the contexts that are used to perform selfreflexion in accordance to MEDIAL REFLECTION. The basic elements of the PsyQ® are formed by following three different contexts:

PsyQ® =
IQ | Intelligence quotient (›What do I think?‹)
EQ | Emotional quotient (›What do I feel?‹)
SQ | Spiritual quotient (›What do I believe?‹)
(see Roethlisberger, 2000: 65f)

In this model self-reflection is performed within the mirrors of personal thinking, feeling and believing. What is more, selfreflection is performed with a technique called ›visualisation‹[1] based on the method of katathym imaginative psychother-

1 The model of TRILOGIC MEDIALITY, PsyQ® is a method of, distinguishes ›Visualisation‹, ›Contemplation‹ and ›Meditation‹: (1) Visualisation is a technique of mind to imagine and make it conscious for a certain period of time. This technique is a form of mental concentration, like autogenic training and based on the method of katathym imaginative psychotherapy. (2) Contemplation means to become (actively) immersed in an idea or an imagined picture. (3) Meditation is a technique of mental mind con-

apy: During visualisation symbols are produced, which are once again seen and used as mirrors for selfreflection[2] (see Roethlisberger, 1999: 149). The aim of visualisation, one method within the broader context of medial mentaltraining (= PsyQ®training), is conscious dreaming (see Roethlisberger, 1999: 140f). This conscious dreaming with its imagined, intuitively, and inspiratively percepted symbols is followed by reflection of the symbols' meaning. The major question is ›What do these symbols mean to me?‹

Now the method of PsyQ®training extends this question to one of the three domains named above. For example: ›What does this symbol mean to me concerning my emotions?‹ or ›Which feelings do come up when I reflect this symbol?‹ – the emotional meaning attributet to a symbol being asked. The result should be a connection to one's everday life. In this way PsyQ®training implies MEDIAL REFLECTION in a differentiated form. Furthermore it also implies the method of strangification, because various contexts are used as media of reflection.

5. PsyQ® as a method of selfreflection for scientists

Which potentials does the PsyQ®training provide for scientists and their scientific work? One presents the following: when a scientist asks ›What does science mean to me?‹, the answer can now be strangified within the three contexts of PsyQ® (IQ + EQ + SQ) (see Roethlisberger, 2000: 65f). The result is a broad horizon, especially due to reflection within the domains of EQ and SQ. This newly gained knowledge influences a scientist in the following ways. On the one hand he/she is able to integrate his/her believes and attitudes more and more into his/her scientific work like an artist into his/her art. And on the other hand the scientist can reflect his/her work within the mirror of his/her community[3].
Concluding, the advantages for science are the following:

---

trol, which often produces a feeling of deep silence and inner peace (see www.trilogos.ch)

2 The PsyQ® planes: IQ, EQ and SQ are the basic-planes of Medial Mentaltraining. In addition there are six planes, which can be differentiated within IQ, EQ and SQ plane. These are: (a) within the mental domain: the psychological, para-psychological and transpersonal (depth psychology) plane; (b) within the material domain: health, relations and profession. For this article the application of the basic-planes of PsyQ® seems to fulfil the needs of the investigation described here. For further readings: Roethlisberger (1999, 2000), www.trilogos.ch

3 In the mirror of other people human's sympathy and honestility are supported: Real change means transformation of collective representations. Percepting, knowing, thinking, feeling, being guided are no longer contradictions, but are going to be mutually conditional.

1. The new produced knowledge gains authenticity, and as a consequence;
2. responsibility of the individual to the community, responsibility of the scientist to science, increases.

Reference

Gissrau, Barbara (2002). *Selbstbilder – Ichbilder. TRILOGOS®; Persönlichkeits- und Bewusstseinsschulung*. Küsnacht/Zürich: TRILOGOS Verlag.

Greiner, Kurt and Wallner, Fritz (Eds.).(2003). *Konstruktion und Erziehung*. Hamburg: Kovac.

Le Van, Alicia (1996). Gorgon Medusa. In www.perseus.tufts.edu/classes/women. html

Pellert, Ada in: Wallner, Fritz (1992a). *Acht Vorlesungen über den Konstruktiven Realismus*. Wien: WUV.

Puntel, Lorenz Bruno (1978). *Wahrheitstheorien in der neueren Philosophie. Eine kritisch-systematische Darstellung*. Darmstadt: Wissenschaftliche Buchgesellschaft.

Roberts, Jane (1988). *Individuum und Massenschicksal. Der Mensch als Urheber allen Umweltgeschehens*. Genf: Ariston.

Roethlisberger, Linda (1999). *Der sinnliche Draht zur geistigen Welt. Ein Lehrbuch zur Entfaltung der medialen Anlagen und der eigenen Persönlichkeit* (3. edition). Freiburg im Breisgau: Bauer.

Roethliserger, Linda (Eds.).(2000). *Der Flug des Quantenschmetterlings*. Petersbert: Via Nova.

Slunecko, Thomas (1997). *The Movement of Constructive Realism*. Wien: Braumüller.

Wallner, Friedrich, & Agnese, Barbara (Eds.).(1997). *Von der Einheit des Wissens zur Vielfalt der Wissensformen: Erkenntnis in der Philosophie, Wissenschaft und Kunst*. Wien: Braumüller.

Wallner, Fritz G. (2002). Die *Verwandlung der Wissenschaft. Vorlesungen zur Jahrtausendwende* (ed. by Martin J. Jandl). Hamburg: Kovac.

Wallner, Fritz (1992a). *Acht Vorlesungen über den Konstruktiven Realismus*. Wien: WUV.

Watzlawick, Paul (2002). *Die erfundene Wirklichkeit. Wie wissen wir, was wir zu wissen glauben? Beiträge zum Konstruktivismus* (15. edition). München: Piper.

Weiss, Michael (2004). *Kann Spiritualität wissenschaftlich sein? Selbst-Erkenntnis als Schnittstelle von Konstruktivem Realismus und TRILOGISCHER MEDIALITÄT*. Hamburg: Kovač.

Wittgenstein, Ludwig (1996). *Ein Reader*. Frankfurt a.M.: Suhrkamp.

Martin J. Jandl

»*Psychology is a social Science.*« Popper and the Subject Matter in Psychology

I will start with some considerations pertaining to the definition of the psychological subject matter and some historical explanations. Then I will show that Popper takes part of the subjectivistic (or mentalistic) definition of the psychological subject matter, but the discrimination of ›world 2‹ and ›world 3‹ prevents him from the individualistic fallacy. Anchoring ›world 2‹ in ›world 3‹ is the opposite to the individualistic fallacy that anchors ›world 3‹ in ›world 2‹. Thus, Popper's definition of the psychological subject matter avoids a frequent mistake, but it does not show psychology the way out of a blind alley. In the following step I will take up Popper's notion of the ›situational logic‹ and I will argue that this notion would be of great advantage to psychology. My argument will be constructivistic, referring to the ideas of Klaus Holzkamp, a German psychologist and philosopher of science. Finally, I will argue that an institutionalized division of basic and applied research in psychology may solve the tension between a subjectivistic definition of the psychological subject matter and an adequate definition of the psychological subject matter that avoids the subjectivistic reduction and the individualistic fallacy.

1. The lack of reflection of the psychological subject matter and its consequences

Without any doubt, psychology is a science of the human individual. The most frequent definition of the psychological subject matter reads that psychology focuses on human behaviour, reasoning and emotion. Psychological research focuses the individual. As far as I see mainstream-psychology does not reflect this definiton. Thus it is not the lack of the definition of the subject matter in psychology that is problematic – even if we bear in mind that the cited definition is very broad and thus unspecified. It is the lack of an adequate reflection of this definition that causes problems, that – to speak more pointed – causes mistakes in psychological theories. The first mistake is the ›subjectivistic reduction‹ of the psychological subject matter, and the second mistake is an ›individualistic fallacy‹.

I define subjectivistic reduction of the psychological subject matter if psychological research is concerned only with the so called ›subjective phenomena‹ (in German: ›das Subjektive‹). The individualistic fallacy is in issue if resulting from this apriori definition of the subject matter it is alleged that subjective phenomena constitute intersubjective phenomena. The individualistic fallacy is not in issue if a science focuses on the individual. It would be paradoxical to claim that a science of the individual should not focus on the individual. The individualistic fallacy will emerge if the relation of individuality to trans-individuality is concepted from the point of individuality, if trans-individual constituents of individuality are not counted and if the relation of the universal to the particular is not reflected. The first component of the individualistic fallacy in psychology is the claim that society is just the sum of individuals. The negation of the cultural impregnation of all psychic phenomena is the second component of the individualistic fallacy in psychology. And the third component results from these both components.

As a striking feature of the individualistic fallacy in psychology the lack of reflection of the subject matter is substituted by a recourse to biological models. It is alleged that experimental results of psychological research is guilty for all individuals because all individuals have the same (or nearly the same) biological constitution (see, for example, Hejl 2001; Barkow 2001; Barkow, Cosmides & Tooby 1992). This argumentation strategy is supported by the predominating statistical methods in psychology.

2. Historical notes on the psychological subject matter

The present situation in psychology has historical roots. First I will dwell on the emergence of the subjectivistic definition of the psychological subject matter and second I will discuss a special aspect of the emergence of the individualistic fallacy in psychology.

For becoming institutionalized as an autonomous science psychology had to become emancipated from philosophy. In this situation dating back to the 19th century it was necessary to define the subject matter not only in a narrow sense, but also in a way that made empirical research feasible. The idea of empirical research of subjective phenomena traces back to the developments in philosophy in the 16th century. I add, but I won't show proof that the turn in philosophy at this time traces back to the change in society and economy since the 14th century (for example the raise of the cities and the new importance of money as a medium of exchange).

The French and English philosophy in enlightment give up the relation of the Greek and medival notion of the soul to a transcendent entity and conceptualized psychic processes in scientific and materialistic models. Thus in the 17th and 18th century a change from the notion of soul to the notion of ›*psyche*‹ takes place (see Geulen 1991, p.532). Hobbes concepts the processes of the soul (perhaps better: mind) as motions of material particles that is triggered by influence of objects in the world on sense organs. These motions transmit as a chain through the body and finally they constitute perception, imagination and memory. In addition to that Hobbes postulates desire and aversion causing usefulness or harmfulness of actions. Locke and Hume continued these thoughts, and the ›invention‹ of an autonomous ›interior‹ is due to Descartes who called it the ›res cogitans‹ (the view that Descartes ›invented‹ the interior is due to Rorty 1997). The subject with its inborn ideas is sharply demarcated from the body, from society and from life-world and it is the basis of guilty knowledge. In Descartes' philosophy the subject is absolut. Enlightment destructs the metaphysical and ontological base of the ancient reign and lead back to the human individual, to human reason (›Vernunftgebrauch‹).

At the end of the 18th century a new motive emerges in the European intellectual history. Individuals come to know that the new-created society unfolds economic-technical and political-social dynamics that catapult them out of the grown and familiar social structures. Thus the individual becomes isolated, and this is a central motive for romanticism. That the subject loses his status as the base of knowledge and becomes itself the object of scientific research is the crucial turning away from the philosophy of enlightment in this time. The raising psychology continues on the one hand the prerequesits of enlightment philosophy (especially the idea of the interior) and is on the other hand ahead in investigating the isolated individual as its object. Thus psychology focuses on the individual, but psychology also takes apart (i.e. analyses) the individual. The more psychology strives for its independence of philosophy, the more psychology focuses on the interior and the analysis of the subject until subjectivity rests as the empirically investigable subject matter.

Enlightment philosophy and Romantic Movement are thus very important for the rise of the psychological subject matter. But a crucial change takes place at the end of the 19th century, the change from romantic to the modernistic conception of the mind – as Kenneth Gergen names it (see Gergen 1990, pp.192). While enlightment made up the idea of the interior but hold up the idea of reason, in romanticism the idea emerges that reason is founded by a deep, mysterious and irrational interior. With the romantic notions fantasy, creativity, passion, genius, moral, freedom of thoughts and mystical longing the interior becomes such a powerful idea like never before. What is deep in the individual is most precious. At the end of the 19th century this powerful idea is replaced by a modernistic principle – the principle of lawful fundaments. The import of the notions of natural sciences to social sciences should guarantee an imposing progress also for social sciences.

Following Gergen (1990, pp.193) this turn shapes the modernistic view of the individual. First, individuals are the result of enviromental influence. Second, the individualistic principle leads to the postulation of personality dispositions. By socialisation the individual should acquire a stable character and traits that enable the individual to be autonomous in regard to its environment. The ›correct‹ socialised individual is the centre of its actions. Third, human actions should be reliable, accessible for scientific research and predictible. Thus, the deep self of the romantic individual is transfered upward; the self is transfered from the deep to just under the surface of the individual.

Sure, the individualistic fallacy is due to this development in intellectual history and is not only found in psychology. The reason for this fallacy in psychology is, as far as I see, that during the 1950ies psychology changed from the ›experimental phase‹ to the ›neo-experimental phase‹ (see Jüttemann 1992, p.32). Since about 1950 psychological experiments have been designed in a way that it is possible to calculate the results statistically. Connected with this statistical orientation is the turn from the trained test person (›geschulte Versuchsperson‹) to the naive test person (›naive Versuchsperson‹) (see Holzkamp 1972b, p.46). The subjects of the ›Würzburger Schule‹ (school of Würzburg) were the assistents of Karl Bühler, the head of this elder cognitive psychological school. But nowadays the subjects are not trained – usually they are not told what the experiment is about. Psychologists want to observe ›pure‹ behaviour; they don't want to observe what persons have already learned – that's the main critic of the introspective procedure used by Bühler. The generalization of the data observed in experiments with untrained subjects is ensured by the statistical handling of the data. The current critics of mainstream-psychology deal with this statistical orientation. Haslam & McGarty (2001) for example argue that the correct handling of data is much more important than the brilliance of the experimental setting. As a consequence psychological results are statistically impeccable, but not very informative. Jüttemann (1992, p.97) points out that in mainstream-psychology ›the universal‹ (›das Allgemeine‹) is identified by plain flattening of ›the indiviual‹ in form of sampling and mean calculation. By these means the ›average person‹ emerges from whom is alleged that she represents the general human being and therefore features the ›universal psyche‹.

Thus the development of the statistical methods enforces the individualistic fallacy in psychology. The statistical procedures should find out the relation the data depend on – but first data are independent. It is alleged that individual behaviour is independent of intersubjectivity like data before calculation.

Reading Popper's works makes obvious that he inclines to the subjectivistic definition of the psychological subject matter, but he avoids the individualistic fallacy. But there is a tension in Popper's philosophy concerning this problem that is due to the problem of the subject matter in psychology itself. It is the problem that individual processes researched by psychology are constitued by intersubjectivity that is not yet part of psychological thinking.

3. Popper's subjectivistic definition of psychology and the avoidance of the individualistic fallacy in Popper's philosophy

In *Logic of Scientific Discovery* a scope for psychology can be found. According to Popper psychology is appropriate to investigate the subjective processes. For the psychologistic theory of knowledge these subjective processes constitute knowledge, but Popper refutes this view. Popper argues his avoidance of psychologism in theory of knowlegde with the comment that psychology as an empirical science can't give an account of knowledge. If an empirical science explains the foundations of knowledge, it will commit a circle vitious; because aposteriori results can't focus on its apriori (see Popper 1984, p.18)

I don't want to dwell on the problematic of psychologism in theory of knowledge, but I want to emphasize Popper's definition of the subject matter in psychology, that is: Psychology has to investigate empirically mere subjective phenomena. This definition is without any doubt conventional. This view is recipated strongly by mainstream-psychology. But Popper avoids the individualistic fallacy that is often found in mainstream-psychology, because Popper does not view the subjective processes as constitutive for intersubjective phenomena like language. This will become evident if we have a short look to the doctrine of the three worlds.

Popper's three worlds are populated by ›real‹ or ›actual‹ entities (in German: ›wirkliche Wesenheiten‹). Usually Popper avoids the questions »What is ...?« or »What do you understand as ...?« because of two reasons. First, these questions push away the discussion of the problems in favour of disputes of words (›Wortstreitigkeit‹) (see Popper & Eccles 1991, p.28) – a hint against analytic philosophy. Second, questions in the form of »What is ...?« are often misunderstood as the philosophical strive for hidden or metaphysical entities. »What is the I?« is counted as a question for a substance. But Popper refutes this essentialism (see Popper & Eccles 1991, p.134). In this point Popper's argumentation meets Wittgenstein's philosophy. (For a discussion of the relation Wittgenstein/Popper see e.g. Wallner 1992).

Dealing with reality makes it even for Popper necessary to ask »What is real?«. Popper's answer is very simple. He takes up the word of Kurt Lewin and states: What has an effect that is real (»Wirklich ist, was wirkt.«). Thus all things of the world we handle with are real. From these things the principle of effect is derived and transmitted to things that are not observable. Atoms are real only if their effects are not put in questions by the majority (see Popper & Eccles 1991, p.28).

According to this definition of reality Popper makes up three worlds. ›World 1‹ is the world of physical objects. ›World 2‹ is the world of subjective phenomena that are perceptions (or animal consciousness), human self-consciousness, and knowledge of death. ›World 3‹ contains products of the human mind, that are language, theories and myths about us and about the death, and the works of art (see Popper & Eccles 1991, p.37). ›World 2‹ is investigated by psychology. It is interesting to note that language is a part of world 3 and not object of psychology. This is in contrast to the fact that since the works of Noam Chomsky language is an object for psychology, especially for cognitive psychology. I suppose that Popper follows the verdict of Wilhelm Wundt who claimed that higher mental processes are not object of experimental psychological research, but object of the so called ›Völkerpsychologie‹ (that's Wundt's notion for ›social psychology‹ – he disliked the combination of ›social‹ that derives from Latin with ›psychology‹ that derives from Greek).

Popper postulates interactions between these worlds. I am not interested in the interaction between world 1 and world 2 that is discussed in philosophy and psychology very detailed – a discussion that blurs the problem of subject matter in psychology. I am interested in the interaction of world 2 and world 3 that counteracts the individualistic fallacy and opens new ways of defining the psychological subject matter.

Popper insists on the autonomy of world 3 in respect to world 2, especially the autonomy of language in respect to world 2. Behaviouristic and physicalistic philosophers or psychologists restrain language to the signal and expression functions, but according to Popper the characteristic features of human language are the propositional and argumentative functions. A reduction of language to verbal behaviour or communication is »disastrous« (see Popper & Eccles 1991, p.87).

Popper states that world 3 is a product of human reason or behaviour (see Popper & Eccles 1991, p.65). If these products are once invented, then they will be autonomous. Popper sets an example. A numerative system is invented or constructed by men, it is not discovered. But the difference between even and uneven numbers is a discovery. ›2+2=4‹ is according to Popper not a convention, but an invariant truth that is discovered. I subscribe Popper's view that there is something like world 3 that is a construction and autonomous, but I don't believe that Popper's inventions in world 3 cease being constructions. At the moment of constructing the constructors can't oversee and forecast all consequences (and perhaps they never will be able to do so), but a new insight in the construction does not show proof that the constructor discovered an invariable truth – he just unfolds the potentials of his constructions, he does not leave the field of construction.

The fundamental learning process in world 3 is the learning of language, and according to Popper this process is not natural, but cultural and social (see Popper & Eccles 1991, p.72). The multitude of languages proofs that they are »work of man« although the competence of speaking is biologically determined (Popper & Eccles 1991, p.76). Learning a language means for personality of children to become a part of world 3 because language enlarges not only the conscious perception of the material environment of the children, but consciousness itself (ibid.). Thus Popper states: »Ein vollkommenes menschliches Wesen zu werden beruht auf einem Reifeprozeß, in dem der Spracherwerb eine außerordentliche Rolle spielt. Man lernt nicht nur wahrnehmen und seine Wahrnehmungen interpretieren, sondern auch eine Person, ein Ich sein. Ich halte die Ansicht, daß uns unsere Wahrnehmungen gegeben sind, für falsch: Sie werden von uns gemacht, sie sind das Ergebnis aktiver Tätigkeit. Ich halte es ebenfalls für einen Irrtum, wenn man nicht sieht, daß das berühmte Descartessche Argument ›ich denke, also bin ich‹ Sprache voraussetzt sowie die Fähigkeit, das Pronomen zu gebrauchen [...].« (Popper & Eccles 1991, pp.76f)

According to Popper the ›I‹ is anchored in world 3 (see Popper & Eccles 1991, p.184). Language enables the individual not only to be a subject that is centre of the own actions, but also to be an object of reflexive reasoning. This is ensured by the social character of language. Conscious human beings emerge from world 3 that is made by men.

Thus it is the conception of world 3 that puts a stop to the individualistic fallacy notwithstanding the subjectivistic definition of the psychological subject matter in Popper's philosophy. But as far as I see, mainstream-psychology didn't recept the doctrine of three worlds. In spite of the fact that there are many points in issue with this doctrine (for example is it the ›I‹ or the ›Me‹ that is socially born?), I will make the next step in my argumentation. Popper's avoidance of the individualistic fallacy is not helpful for psychology because of his view that psychology has to investigate world 2 by falsification of empirical hypotheses.

4. Psychology as a social science and situational logic – Popper's reduction of psychology

In *Logic of Social Sciences* Popper classifies psychology as social sience that has the individual subjectivity as its subject matter, but psychology can't focus the constitutives of its subject matter methodologically. But Popper unfolds a sociological methodology to deal with these constitutives. Thus the tension that forms the subject matter of psychology and that is located between subjectivity and intersubjectivity (or between world 2 and world 3) is to be found within Popper's philosophy of social sciences. However, Popper's definition of the psychological subject matter overcomes what Campbell (1994, p.141) calls the ›Comptean division‹. In his hierachical developmental division of the sciences, August Compte provided no room for psychology, dividing its contents between biology and sociology that is between world 1 and world 3. Popper emphasizes not only the importance of world 2, but unfortunately he reduces psychology to an empirical research project of world 2.

Popper's 22nd thesis of *Logic of Social Sciences* reads: »Die Psychologie ist eine Sozialwissenschaft, da unser Denken und Handeln weitgehend von sozialen Verhältnissen abhängt. [Psychology is a social science because our reasoning and acting depend largely on social circumstances.]« (Popper 1993, p.119). Popper argues that categories as imitation, language, and family are obviously social categories and that the psychology of learning and reasoning, but also psychoanalysis depend on one or more of these categories. Psychology refers to social notions and Popper follows that it is impossible to explain society completely psychologically and that it is impossible to reduce society to psychology (Popper 1993, p.119). Thus psychology is out of the question of being the fundamental science of social sciences.

For my argumentation it is important to underline Popper's view that the subject of psychology is a result of social processes. This view does not only avoid the individualistic fallacy, but it relativizes also the subjectivistic reduction of the psychological subject matter. That becomes obvious in the sentence that I judge as pioneering: »Das, was wir prinzipiell nicht psychologisch erklären können, und das, was wir in jeder psychologischen Erklärung voraussetzen müssen, das ist die soziale Umwelt des Menschen. [What is in princip not psychologically explainable and what we have to presume in every psychological explanation is the social environment of men.«] (Popper 1993, p.119)

In the 23rd thesis Popper states that on the one hand sociology is autonomous in respect to psychology, but on the other hand psychology is not autonomous in respect to sociology. The reason for this dependency lies in the fact that in sociology there is an approriate method to explain the social environment, the ›situational logic‹. To quote Popper: »The objective understanding consists in the insight that an action was appropriate to a situation. In other words, the situation is analysed to a point that shows that psychic moments like wishes, motives, memory, and associations are transformed to situational moments.« (Popper 1993, p.120; translated by M.J.) Thus the method of situational logic is individual, but not psychological because psychic moments are eliminated and replaced by situational moments (see Popper 1993, p.121). It will hardly be necessary to note that for Popper there is no pure description of a situation; there are only explanations that can be true or wrong (see Popper 1993, p.119).

Situational logic is individual and seizes the constitutives of subjectivity – this is the gist of Popper's notion of situational logic. In my next step of argumentation I will show that this method must become part of psychology to avoid its subjectivistic reduction.

5. Discourse of nomological causation and discourse of subjective foundation

It is due to the German psychologist Klaus Holzkamp to point out that in all psychological experiments the dialogue between psychologist and test person (›Versuchsperson‹) is restricted by reasons of social role-taking (see Holzkamp 1972a, p.41). In a psychological experiment not nature is observed, but the social interaction between psychologist and test person (see Holzkamp 1972a, p.39) Thus psychological experiments do not discover natural laws, but a technical knowledge of disposal (›Verfügungswissen‹) of men who act in self-determination (see Janich 1996, p.285).

To make a clear difference between the experiment in natural sciences and in psychology Holzkamp (1995) differentiates between the ›discourse of nomological causation‹ and the ›discourse of subjective foundation‹ (in German ›nomologischer Bedingtheitsdiskurs‹ and ›subjektiver Begründungsdiskurs). The discourse of nomological causation investigates causal relations that are given if and only if two independent entities interact when they are put in reciprocal action. The prerequesite of the investigation of causal relations is the independency of the ›if-component‹ and the ›then-component‹ in the hypothesis. In contrary, the discourse of subjective foundation is based on subjective reasons for actions (›subjektive Handlungsbegründung‹). That means individuals act according to subjective reasons and there are no compelling causal conditions for actions. A stone can't choose falling down to earth or not, individuals can choose what they will do or how they will act. Reasons of actions are related to the premises of actions not contingentically (or accidentally), but they are related by discoursive evidence (›diskursive Schlüssigkeit‹).

Psychological theories are alleged to be empirically falsifyable or verifyable, and it is furthermore alleged that the ›if-component‹ and the ›then-component‹ in psychological hypothesis are independent. But according to Holzkamp psychological theories are »implicite and by logical reasons self-evident structures«. Holzkamp shows proof for this claim by two criteria. I want to list only one of them, and that is the insertion of the word ›reasonably‹ into a proposition. If the insertion ›reasonably‹ is logic stringent in the proposition that formulates a hypothesis, then ›if-‹ and ›then-component‹ are not independent and then there is an implicative relation of the both components (see Holzkamp 1994, p.34)

Let me set an example. Have a look to the following sentence: »If it is cold outside, then you will put on warm clothes.« This sentence with the insert ›reasonably‹ makes sense, it reads: »If it is cold outside, then you will reasonably put on warm clothes.« Thus this sentence is a part of the discourse of subjective foundation. Now have a look to this sentence: »If it is cold outside, you will catch a chill.« This sentence with the insert reads: »If it is cold outside, you will reasonably catch a chill.« In this case the insert makes the sentence nonsensical. Thus this sentence is part of the discourse of nomological causation.

Theories of social psychology like consistence theory, decision theory, attitude theory, theories concerning processes of group interaction, theories about social perception and cognition are usually understood as nomological ›if-then-propositions‹ (›Wenn-dann-Aussagen‹) that are empirically falsifyable. But Holzkamp emphasizes that these theories are foundational theories (›Begründungstheorien‹) with ›relation of application‹ (›Anwendungsbezug‹) to the experimental findings, i.e. these theories imply relations of reasonable foundation (and not causal relation as in the nomological discourse) between the ›if-‹ and the ›then-component‹. Holzkamp uses the notion ›typical foundational pattern‹ (›typisches Begründungsmuster‹ or, in short, ›BGM‹) and he states pertaining to the psychological experiment that the ›if-component‹ is not an empirical antecedens condition for behaviour that is caused by it, but it is a premise for the subjective foundation of action for test persons in the experimental situation. Furthermore, the ›then-component‹ is not caused by the antecedens conditions, but the ›then-component‹ is an action that realises the intentions of test persons – an action that is a reasonable consequence out of the premises. Thus the variables in between the ›if-component‹ and the ›then-component‹ are not hidden physiological or subjective transmission instances, but implicite or explicite intentions of test persons by that they determine what is a reasonable action in respect to the constellation of premises in the experimental setting (see Holzkamp 1995, p.35).

6. A new view of basic and applied research in psychology

I see the contradiction between Popper and Holzkamp in the point that Popper writes experimental investigations of world 2 out for psychology and states that the situational logic is part of sociology, while Holzkamp does not omit social environment of the psychological subject matter. Popper tends to a subjectivistic reduction of psychology because obviously world 2 resembles Descartes' ›res cogitans‹ – notwithstanding Popper rejects the sensualistic philosophy of knowledge. It is due to Descartes to divide consciousness from the body, the objects in the world and lifeworld. Thus Popper's definition of the psychological subject matter is based on the birth of consciousness in modern philosophy and on the idea of an autonomous interior. That Popper overcomes the idea of the absolute subject with his notion of world 3 has no importance for psychology, because world 3 is not the scope of psychological investigations. Even the situational logic that would avoid subjectivistic reduction in psychology is reserved for sociology. Thus it is not astonishing that the reception of Popper's philosophy of science in mainstream-psychology does not help psychology out of the individualistic fallacy.

The common point of Holzkamp's notion of the typical foundational matter and Popper's notion of situational logic is the claim that individuals act and that the reality of laboratory gives the reasons for this acting. A situational analysis in the sense of Popper would show proof that Holzkamp's idea is a worthful constructivistic idea, including that we have to take into account the social prescripted role-taking and as a result the fact that test persons act reasonably in respect to what they find as premises for their actions. Granted this point we have to make a further step and give a new defintion of basic research and applied research in psychology – an idea that is due to the German psychologist Jüttemann (1992). According to Holzkamp's notion of the typical foundation patterns that shows that test persons don't discard the interior or the world 2, but that test persons acts according to reasons, the applied research is the current mainstream-psychology. It is the aim of the applied research to develop useful tools for understanding psychic phenomena and for helping individuals to cope with their problems.

What is to be new founded is the psychological basic research. According to Jüttemann (1992, p.111) basic research is not practice centred, but it aims at a ›higher‹ interest of knowledge (›Erkenntnisinteresse‹) that is for its own sake. (But Jüttemann also points out that this being for its own sake is not absolute, the ›search of the truth‹ is embedded in lifewords.) Literally quoted: »Grundlagenforschung hingegen arbeitet nicht praxiszentriert, sondern sie dient dazu, eine allgemeines, nicht unmittelbar anwendungsbezogenes und deshalb einer ›höheren‹ Wertorientierung verpflichtetes Erkenntnisinteresse zu befriedigen. Insofern stellt das grundlagenwissenschaftliche Erkenntnisinteresse eine Art Selbstzweck dar. Dennoch ist dieser Selbstzweckcharakter nicht verabsolutierbar, weil auch die Suche nach der ›reinen‹ Wahrheit nur aus einem grundlegenden Lebens- oder Weltinteresse oder einem generellen gesellschaftlichen Fortschrittsinteresse heraus verständlich wird. [...] Das bedeutet zugleich, daß das, was im Rahmen einer Grundlagenwissenschaft zum Gegenstand der Forschung erhoben werden kann, nicht einfach ›gegeben‹ ist, sondern bereits eine darauf ausgerichtete Motivation voraussetzt.« (Jüttemann 1992, p.111)

Thus I suggest that psychological basic research should deal about the subject matter. Psychology should not pragmatically put up an old philosophical idea – the idea of the interior – and should not believe that empirically generated data relieve from reflection. In this way psychology depends strongly on philosophical ideas, but psychology does not reflect this fact, or better: psychology denies its roots. I hope not to be misunderstood. I don't claim that psychology should become a part of philosophy, and I don't claim that psychology should give up its empirical research. But empirical research is part of psychological applied research, and I claim that psychology should reflect its subject matter as basic research. Every reflection in this way is philosophical – if a physicist reflects about his science, he does not think physically, but philosophically. In my view it is necessary that the reflection of the subject matter has to become a part of psychology. I don't believe that this is necessary for other sciences, but in psychology it is necessary. Psychological basic research should inspire psychological applied research, and this will be feasible only if the basic researchers are psychologists – they know the problems, but also the methods of psychology.

According to my view psychological basic research is interdisciplinary because different sciences contribute to the investigation of the ›psyche‹. In short, there should be philosophy, historical psychology, psychohistory, history of psychology, but also scopes of sociology, and social history parts of the psychological basic research. The disciplines that I propose as parts of psychological basic research just subsist, but they are not considered in mainstream-psychology. Historical psychology for example that is concerned with the historical development of the psyche is a wallflower in mainstream-psychology.

This new defintion of basic and applied research in psychology is due to two ideas. First, it seems to be possible to bridge the gap between psychological theory and practice if the theorists reflect more on their subject matter – then they will become aware of the artificial components of psychological theories what will lead to ›ecological validity‹ (the claim of Ulric Neisser since about 20 years, for example see Neisser 1981). Second, this new definition is due to the claim of Constructive Realism to counteract instrumentalism in science. An instrumentalistic reduced psychology would be concerned only with ways of ›correcting‹ problems in the ›individual sector‹. In other words, an instrumentalistic reduced psychology is a social technique. This is a strong tendency in psychology (remember Behaviourism and its broad acceptance by the majority of psychologists in the 1960ies and 1970ies), but the potentials of psychology to be a science beyond social techniques, to be a science that deepens our knowledge of the ›conditio humana‹ should not perish.

The consequences of this new view of psychology are, following the words of Kvale (1992a, p.53): »This would involve facing the rootedness of human existence in specific historical and cultural situations, and being open to the insights into the human condition provided by the arts and the humanities. Main topics of study would include the linguistic and social construction of reality, and the interrelations of a local context and the self in a network of relationships. And this would require accepting the open, perspectival and ambiguous nature of knowledge and validation of knowledge through practice. It would involve a multimethod approach to research, including qualitative descriptions of the diversity of a person's relation to the world and a deconstruction of texts that attempts to describe this relation. The question remains whether such changes are too radical to find their place within a psychological sciene with strong individualistic and rationalistic roots.«

Reference

Adorno, Theodor W. (1993). Soziologie und empirische Forschung. In Th. W. Adorno, H. Albert, R. Dahrendorf, J. Habermas. H. Pilot, K. R. Popper (Eds.), *Der Positivismusstreit in der deutschen Soziologie* (pp.81-102). München: dtv.

Albert, H. (1971). Konstruktivismus oder Realismus? Bemerkungen zu Holzkamps dialektischer Überwindung der modernen Wissenschaftslehre. In *Zeitschrift für Sozialpsychologie 2*, 5-23.

Barkow, Jerome H. (2001). Universalien und evolutionäre Psychologie. In Peter M. Hejl (Ed.), *Universalien und Konstruktivismus* (pp.126-138). Frankfurt a.M.: Suhrkamp.

Barkow, Jerome H., Cosmides, Leda, & Tooby, John (Ed.). (1992) *The Adapted Mind. Evolutionary Psychology and the Generation of Culture*. New York: Oxford University Press.

Campbell, Donald T. (1994). The Social Psychology of Scientific Validity: An Epistemological Perspective and a Personalized History. In William R. Shadish, & Steve Fuller (Eds.), *The Social Psychology of Science* (pp.162-178). New York: The Guilford Press.

Gergen, Kenneth J. (1990). Die Konstruktion des Selbst im Zeitalter der Postmoderne. In *Psychologische Rundschau, 41*, 191-199.

Geulen, Dieter (1991). Das Gesellschaftliche in der Seele. In G. Jüttemann, M. Sonntag, & Ch. Wulf (Ed.), *Die Seele. Ihre Geschichte im Abendland* (pp.528-552). Weinheim: PVU.

Habermas, Jürgen (1993a). Analytische Wissenschaftstheorie und Dialektik. In Th. W. Adorno, H. Albert, R. Dahrendorf, J. Habermas. H. Pilot, K. R. Popper (Eds.), *Der Positivismusstreit in der deutschen Soziologie* (pp.155-192). München: dtv.

Habermas, Jürgen (1993b). Gegen einen positivistisch halbierten Rationalismus. In Th. W. Adorno, H. Albert, R. Dahrendorf, J. Habermas. H. Pilot, K R. Popper (Hg.), *Der Positivismusstreit in der deutschen Soziologie* (pp.235-268). München: dtv.

Haslam, S. A., & McGarty, C. (2001). A 100 years of certitude? Social psychology, the experimental method and the management of scientific uncertainty. In *British Journal of Social Psychology, 40*, 1-21.

Hejl, Peter M. (2001). Konstruktivismus und Universalien – eine Verbindung contre nature? In P. M. Hejl (Ed.), *Universalien und Konstruktivismus* (pp.7-67). Frankfurt a. M.: Suhrkamp.

Holzkamp, Klaus (1972a). Verborgene anthropologische Voraussetzungn der allgemeinen Psychologie. In K. Holzkamp, *Kritische Psychologie. Vorbereitende Arbeiten* (pp.35-74). Frankfurt a.M.: Fischer.

Holzkamp, Klaus (1972b). Verborgene anthropologische Voraussetzungen der allgemeinen Psychologie. In K. Holzkamp, *Kritische Psychologie. Vorbereitende Arbeiten* (pp.35-74). Frankfurt a.M.: Fischer.

Holzkamp, Klaus (1972c). Kritischer Rationalismus als blinder Kritizismus. In K. Holzkamp, *Kritische Psychologie. Vorbereitende Arbeiten* (pp.173-206). Frankfurt a.M.: Fischer.

Holzkamp, Klaus (1995). *Lernen. Subjektwissenschaftliche Grundlegung* (Studienausgabe). Frankfurt a.M.: Campus.

Janich, Peter (1996). Das Experiment in der Psychologie. In P. Janich, *Konstruktivismus und Naturerkenntnis. Auf dem Weg zum Kulturalismus* (pp.275-289). Frankfurt a.M.: Suhrkamp.

Jüttemann, Gerd (1992). *Psyche und Subjekt. Für eine Psychologie jenseits von Dogma und Mythos*. Reinbek bei Hamburg: Rowohlt.

Kvale, Steinar (1992). Postmodern Psychology: A Contradiction in Terms? In S. Kvale (Ed.), *Psychology and Postmodernism* (pp.31-57). London: Sage Publications.

Neisser, Ulric (1981). L'approccio ecologico in psicologia cognitiva. Edizioni Scientifiche Italiane.

Popper, Karl R. (1965). *Das Elend des Historizismus*. Tübingen.

Popper, Karl R. (1984). *Logik der Forschung* (8. Aufl.). Tübingen: J.C.B. Mohr (Paul Siebeck).

Popper, Karl R. (1993). Die Logik der Sozialwissenschaften. In Th. W. Adorno, H. Albert, R. Dahrendorf, J. Habermas. H. Pilot, Karl R. Popper (Eds.), *Der Positivismusstreit in der deutschen Soziologie* (pp.103-124). München: dtv.

Popper, Karl, & Eccles, John (1991). *Das Ich und sein Gehirn* (10. Aufl.). München: Piper. [Originalausgabe: *The Self and Its Brain*, 1977]

Rorty, Richard (1997). *Der Spiegel der Natur. Eine Kritik der Philosophie* (4. Aufl.). Frankfurt a.M.: Suhrkamp. [Originalausgabe: *Philosophy and the mirror of nature.*]

Wallner, Fritz (1992). The Split in Austrian Philosophy: Wittgenstein and Popper. In F. Wallner, & M. Peschl (Eds.), *Konstruktion der Realität. Von Wittgenstein zum Konstruktiven Realismus* (pp.45-61). Wien: WUV.

D. Physics, Informatics

Herbert Pietschmann

Complementarity in Quantum Mechanics and in Life[1]

Abstract

It is claimed that in the 17th century science replaced the physics of Aristotle, but not his frame of thinking (logic). Only in the 20th century Quantum Mechanics broke this frame and replaced the Aristotelian Either-Or by complementarity. It is further claimed that Platonian dialectic is better suited for problems with complementary aspects. A simple model to cope with dialectic situations is presented. It is applied to some typical problems of science and culture in general.

The challenge of quantum mechanics

It is well known that five outstanding physicists who obtained the Nobel Prize for their essential contribution to the development of quantum physics did not accept the final version of current quantum mechanics: Max Planck, Albert Einstein, Max von Laue, Louis de Broglie and Erwin Schrödinger. The reason was a deep resistance to give up familiar notions of »reality« which used to be the basis for all new developments in physics. (This is particularly surprising in the case of Albert Einstein, who did the first step away from classical realism with his criticism of absolute time and his development of special relativity.) Albert Einstein said to Wolfgang Pauli[2]: »With only ›perhaps‹ you can't make a theory. Physics is the description of reality or shall I say physics is the description of what I just imagine?« Einstein feared if quantum mechanics prevails, that the difference between physical reality and dream or hallucination may be blurred! He wrote to Schrödinger: »Except for Laue you are the only one who realises that you cannot avoid accepting reality if you are honest. Most of the others don't even see what kind of a dangerous game they play with reality.«

However, Einstein's resistance was very fruitful for the further development of quantum mechanics. Niels Bohr wrote[3]: »Einstein's objections were the reason I tried to clarify the role of measuring and complementary phenomena.« And he designed the famous double slit experiment which proves that all microscopic ob-

1 Dedicated to Fritz Wallner on the occasion of his 60th birthday.
2 W. Pauli: *Physik und Erkenntnistheorie*. Vieweg Verlag, Braunschweig (1984) p.89
3 P. A. Schilpp (Ed.): *Albert Einstein als Philosoph und Naturforscher*. Vieweg Verlag, Braunschweig (1983) p.99

jects show both discrete (particle like) as well as continuous (wave like) properties. This »dualism« of particle and wave is more generally described by objects showing *complementary* properties, i.e. properties which are contradictory but nevertheless have to be attributed to one single object. This phenomenon which is completely new in the history of science is called *complementarity*!

The double slit experiment was well known in optics. A light wave sent through a double slit will show a typical interference pattern on a screen behind the double slit, i.e. a row of alternating dark and bright stripes. This is a typical proof of the wave nature of light for we know this phenomenon also for example from water surface waves if two rocks are thrown into water with a still surface and thereby create an interference pattern of the two circular waves emanating from the impact points of the rocks. But for quantum objects, e.g. photons, neutrons, or electrons, this is no longer obvious because these objects show discrete particle nature and – classically – should follow a definite path. Such a path can go through one of the two slits but certainly not through both! Nevertheless the objects arrive only at locations were the bright stripes in the case of light were found and never at the dark spots. If one of the slits is closed, the pattern will change completely and the stripes will disappear. Thus it seems that either the objects do pass both slits or they pass only one and »know« whether the other one is open or closed. Both alternatives are not acceptable! Quantum mechanics found another alternative and was able to support it by experiments: If we cannot know the path of the object in principle, we obtain the interference pattern (like from waves); if we somehow observe the path, it is always either through one slit or through the other, but the interference pattern disappears (like from particles). Thus we arrive at a new kind of complementarity between path and interference! Either we know the path or we observe interference with the same objects.

A consequence of this observation can be phrased in the following way[4]: In quantum mechanics, by measuring an object, its properties are not *determined* but *produced*! Clearly, this contradicts the classical notion of a given reality independent of its observation. There are even more surprising consequences of quantum mechanics when we consider states of more than one particle. The notion of »entanglement« of two or more particles leads to antinomies (Schrödinger[5]) or to paradoxes (Einstein[6]). We shall not go into this fascinating chapter for it suffices for our purposes to accept the simpler notion of complementarity.

---

4 For further details see e.g. H. Pietschmann: *Quantenmechanik verstehen!* Springer Verlag Berlin (2003) or the Video »Aufbruch in die Quantenwelt« (lhotsky-film@netway.at)

5 E. Schrödinger: Die gegenwärtige Situation in der Quantenmechanik. *Die Naturwissenschaften Vol.23* (1935) pp.844-849

6 A. Einstein, B. Podolsky, N. Rosen: Can quantum-mechanical description of physical reality be considered complete? *Physical Review Vol.47* (1935) pp.777-780

Today, these complementary aspects are no longer restricted to elementary objects as mentioned above; experiments have been performed[7] which prove the dual nature of so called Buckey-balls, sphere shaped molecules of 60 or 70 carbon atoms! The (as yet unpublished) record lies at so called fluorinated fullerenes with the chemical formula $C_{60}F_{48}$, i.e. large molecules of 108 atoms and a mass of 1682 amu (atomic mass units)[8].

Quantum mechanics versus Aristotelian logic

At first glance, it may seem surprising that so many eminent physicists could not accept the experimentally well founded ideas of quantum mechanics. However, as we have clearly pointed out, these ideas cannot be reconciled with the axioms of Aristotelian logic. This becomes evident, when we recall some of the original quotations from Aristotle[9]:

»[T]he most certain principle of all is that about which one cannot be mistaken; for such a principle must be both the most familiar [...] and not based on hypothesis. For the principle which the student of any form of Being must grasp is no hypothesis [...]. Clearly, then, it is a principle of this kind that is the most certain of all principles. Let us next state what this principle is. ›It is impossible for the same attribute at once to belong and not to belong to the same thing and in the same relation‹; and we must add any further qualifications that may be necessary to meet logical objections. This is the most certain of all principles, since it possesses the required definition; for it is impossible for anyone to suppose that the same thing is and is not, as some imagine that Heraclitus says – for what a man says does not necessarily represent what he believes.«

It is quite obvious that this contradicts the experimentally established facts we have described above. But it is a general believe that Aristotle – at least his physics – has been overcome in the 17th century when science as we know it today has been created. Why, then, did the five above mentioned Nobel laureates rather back away from quantum mechanics than from Aristotle?

My thesis, which I want to expose in this paper, is that only the factual content of Aristotelian physics has been overcome; his logic remained part of our *frame of thinking* as I chose to call it[10]. But the development of science was not so simple. Galilei is generally assumed the most prominent father of »nuova

---

7 O. Nairz, M. Arndt, A. Zeilinger: Quantum interference experiments with large molecules. *American Journal of Physics Vol.71* (2003) p.319

8 M. Arndt (Vienna), private communication.

9 Aristotle: *Metaphysics* 1005b

10 H. Pietschmann: *Phänomenologie der Naturwissenschaft*. Springer Verlag Berlin (1996) p.110

scienza«, of modern science. This is certainly right for he designed the experiment as crucial test for any hypothesis and it remains the method of science till today[11]. But he was not the first to refute Aristotelian physics. According to Aristotle, physics was different below and above the sphere of the moon. Below was terrestrial physics were every motion comes to a halt; above was celestial physics with eternal, circular motion and never changing perfection. Already Tycho de Brahe[12] questioned this system when he observed a supernova in the 16th century and when he noted that comets could not very likely be below the sphere of the moon. So what was the contribution of Galilei that made him the founder of modern science?

One aspect was certainly his open fight for a change of paradigm. However, I think that his main contribution was more subtle! Let us quote from Aristotle again[13]: »... it is clear that Wisdom is knowledge of certain principles and causes. Since we are investigating this kind of knowledge, we must consider what these causes and principles are whose knowledge is Wisdom.« Whereas Aristotle searched for principles which are self-evident, the new method of science according to Galilei discarded the request of self-evidence and replaced it by experiment as the criterion for validity. This is the crucial new idea of science! It is radical, because these new principles cannot be derived in any systematic way; they rely on intuition and creativity of talented men or women. In a letter to his friend Solovine from May 7, 1952 Albert Einstein wrote[14]: »Psychologically the axioms are based upon the experiences. There is however no logical path from the experiences to axioms, but only an intuitive (psychological) connection, which is always subject to revocation.« Nobel laureate Richard Feynman, in writing about his way of thinking, also emphasizes instinct rather than rationality[15]: »He thinks I'm following the steps mathematically, but that's not what I'm doing. I have the specific, physical example of what he's trying to analyse, and I know from instinct and experience the properties of the thing.«

---

11 see e.g. R. P. Feynman: What is and what should be the role of scientific culture in modern society. *Nuovo Cimento Supplemento Vol.4* (1966) pp.492ff

12 J. R. Christianson: *On Tycho's Island – Tycho Brahe and his Assistants 1570-1601*. Cambridge University Press (2000) pp.64, 103

13 Aristotle: *Metaphysics* 981b – 982a

14 P. C. Aichelburg and R. U. Sexl (Eds.): *Albert Einstein – His Influence on Physics, Philosophy and Politics*. Vieweg Verlag Braunschweig (1979) p.113

15 R. P. Feynman: *Surely you'r joking, Mr. Feynman*. Norton & Co., New York (1985) p.245

We have demonstrated clearly that Aristotelian logic is refuted by the experimentally founded quantum mechanics. How shall we extend our frame of thinking in order to incorporate complementary aspects in our world? For we can never simply ignore Aristotelian logic, it has proven to be powerful and remains to be the basis of our construction of reality. But we may try to complement it with another kind of thinking which is appropriate whenever the »either-or« of Aristotle is not satisfactory. This is not to be restricted to quantum mechanics since there are many aspects in life which are better understood in terms of complementarity. Thus, from now on I shall open my view and consider complementary phenomena in life at large. I am following the great physicist with philosophical interest Wolfgang Pauli, who wrote[16]: »The author belongs to those physicists who believe that the new epistemological situation which is the basis of quantum mechanics is satisfactory; both from the point of view of physics and as well from the broader point of view of human perception.«

My suggestion is – in spiritual agreement with Wolfgang Pauli – to turn to the teacher of Aristotle, Plato. That Plato's way of thinking may be more appropriate for complementary phenomena is born out from a comparison of their attitude towards being. Aristotle said[17]: »To say, that *what is* is not, or to say that *what is not* is, is false; but to say that *what is* is, and *what is not* is not, is true.« Whereas Plato formulates more softly[18]: »In order to defend ourselves, we will be compelled to test the statement of our father Parmenides and force *what is not* to be in a certain aspect, and on the other hand force *what is* in some sense not to be.« Aristotle – pupil of Plato – formulated his logic in opposition to some of Plato's methods. He said[19]: »In his youth Plato first became acquainted with Cratylus and the Heraclitean doctrines – that the whole sensible[20] world is always in a state of flux and that there is no scientific knowledge of it – and in after years he still held these opinions. And when Socrates, disregarding the physical universe and confining his study to moral questions, sought in this sphere for the universal and was the first to concentrate upon definition, Plato followed him and assumed that the problem of definition is concerned not with any sensible thing but with entities of another kind; for the reason that there can be no general definition of sensible things which are always changing. These entities he called ›ideas‹.« Whereas Aristotelian philosophy is based on logic, Plato called his way of thinking »dialectic«; it is dedicated to problems with complementary aspects. Aristotle

16 W. Pauli: *Physik und Erkenntnistheorie.* Loc.cit., p.61

17 Aristotle: *Metaphysics* 1011b

18 Plato: *Theaitetos*

19 Aristotle: *Metaphysics* 987a-b

20 »Sensible« is the term for »experienced with our senses« (as opposed to reason).

naturally criticized it[21]: »Dialecticians wear the same appearance as the philosopher, for dialecticians discuss all subjects, and being is a subject common to them all; but clearly they discuss these concepts because they appertain to philosophy. Dialectic is concerned with the same class of subjects as philosophy, but philosophy differs from it in its outlook on life. Dialectic treats as an exercise what philosophy tries to understand.«

Richard Feynman has said about quantum mechanics[22]: »Even the experts do not understand it the way they would like to, and it is perfectly reasonable that they should not [...].« Hence dialectic is more appropriate when understanding (in the traditional sense of the word) is no longer possible. The Aristotelian approach leads all too often into a dilemma: Either we understand something scientifically or we can just have (valueless) opinions about it[23]. Plato, on the other hand, proclaimed that dialectic is less than science but more than opinion! In a way, it is very modest for it accepts the limitations of our knowledge in the same way as Socrates, who said[24]: »So it seems at any rate that I am wiser in this one small respect: I do not think I know what I do not.«

A practical model for dialectic

We are not trained in dialectic thinking; and in philosophy books dialectic is often explained in very cumbersome phrases. Therefore, I have made a simple model[25] which should serve as introduction to the way, complementary phenomena can be handled. Let us choose – as typical example – a situation in which two contradictory goals yearn for harmonization: Unity and Diversity. (The process of unification of Europe is an example, but any human community may have to handle this problem also.) If we want to achieve a kind of unification which does not exclude diversity, we have to transcend the frame of thinking of Aristotle.

The first step is to realise, that complementary notions (such as unity and diversity) cannot be *defined* in the same way as in logic. Both notions include aspects which we appreciate and aspects which we want to avoid. I call the latter *shadow* of the notion (in the same way as Carl G. Jung used this expression). We recognise the shadow of each notion when we try to separate it from its complementary counterpart; Unity without Diversity becomes Uniformity thus Uniform-

---

21 Aristotle: *Metaphysics* 1004b

22 R. P. Feynman: *Lectures on Physics – Quantum Mechanics*. Addison-Wesley, Reading MA (1995) 1-1

23 An example is the struggle about the Kyoto-protocol: Some claim, as long as we do not have scientific proof that greenhouse gases lead to global warming, we deal with mere opinions that can be discarded.

24 Plato: *Apology* 21d

25 for more details see H. Pietschmann: *Eris&Eirene*. Ibera Verlag Wien (2002)

ity is the shadow of Unity. Likewise, Diversity without Unity becomes Arbitrariness and this is the shadow of Diversity. Let us order these four notions at the corners of an H (standing for the wanted harmony):

Unity	Diversity
H	
Uniformity	Arbitrariness

If we are able to exclude the shadows (Uniformity and Arbitrariness), we will be able to bring Unity and Diversity together in harmony (a synthesis). However, as a general rule, this is never immediately possible; in any situation like this, there will soon be a split into two parties, one fighting for Unity, the other one fighting for Diversity. The first group will fight against Arbitrariness, the second against Uniformity. Both of them are right, for we do not want the shadows! I call this state of affairs the »HX-confusion« for we can represent it by an X instead of the wanted H[26]:

Unity	Diversity
X	
Uniformity	Arbitrariness

The sad observation is that this fight (the HX-confusion) can endlessly go on because both parties are right! Even more, it would not be desirable that one of them wins the fight, because it would negate the complementarity and we would end up with a rational solution, i.e. one side is right, the other one wrong; instead of harmony between Unity and Diversity we would have *either* Uniformity *or* Arbitrariness!

A possible way out of this dilemma can be found when both parties realise that they are fighting the wrong enemy! It is not the shadow of the other side, but their own shadow which each of them should consider enemy! When the defenders of Unity realise, that they should fight (or at least suppress) Uniformity and the defenders of Diversity realize that their enemy is Arbitrariness, a solution is to be achieved. Both sides can arrange themselves in harmony with the others. But there is the obstacle of simultaneity! *Both* sides must be ready to switch enemy, otherwise there is no harmony and the fight must go on. The way to the insight

26 The HX-confusion in quantum mechanics can be observed from many conferences on »Interpretation of Quantum Mechanics«, e.g. P. Mittelstaedt and E. W. Stachow (Eds.): *Recent Developments in Quantum Logic*. B.I.Wissenschaftsverlag, Mannheim (1985)

goes via the realization that fighting the shadow of the opponent will invariably induce a fall into ones own shadow. Fighting Arbitrariness from the standpoint of Unity leads to Uniformity and vice versa.

On the way from HX-confusion to harmony (or synthesis) we thus have to pass two essential barriers: Both sides must realize that the fight is to their own disadvantage and both sides must *simultaneously* declare that they were fighting the wrong enemy.

Some other important examples

By comparing logic of Aristotle and dialectic of Plato we ran into their main focus of contemplation: Being versus Becoming. This is a complementary aspect in everybody's life as well as in any company, production plant and the like. We always have to balance preserving and changing (or renewing) and to avoid rigidity (a kind of death) and loss of identity. Thus we have the following H and X:

preserve change

H

rigidity loss of identity
death

preserve change

X

rigidity loss of identity
death

This situation has its counterpart in science. The wanted scientific attitude is both critical and open simultaneously, hence it requires synthesizing two complementary attitudes! If we are too critical, there is no progress and science becomes rigid. If we are too open, we will take as facts what is not shown to exist properly, scientists become credulous. We can thus reiterate the above H and X as applied to science:

critical open

H

rigid credulous

critical open

X

rigid credulous

This is a problem for every scientist individually, but also for science as a whole, as social product. Historically, science seems to swing between the two extremes like a pendulum. At the turn of the 18th century, science was too critical, i.e. it became rigid. It declared publicly that meteorites could not fall from the sky[27]! And

27 See e.g. W. Gentner: Irdische und meteoritische Materie. *Die Naturwissenschaften Vol.50/6* (1963)

at the turn of the 19th century, when all of a sudden so many unexpected forms of radiation were discovered, science wanted to be open for everything new and thus became credulous; many experiments were performed (and published) on so called »N-rays« which turned out not to exist[28]!

Let us dare to tackle even more pressing problems in conjunction with science and society: The so-called »two culture problem«. Very often, science is unfortunately considered in opposition to humanics, say. Rather, we should take it as a dialectic situation where harmony between the opponents is to be attempted. It is rather easy to find the »X« in the state of HX-confusion: Humanists lament the materialism of science and scientists complain about the subjective and thus arbitrary nature of humanics. Neither side is as yet willing to admit that there is some grain of truth in the arguments of the opponents. Thus we have the HX-confusion

Science Humanics

X

materialistic arbitrary, subjective

Personally, I deplore this situation for as a particle physicist I am deeply attached to science; but at the same time I have benefited greatly from my interest in philosophy. Thus I would appreciate any small step taken in this dialectic process towards mutual acceptance of the two sides.

Last not least let me mention a problem which is less urgent in Europe, but very open in the United States: The fight between creation and evolution. It is my personal conviction, that also this problem could be handled in a dialectic fashion rather than risking an endless fight from which nobody benefits. Let me first draw the X of the present state:

evolution creation

X

atheistic anti-scientific

I should repeat what I said above: Both sides are right, i.e. science cannot accept the picture of creation *without any change*! But it should also understand the other side, which cannot accept that there is »scientific proof« that our world is the product of mere accident. Obviously, creation can never replace evolution and has no place in scientific curricula. However, if the dialectic process gets under way, we may extend our view of life to also incorporate spiritual (or religious) aspects which deal with *meaning* rather than *existence* and thereby allow for a broader

---

28 See e.g. I. M. Klotz: The N-Ray Affair. *Scientific American* (May 1980) pp.122ff

view including complementary aspects. Both sides will have to recognize the negative influence of their own shadow!

evolution   creation

H

atheistic   anti-scientific

It is clear, that the first step – accepting the right of existence of the other side – can only be done simultaneously by both. Thus, as long as creationists want to *replace* evolution by creation, we scientists have to continue the fight but we should not give up the hope that one day our materialistic world view will – without any loss of acceptance and prestige – be complemented by the meaning of all the wonderful experiences we are allowed to meet in our life.

Kambiz Badie

Generating New Ideas through Strangifying Frames of Concepts into Each other

Abstract

In this paper, it is shown that linking the frames of concepts can be viewed as an approach to strangifying them into each other. Concepts considered by us are either a methodology, or a theory, or a context. As a conclusion of this approach, strangification should not only be viewed as strategy for understanding the inherent capabilities of a concept, but in the meantime should be viewed as a systematic method for realizing the inherent capabilities of the concept within which this process is performed.

1. Introduction

Adopting that a scientific school of thought, or in its particular form a scientific theory, is a new idea in the realm of science, it would be reasonable to think of development of new schools of thought and new theories as a process of generating new scientific ideas. This can be of particular significance, since constructivistic approaches to epistemology have supported the fact that, scientific theories/schools of thought, despite their external objectivistic manifestations, are deeply rooted in the way scientists or researchers look at their surrounding world and presuppose the surrounding facts; i.e. their world views. Under such circumstances, all entities like paradigms, theories, methods, etc. can be viewed as some ideas, which emerge based on some sort of interaction between the scientist or the researcher's presuppositions and his/her perception toward the external facts. On the other hand, it may happen that within such a process of idea generation, the scientist may tend to put into composition, some previously generated and examined concepts, to produce some new concepts, which can enjoy a higher capability/competence with respect to more complex situations. Taking this point into view it will undoubtedly be beneficial to think that an advanced science theory should have the ability to explain how new scientific concepts can emerge based on those previously generated and examined. This can help us make a bridge between the existing scientific concepts for a more comprehensive understanding of the nature of science. We found out in practice that, strangification as the main strategy of the science theory of Constructive Realism [1], has the potential to justify the process of idea generation, based on putting into composition the previously generated concepts. Based on this fact, in this article, we will demonstrate how concepts can be strangified into each other, leading to composite concepts, which can enjoy higher capability/competence compared to their own compatibility/competence.

2. What do we mean by strangifying concepts into each other?

Strangification, as the key strategy of the epistemological theory of Constructive Realism, is mainly concerned with the way a proposition system (PS) reacts toward a new context, which itself can be described in terms of another PS. The final objective behind such a process is to see the potential of the first PS as a meaningful entity with respect to the second PS; let say to see whether or not and how the first PS can act meaningfully respecting the second one. Within this process, it is possible to see (i) how fittable the first PS; can be regarding the second PS, (ii) what are the biases in the first PS, and (iii) what considerations should be made to make the entire process more practical for future trials [2].

Taking the above point into account, a variety of intellectual and innovative tasks like »enhancing/improving the capability of an entity«, »justifying the role/utility of an entity within the scope of another entity«, »anticipating the impact/prospect of using an entity in the domain of another entity« and »characterizing or formulating new concepts for scientific formulation« all can be regarded as the issues of strangifying a concept into another. An interesting point is that, such a process can be equally regarded as a process for innovating or generating new ideas, taking into account the fact that ideas are frequently generated to achieve these tasks. For instance in the domain of methodology, innovation occurs at the place where a variety of pre-known methods, together with a number of predefined concepts, interact with each other in certain directions, to finally yield a composite or blended method which is characteristically novel compared to each of these methods and concepts. Obviously, the final product is expected to be benefited by the advantages of each participating element while trying to avoid their disadvantages.

3. Linking contents of concepts as an approach to strangification

To see how a PS of a concept may behave toward the PS of another concept, each PS is represented in terms of a frame, which is structured and hierarchical in its nature[3] and the contents (attributes' values) of the two frames are linked with each other using some conjunction structures preferably with a compound nature. Role of a conjunction structure is to make a fluent and comprehensible conjunction between the related attributes' values. They might be variant, based on the situations in these values, and it is thus important to consider the possibility of setting the appropriate conjunction structures on-line. The idea on the type of conjunction structures and the formats for expressing them depends on both the type of the concepts participating in strangification that in turn leads to selection of the attributes, as well as the role of each attribute. Here, concept linking is performed for the purpose of (i) enhancing/improving the capability of an entity, (ii) justifying the role/utility of an entity within the scope of another entity, (iii) anticipating the impact/prospect of using an entity in the domain of another entity, or (iv) characterization/formulation of scientifically significant concepts.

To see how strangification through concept linking works, we elaborate the following scenarios:

- Strangifying the PS of a concept indicating a state (as an epistemological entity) into the PS of another concept to show how an idea can emerge respecting the specific situation for this state.
- Strangifying the PS of a concept indicating a methodology in general, and a method or technique in particular, into the PS of an entity to show how the idea of applying that methodology to the entity under study can mean.
- Strangifying the PS of a theory into the PS of another theory, which means to show how far a theory may be capable of enhancing/improving the capabilities of another theory to make it capable of responding to more specific situations.

Before getting into the examples we draw the reader's attention to the point that two types of linguistic operators are responsible for linking the attributes' values in the corresponding frames; (i) simple substitution operators that are responsible for replacing a part of the text belonging to an attribute value in the first PS, with the nouns or phrases belonging to an attribute value from the second PS, and (ii) conjunction structures preferably with compound nature, that are in charge of incremental linking of the attributes' values, respectively belonging to the first and the second PSs. It would later be explained in the example that, the process of linking is to be performed in a hierarchical manner, thus making an environment within which both types of the operators can at the same time be used to link the contents of the two PSs, based on the type of the attribute (in the final composite concept) whose value is to be assigned.

In this respect, frame as a structured means for representing knowledge, has been selected as the means for representing the knowledge content of the concepts.

4. Linking contents of two frames as an approach for strangifying them into each other

4-1 Basics

Before getting into the actual process of linking the contents of two concepts frames for generating novel ideas, we should briefly mention the operators which are essential to this process. Regarding this, it is first necessary to make distinction between two types of noun concepts; action-type noun and non action type noun, from the standpoint of the attributes, which are essential to their description. Once some partial texts were generated as the result of the first stage in linking, a new stage of linking will start, this time replacing a prime item in an attribute value of the first concept with those belonging to an attribute value in the second concept. This process will continue until the stage where the content obtained through this hierarchical process can be sufficiently sound for the human mind. This is a process, which is supposed to be performed automatically in the expert's mind, when it comes to tasks such as innovation or idea generation [4,5,6].

4-2 Linking the concept of two nouns in general

Regarding what mention in 4-1, some similar attributes can be proposed for both action-type and non-action type nouns, which can cover the requirements of each type. The nouns, which are of major interest to us, include »methodology«, »theory« and »context«. Here, from strangification point of view, »methodology« and »theory« can be mutually strangified into each other, while each can also be strangified into a »context«. Obviously, a »context« due to its particular status, has no chance to be strangified into neither a »methodology« and nor a »theory« as well.

The linking operators for the contents of those noun-type entities can then be conceptualized as follows:

- Value for »Major Concern« = Value for »Major Concern« in Concept A + »when it comes to« (or »with respect to«) + Value for »Basics« in Concept B
- Value for »Basics« = Value for »Basics« in Concept B + »Based on« + Value for »Basics« in Concept A
- Value for »Advantage« = Value for »Advantage« in Concept A + »in order to« + Value for »Advantage« in Concept B, or Value for »Advantage« in Concept A + »in order to solve the problem of« + Value for »Disadvantage« in Concept B
- Value for »Disadvantage« = Value for »Disadvantage« in Concept A + »regarding« + prime items in the value of »Disadvantage« in Concept B

4-3 Some examples

Example 1: Linking the frames of the two concepts of »Fuzzy« and »Clustering« as two methodologies

An example is presented in figure 1 where the frames of the two concepts of »Fuzzy« (figure 1(a)) and »Clustering« (figure 1(b)) including the attributes discussed in 3 are linked in two different directions (figure 1(c)) and figure 1(d)).

Each direction indicates the way PS of the first concept is strangified into the PS of the second concept to remove in this case the drawbacks of the second concept, thus turning it into a more capable methodology. As it is seen from figure 2(c) and figure 2(d), »action-type nouns«, »non-action type nouns«, and the conjunction structures are appropriately used as discussed to determine the final content of the corresponding attributes in the final composite concept.

For instance, the value of the attribute »Major Concern« in »Fuzzy Clustering« is determined through linking »Fuzzy«'s »Major Concern« with some prime items in the value of »Clustering«'s »Basics« via using the conjunction structure »with respect to«, while the value of »Basics« for »Fuzzy Clustering« is determined through linking »Fuzzy«'s »Basics« with the value of »Clustering«'s »Basics« using »Based on« as the conjunction structure.

The reason for picking out the prime items in the value of the concept B's »Basics« (in case of determining the value of the attribute »Major Concern« in the composite concept), goes back to the related conjunction structure, which is »with respect to« in this case. When a phrase comes after such a conjunction structure, it is obvious that some prime items in this phrase are to be highlighted as the alternatives, with respect to which the entire sentence makes sense. In the example above, »sufficiently close points in the feature space« are the prime items in the value of the attribute »Basics« in the frame of Clustering as the Concept B. Let say, in this way this sense will appear that the major concern of the composite (or blended) concept of »Fuzzy Clustering« would be to manage uncertainty with respect to those points that are close enough to each other in the feature space. This together with the value of the attribute »Basics« in »Fuzzy Clustering« will eventually lead to the idea that Membership Functions (MFs) can be used to handle uncertainty regarding the distance between those points in the feature space, which are sufficiently close to each other. Also, regarding the composite (or blended) concept »Clustering Fuzzy«, the eventual idea is that, clustering techniques can be applied to MFs in order to turn them into more efficient structures for uncertainty handling purposes. In this case, a variety of ideas may subsequently be generated for clustering MFs, each depending on its own interpretation of MF as a pattern. One way is to regard MF as a geometric shape consisting of some geometrically significant points. Regarding this case, these points would become subject to clustering. The other way is to regard MF as a mathematical function like a Gaussian Distribution Function with some basic parameters such as variance and mean value. In this case, the total vector comprising of the values of these parameters would be a subject for clustering. Regarding the above discussion, application of Clustering as a technique, to Fuzzy (Processing) as another technique, may yield some new ideas as follow:

- Generating class structures for classifying the geometrically significant points of a fuzzy membership function.
- Generating class structures for classifying the (mean value, variance) vector, which represents the Gaussian Distribution for fuzzy membership function

This can be quite interesting from research & development viewpoint, since the researcher/developer can in this way become aware of the possibilities behind different compositions of the existing techniques, and choose the one that can best fit his/her current problem requirements.

It is worth noticing that the very ideas to be obtained through concept composition, as discussed in the above example, are propounding new problems, and do not point out the way these problems can be solved. Let say, the generated ideas look at the problems, but not the solutions. For example, the value for the attribute »Basics« in the composite concept of »Clustering in Fuzzy Processing« is: Utilizing MF to determine the status of assigning a pattern to different classes based on determination of sufficiently close points in the feature space...

Referring to this content, the researcher, despite getting the idea that determination of sufficiently close points in the feature space can be a ground for utilizing fuzzy membership functions for the purpose of classifying patterns, gets no clue regarding its »how to« (the way it can come true). An alternative to circumvent this problem is to add the essential procedure for the value of »Basics« in the Concept A to its corresponding frame. For example, beside the value of »Basics« in »Clustering«, one can add its essential procedure together with the essential tools, to the structure of the frame. It is well known that, Distance Function is a suitable alternative in this regard. In this way, the very ideas generated through concept composition can be enhanced.

Going back to the example discussed above, the researcher may acquire the idea that fuzzy membership function can be used to assign a pattern to possible classes if it is somewhat considered in a distance function. It is possible that, at this stage, the researcher, according to his/her past experiences, gets to find out that one way of materializing this idea is to consider fuzzy distance function. In case that the researcher has no sense toward the above idea, »fuzzy distance function« itself can be propounded as a frame (with the same attributes discussed above), and concept composition can then be repeated for this new frame.

We therefore observe that generating a new idea can cover all the necessary stages from the way a problem is propounded to its solution, if the linking process considered hierarchically.

Fuzzy (a)

Super Class	Logic of uncertainty
Sub Class	T-Norm, …
Major Concern	Uncertainty management
Basics	Utilizing *MF* to determine the status of assigning a pattern to different classes, Using some *operators* for decision making
Advantage	Enhancing DM performance through considering the affiliation of a pattern toward different classes
Disadvantage	*MFs* may not be defined properly

Clustering (b)

Super Class	Category theory
Sub Class	Model-based, adaptive, neural, self-organizing, …
Major Concern	To generate class structures for *classification* purposes
Basics	*Determination* of sufficiently close points in the feature space
Advantage	Optimizing search with respect to Decision Making
Disadvantage	Defining distinct classes

Fuzzy Clustering (c)

Super Class	Category theory
Sub Class	Fuzzy model-based clustering
Major Concern	Uncertainty management *with respect to* sufficiently close points in the feature space
Basics	Determination of sufficiently close points in the feature space *based on* utilizing MF to determine the status of assigning a pattern to different classes
Advantage	Enhancing Decision Making performance through considering the affiliation of a pattern toward different classes *in order to* optimize search, Enhancing … *in order to solve the problem of* distinct classes
Disadvantage	MFs may not be defined properly *regarding* Decision Making, MFs may not be defined properly *and* define distinct classes

Clustering Fuzzy (d)

Super Class	Logic of uncertainty
Sub Class	Clustering T-Norm
Major Concern	To generate class structures for classification *with respect to* MF
Basics	Utilizing MF to determine the status of assigning a pattern to different classes *based on* determination of sufficiently close points in the feature space
Advantage	Optimizing search with respect to Decision Making *in order to solve the problem of* MFs, Optimizing search with respect to Decision Making *in order to* enhance DM
Disadvantage	Defining distinct classes may be problematic *regarding* the decision making process, Defining distinct classes may be problematic *and* MFs may not be defined properly

Figure 1 (a-d). Linking the frames of the concepts »Fuzzy« and »Clustering«

Example 2: Linking the frames of the two concepts of »Functionalism« and »Historical Particularism« as two theories (in the domain of cultural anthropology as a dominant research area)

In this example, a theory as a concept is composed with the concept of another theory in order to identify its further capabilities in specific situations [7]. Regarding the present example, both theories are represented in terms of frames, just like the same way in the previous example, taking into account the point that some of the premises explaining a theory stand for the attribute »Major Concern«, while the others stand for the attribute »Basics« [3] (figures 2(a) and (b)). Taking into account the above fact, the values of the attributes »Major Concern« and »Basics« for the two theories of Historical Particularism and Functionalism are illustrated in figure 2(c), respectively.

It is interesting to see that, contribution of Functionalism to Historical Particularism includes many aspects, in which, for instance, seeing a society as a system of inter- related parts can be propounded as a basic perspective in handling some of the basic concepts in Historical Particularism, such as incorporation of prehistory, linguistics and physical anthropology, collection of anthropological data and field experiences, as well as documenting and studying vanishing cultures. This, of course, can be quite interesting from an idea generation viewpoint, since it can systematically draw the attention of the researcher in this field to some specific viewpoints, whose interpretation may finally lead to some new strategies, tactics and techniques for handling more complex cultural anthropological issues;

a matter which is of particular importance for a newly-developed theory. For instance, results of applying the ideas of Functionalism to Historical Particularism in terms of the attributes' values will offer some clues to the researchers, which upon interpretation will yield new strategies and tactics that can help a broader range of expectations within Cultural Anthropology.

It is interesting to notice that, in case that the prime terms in the newly-developed contents (either action-type or non-action type nouns) are considered in some way, the same approach to concept framing and linking the frames can be continued until the stage where the contents determined in the above manner, can be transparent enough to the researcher. For instance, assuming that prehistory, linguistics and physical anthropology are the prime terms respecting the concept »Historical Particularism«, through considering them as separate frames, the researcher may find out ultimately that the above value can be interpreted in the following manner: seeing society as a system of interrelated parts that operate independently, when it comes to incorporating preliminary style of living (obtained from expanding the frame of »prehistory«), patterns of interpersonal communication (obtained from expanding the frame of »linguistics«), and style of nutrition (obtained from expanding the frame of »physical anthropology«). The above interpretation may lead the researcher in the field to the point that a major concern behind applying Functionalism to Historical Particularism, can lie in the way that all the elements of prehistory, linguistics and physical anthropology in terms of »preliminary style of living«, »interpersonal communication« and »style of nutrition«, are considered in the process of seeing a society as a system of interrelated parts. This can help upgrade the efficiency of applying Functionalism tactics within the framework of the latter.

It should however be noted that, the ideas, which are systematically generated through concept composition, should be assessed in some way. At this stage, we assume that the intuitive opinion of the human expert on the generated ideas would be sufficiently capable of performing this assessment. It is however expected that an intelligent program making use of natural language processing, can be constructed to perform this assessment in some way. Obviously, the deficiencies found out, should somehow be overcome through modulation of the conjunction structures, which are required for linking these values. Moreover, assuring the quality of the final composition calls for a basic compatibility in the participating concepts from the viewpoint of the minimum requirements for such a process. This necessitates an approach to detecting the domain compatibility between the participating concepts before initiating the composition process. This again is a matter, which is to be studied in future, for overcoming the probable deficiencies of concept composition. Finally, propounding multiple conjunction structures for linking the attributes' values can increase the performance of the composition in the situations where these values are complex enough not to be linkable through simple conjunction structures.

Functionalism (a)

⋮	
Major Concern	• Seeing society as a system of interrelated parts that operate independently
Basics	• Particular social forms functioning from day to day, to reproduce the traditional structure of the society
⋮	

Historical Particularism (b)

⋮	
Major Concern	• Emphasizing on particulars as opposed to universals • Focusing on individuals • Challenging ethnocentric assumptions of the environments
Basics	• Incorporating prehistory, linguistics, and physical anthropology • Collection of ethnographical data and field experience (as opposed to the comparative methods of unilineal cultural evolutionists) • Documenting and studying vanishing cultures
⋮	

Functional Historical Particularism (c)

⋮	
Major Concern	• Seeing society as a system of interrelated parts that operate independently, ***when it comes to*** incorporating prehistory, linguistics, and physical anthropology • Seeing society as a system of interrelated parts that operate independently, ***when it comes to*** collection of ethnographical data and field experience (as opposed to the comparative methods of unilineal cultural evolutionists) • Seeing society as a system of interrelated parts that operate independently, ***when it comes to*** documenting and studying vanishing cultures
Basics	• Incorporating prehistory, linguistics, and physical anthropology, ***based on*** particular social forms functioning from day to day, to reproduce the traditional structure of the society • Collection of the anthropological data and field experience, ***based on*** particular social forms functioning from day to day, to reproduce the traditional structure of the society • Documenting & studying vanishing cultures, ***based on*** particular social forms functioning from day to day, to reproduce the traditional structure of the society
⋮	

Figure 2 (a-c): Composing the concepts of theories for generating further ideas

5. Concluding remarks

It was discussed in the paper that, linking the contents of the frames of concepts can be viewed as an approach to strangifying one concept into the other, and in the meantime an approach for generating new ideas. Here, the concepts can be either a methodology, or a theory, or a context as well. The process of strangification based on such an approach, is principally capable of clarifying a variety of facts with respect to the possible roles that a concept may achieve toward the other concepts. This makes it quite promising for a variety of real-world applications in the era of Information & Knowledge Technology, such as cyber-learning, research and development, as well as cyber planning, where the user needs some new ideas to be generated based on his/her desired application. It was shown in the paper that, strangifying the frame of a methodology/theory into another methodology/theory can lead to understanding of a composite configuration, within which the capability of the latter is reinforced (or enhanced) through the contribution of the former. This observation leads us to the conclusion that, strangification should not only be viewed as a strategy for understanding the inherent capabilities (as well as biases) of the construct which is strangified, but in the meantime should be viewed as a systematic method for realizing the inherent capabilities (as well as biases) of the construct within which this process is performed. Let say, if we consider the metaphors of »content« and »vessel« respectively for the construct which is strangified, and the construct within which strangification is performed, the final objective behind strangification is understanding both the capabilities (as well as the biases) of the »content« and the »vessel«.

References

[1] F.G. Wallner (1994). *Constructive Realism: Aspects of a New Epistemological Movement.* Vienna: Braumüller.

[2] K. Badie (1999). *Artifical Intelligence, Strangification and Innovative Design.* Vienna: Braumüller.

[3] M. Minskey (1975). A Framework for Representing Knowledge, MIT-AI Laboratory Memo306, 1974. Reprinted in P. Winston (ed.) (1075), *Psychology of Computer Vision.* McGraw-Hill. Shorter versions in Haugland (ed.) (1981), *Mind Design.* MIT Press. And in Collins, Allen and Edward E.Smith (eds.) (1992), *Cognitive Science.* Morgan-Kaufmann.

[4] K. Badie and M.T. Mahmoudi (2004). *An Approach to Generating New Ideas Based on Liking the Frames of Concepts*, ECCBR 2004. Workshop on Computational Creativity, Madrid 2004.

[5] K. Badie and M.T. Mahmoudi (2004). *Correlation Justification as an Approach to Generating New Ideas*, CSCC2004, 8th WSEAS Intl. Conf. on Computers, Vouliagmeni, Greece 2004.

[6] M.T. Mahmoudi and K. Badie (2004). *Content Determination for Composite Concepts Via Combining Attributes' Values of Individual Frames*, IKE'04, Intl. Conf. on Information & Knowledge Engineering, Las Vegas, USA 2004.
[7] K. Badie and M.T. Mahmoudi (2005). *Generating Composite Theories Based on Linking Frames of Concepts*. [Accepted for publication in »Lecture Notes in Computer Science« of Springer, SMI05, 3rd Conference Professional Knowledge Management Experiences and Visions, Kaiserslautern, Germany 2005]

Kurt Greiner

Knowledge of Life World by Functional Strangification of High-Tech Equipment: Instruction for a Thought Experiment

Translated by Martin J. Jandl

Primarily remark

We live in high-tech life worlds – this statement may be trivial, but nevertheless it characterises truly the existential situation in the Western world. It seems that we manage our high-tech everyday life well re-producing it as a social-cultural product day in, day out when we strive to reach our goals as well as possible. We are right in the middle of this special high-tech life world or, in other words, we exist concentrically in and with it, but we are not able to recognise it because of the special existential indifference between us and our life world as long as we don't learn to dissociate ourselves from it. Pointedly speaking: The less the distance to the technified everyday life, the less it will be the matter of successful reflection.

Reflecting methodologically on the status quo of life world is possible by means of the epistemological method called ›strangification‹. This special method of achieving knowledge was developed by the constructive-realistic philosophy of science for the purpose to initiate reflection of science done by scientists. I will sketch this method briefly, and then I will strangify it by transferring it in the context of life world existence.

Strangification. Notes on the knowledge technique in Constructive Realism

The Viennese school of constructivist philosophy of science, Constructive Realism, is interested in the issue: What do scientists actually when they produce scientific knowledge? In respect to natural sciences the answer of Constructive Realism reads: »The work of natural scientists is to construct worlds. Natural science is not a description, but a construction. [*Naturwissenschaftliche Arbeit stellt Konstruktion von Welten dar. Naturwissenschaftliche Arbeit stellt nicht eine Beschreibung von etwas dar, sondern ist immer konstruktiv.*]« (Wallner 1997, p.21) The Viennese philosopher of science, Fritz Wallner who is the founder of Constructive Realism names the results of scientific construction simply ›microworlds‹ continuing Wittgenstein's theory of language games. Wittgenstein claims that the world or reality that is the objective of scientifice is pre-structured by the views of special scientific communities; hence cognition of the world is determined by a linguistic context and thus depends on this context in principle (see Wallner 1997, pp.23ff).

A famous proponent of this view beside Constructive Realism is the constructivist philosophy of science supported by the ›School of Erlangen‹ arguing that modern physicists (apart from few exceptions) don't share the naive-realistic correspondence theory of truth. Science as an activity of producing knowledge is not loaded with the claim that the results of this knowledge production are the so called ›natural laws‹ as a fix representation of the one and homogenous reality. On the contrary, current physicists deal with self-produced constructions and not with objects existing without human actions that can't be thus discovered. Physicists are no longer naturalists deciphering the world and its code, but according to this view and self-understanding their core task is making technology possible (see Zitterbarth 1991, pp.82f). Modern physics don't draw the divine construction plan of the world-machine, but rather generate knowledge (called ›language games‹, ›constructions‹, ›micro-worlds‹, or whatever) that allows to construct machines to facilitate our lifes.

From the viewpoint of philosophy of science the instrumentalistic dimension of science is not problematic, but what is problematic in natural sciences is its self-reflexive dimension (see Wallner 1997, p.25). That's why I will deal with the issue of a technique of understanding that is relevant to understanding, and not with the issue of technology that is relevant to actions. Or, in other words, I will discuss the issue of knowledge, or more exactly, of self-knowledge. According to the constructive-realistic viewpoint it is a fact that scientists are not able to recognise what they do in the course of micro-world construction. Enclosed in their scientific language games – to quote Wittgenstein once more – it is not possible to obtain the necessary distance to this language game, and without distance it isn't possible to achieve knowledge (see Wallner 1997, p.26). »A language game structures the world in any sense […], but it is not possible to understand it. My idea is: We must transfer one scientific proposition system in the context of another one to achieve knowledge. [*Ein Sprachspiel strukturiert die Welt in irgendeinem Sinn (...), es kann aber nicht verstanden werden. Es kann von sich aus nicht verstanden werden. Aber, wie ist es denn, habe ich mich gefragt, wenn wir ein Satzsystem aus einer Spezialdisziplin in eine andere übertragen*?]« (Wallner 1997, p.26)

As a consequence Wallner developed a hermeneutical technique called ›strangification‹ claiming to take a proposition system X out of its original context K and to place in another context R (e.g. see Wallner 1992, pp.82ff). This method causes the scientist to place his theory in a different and strange context. From the viewpoint of this context R the theory X is considered, assessed, etc. newly and, that's for sure, differently. Strangification means hence to leave the ways of thinking of a special discipline. Without referring to any meta-theoretical instances the procedure of strangification reveals implicit prerequisites of a theory unknown and unrecognised by scientists before strangification. Mostly strangification gives rise to a relativation of the original theory (see Peschl 1991, p.6). Strangification opens a new understanding of a scientific method – insights that wouldn't be disclosed in the manner of instrumentalistic work.

Conclusion: Strangification has a self-reflection motivating and knowledge encouraging effect on micro-world constructors. Hence, strangification is an instrument or tool that leads to scientific (self-)knowledge and (self-)understanding.

Knowledge of life worlds by functional strangification of high-tech equipment

Instructions for a thought experiment

The following considerations should invite to a thought experiment concerning self-reflective intentions with regard to constructive knowledge of life world circumstances. For that purpose I suggest to view the own flat including the high-tech equipment as items exhibited in a fictitious museum of contemporary everyday life. From this consciously imagined perspective we look at the usual things of our everyday environment. The objects of everyday life leave the usual context of employment and dive into the contemplation context of the imagined museum.

Strangification

According to the German philosopher Peter Sloderdijk the context of a museum implies potentially a ›xenological function‹. Thus every museum context can be interpreted as a ›place of encounter with aliens‹ that possibly evokes amazement caused by the alienation effects and that is understandable as a place of functional alienation. The imaginary museum-procedure functions analogous to the constructive-realistic method of strangification (that is, however, developed for the scientific scope) taking a theory out of its original context and putting into a heterogeneous context. The installation of everyday objects (like machines, instruments, apparatus, etc.) within a fictitious context of contemplation changes them functionally. In both cases objectified matters are taken out of their specific action and employment context and transferred to a reflection context, or, in short, in both cases alienation takes place. In as far I suggest interpreting the museum experiment as a functional alienation/strangification action.

Astonishment

The functional action of alienation/strangification is now the condition that bursts the ›varnish of familiarity‹ (Sloterdijk) covering the everyday objects. This fictitious ›frame of view‹ as ›object alienating space‹ in which the same items show by their state of totally difference an abyss of strangeness can be interpreted as a place of astonishment. It is a place of encounter opening the way to a therapy of ›routine-blindness of the objects owners and objects users‹ (Sloterdijk). Curing of the usual shortsightedness caused by life world determined usage of items can start now: Detaching items from their usage context, these high-tech-life-world items lose their everyday action relevance. Now they appear misused-alienated and simultaneously loaded with the contemplative value of the museum. In this situation we will have a ›second look‹ (in the sense of Sloterdijk) at the items and we will be astonished about them. But astonishment causes amazement and at best self-reflection. Thus the imagined safekeeping place for tools of life mastering turns out to be a place of life world knowledge.

Life world knowledge

The constructive-realistic strangification practice understood as exchange of contexts possibly gives rise to reflexive self-knowledge – implicit prerequisites, unconsidered and unconscious presuppositions of theoretical specifications and structuring become visible, recognisable, and understandable by meaning alienation. Sure, the scientist who applies the constructive-realistic method of strangification must be willing to question the results he gained by applying certain methods of his science. His prize will be a better understanding of his own actions because he is confronted with issues that have not been taken into account up to now. In other words, the scientist will gain insight in theories and in methods he applied like a robot. With it he will obtain the insight that it is possible to handle constructs (theories, micro-worlds, etc.) differently.

The imagined museum procedure has the similar horizon broadening and shortsightedness curing effect. Functional strangification by fictitious changing everyday tools into museum pieces entails an act of reflexive self-knowledge at the side of the contemplative astonished leader of the self-experiment by the second look. Some behavioural and handling forms, implicit points, partly unconscious and partly unconsidered perspectives in context of functional strangified apparatus and machines of the high-tech life world will possibly emerge by reflective confrontation and hence they will be understood. Sure, the experimentator disassociating himself contemplatively from his own life world by taking the perspective of a fictitious museum visitor must be willing to question his manner of behaviour and thinking. The advantage of this shattering the varnish of familiarity is to understand better life world because issues are provoked by the ›museum relation‹ that are usually not considered and discussed.

In other words: If the instrumental everyday action is replaced by the self-referential reflection-action, self-reflection will take place – the imaginary procedure of viewing everyday high-tech equipment as museum pieces may lead potentially to life world knowledge.

Reference

Peschl, Markus F. (1991). Wissen, Wirklichkeit und Handeln. In M.F. Peschl (ed.), *Formen des Konstruktivismus in Diskussion. Materialien zu den »Acht Vorlesungen über den Konstruktiven Realismus«* (pp.1-16). Wien: WUV.

Sloterdijk, Peter (1989). Museum: Schule des Befremdens. *In Frankfurter Allgemeine Magazin, 17th march 1989.*

Wallner, Fritz (1992). Das Verfahren der Verfremdung. In F. Wallner (ed.), *Wissenschaft in Reflexion*. Wien: Braumüller.

Wallner, Fritz G., & Agnese, Barbara (ed.). *Von der Einheit des Wissens zur Vielfalt der Wissensformen. Erkenntnis in Philosophie, Wissenschaft und Kunst.* Wien: Braumüller (Philosophica 14).

Zitterbarth, Walter (1991). Der Erlanger Konstruktivismus in seiner Beziehung zum Konstruktiven Realismus. In M. F. Peschl (ed.), *Formen des Konstruktivismus in Diskussion. Materialien zu den »Acht Vorlesungen über den Konstruktiven Realismus«* (pp.73-87). Wien: WUV.

Kolibri 360 GmbH
Ferdinand-Jühlke-Straße 7
99095 Erfurt, Deutschland
produktsicherheit@kolibri360.de

Druck:
CPI Druckdienstleistungen GmbH
im Auftrag der
Kolibri 360 GmbH
Ferdinand-Jühlke-Str. 7
99095 Erfurt